Small Animal Ear Diseases: An Illustrated Guide

Small Animal Ear Diseases: An Illustrated Guide

Louis N. Gotthelf, DVM
Animal Hospital of Montgomery
Montgomery, Alabama

SECOND EDITION

with 302 illustrations

ELSEVIER

ELSEVIER
SAUNDERS

11830 Westline Industrial Drive
St. Louis, Missouri 63146

SMALL ANIMAL EAR DISEASES: AN
ILLUSTRATED GUIDE, SECOND EDITION   ISBN 0-7216-0137-5

NOTICE

Veterinary Medicine is an ever-changing field. Standard safety precautions must be followed,
but as new research and clinical experience broaden our knowledge, changes in treatment and drug
therapy may become necessary or appropriate. Readers are advised to check the most current
product information provided by the manufacturer of each drug to be administered to verify the
recommended dose, the method and duration of administration, and contraindications. It is the
responsibility of the treating veterinarian, relying on experience and knowledge of the animal to
determine dosages and the best treatment for the animal. Neither the publisher nor the editor
assumes any liability for any injury and/or damage to animals or property arising from this
publication.

The Publisher

Previous edition copyrighted 2000

International Standard Book Number 0-7216-0137-5

Publishing Director: Linda Duncan
Acquisitions Editor: Anthony J. Winkel
Developmental Editor: Shelly Dixon
Publishing Services Manager: Linda McKinley
Senior Project Manager: Jennifer Furey
Designer: Amy Buxton

Printed in China.

Last digit is the print number: 9 8 7 6 5 4 3 2 1

Contributors

John C. Angus, DVM, Diplomate ACVD
Staff Dermatologist
Southern Arizona Veterinary Specialists
Tucson, Arizona
Cytology of the Ear in Health and Disease

Margo Ruth Roman-Auerhahn, BS, DVM
Staff Clinician and Owner Veterinarian
MASH Main St. Animal Services of Hopkinton
Hopkinton, Massachusetts
Anatomy of the Canine and Feline Ear

Todd W. Axlund, DVM, Dipl ACVIM
Assistant Professor
Veterinary Clinical Sciences
Auburn University
Auburn, Alabama
Otitis Interna and Vestibular Disease

Noel Berger, DVM, MS
Boston Road Animal Clinic
Sutton, Massachusetts
Laser Ear Surgery

Paul Bloom, DVM, DACVD, DABVP
Assistant Adjunct Professor
Department of Dermatology
Michigan State University
East Lansing, Michigan
Adverse Food Reactions

Peter H. Eeg, B.Sc., DVM
Poolesville Veterinary Clinic, LLC
Poolesville, Maryland
Laser Ear Surgery

Louis N. Gotthelf, DVM
Animal Hospital of Montgomery
Montgomery, Alabama
Examination of the External Ear Canal; Primary Causes of Ear Disease; Factors that Predispose the Ear to Otitis Externa; Factors that Perpetuate Otitis Externa; Failure of Epithelial Migration: Cerumenoliths; Diagnosis and Treatment of Otitis Media; Healing of the Ruptured Eardrum; Inflammatory Polyps; Ototoxicity

A. Kumar, BVSc, MVSc, MS, PhD
Professor, Department of Biomedical Sciences
Course Director, Small and Large Animal Gross Anatomy
Co-Director, Clinical Anatomy
Tufts University School of Veterinary Medicine
North Grafton, Massachusetts
Anatomy of the Canine and Feline Ear

Geneviève Marignac, DVM
Unite de Parasitologie-Mycologie-Dermatologie
Ecole Nationale Veterinaire d'Alfort
Maisons-Alfort, France
Diseases that Affect the Pinna

Steven A. Melman, VMD
Founder
Dermapet, Inc.
Potomac, Maryland
Simple Diagnosis and Treatment of Pruritic Otitis

Sandra R. Merchant, DVM, Dipl ACVD
Professor of Dermatology
Department of Veterinary Clinical Sciences
School of Veterinary Medicine
Louisiana State University
Baton Rouge, Louisiana
Microbiology of the Ear of the Dog and Cat

Jeffrey R. Moll, DVM
Christensen Animal Hospital
Wilmette, Illinois
Laser Ear Surgery

Mauricio Solano, MV, DACVR
Assistant Professor of Clinical Sciences
Tufts University School of Veterinary Medicine
Hospital for Large Animals
North Grafton, Massachusetts
Radiology and Diagnostic Imaging in the Ear

Norma White-Weithers, MS, DVM, Diplomate ACVD
Staff Dermatologist
Center for Specialized Veterinary Care
Westbury, New York
Ceruminous Diseases of the Ear

Ronald E. Whitford, DVM
Chief of Staff
St. Bethlehem Animal Clinic
Clarksville, Tennessee
Marketing Ear Service

Preface

As a full-time veterinarian in a small animal practice, working every day on the front lines of veterinary medicine, I am always asked, "How can you find the time to write a book?" My answer is that I truly believe that one of the most important challenges of being a doctor is that we should each share the knowledge that we acquire with our colleagues. I have found that I read everything I can find in books and journals, as well as on the Internet, pertaining to dog and cat skin and ear diseases. So, writing a book to share the information I have gathered about ear disease seems to be a logical progression.

Since the introduction of the first edition of *Small Animal Ear Diseases: An Illustrated Guide,* the awareness of otic disease as a serious ailment has been brought to the forefront of veterinary medicine. Veterinarians worldwide have embraced the use of video otoscopic diagnostics for ear disease, and we are now more often identifying treatable ear disease as a result. For example, recognizing otitis media in our patients and properly treating it has helped to relieve the misery and suffering that accompanies this painful disease.

The body of knowledge about ear disease is ever increasing. The number of published papers on the diagnosis and treatment of external and middle ear diseases has grown. Today, almost every small animal seminar or conference now includes lectures on ear disease and provides hands-on laboratory sessions using video otoscopy. New treatment modalities are being used in ear disease, and that has increased therapeutic options. Treating the tympanic bulla with infused topical medication is one example. Newly improvised intra-otic surgical procedures using the CO_2 laser and the diode laser, as well as radiofrequency surgery through the video otoscope, have decreased the number of lateral ear canal resections and ear canal ablations.

Many questions remain unanswered, but there are currently many ongoing studies that are attempting to answer the questions of why the ears become infected and what therapeutic options are the best for treatment. Exciting new drug classes and nutritional products may prove to be valuable in the prevention and treatment of ear diseases.

In this second edition, I have added new, useful information to the body of knowledge. Obviously, some of the information has not changed since the first edition, but based on the feedback that I received from readers, many of these topics have been expanded to give an in-depth review. The new chapters are enlightening. One of my goals in the second edition was to bring a better discussion of otic cytology and a photographic manual of ear cytology to the practitioner. In addition, the chapter on diagnostic imaging is superior to anything I have ever seen relating to diagnosing ear disease.

Many new photos in the second edition illustrate the vast number of ear conditions that are being commonly identified in dogs and cats by veterinarians. I have received many photos of interesting cases from practitioners and I have included several in this volume where appropriate.

My hope is that by presenting an expanded review of ear disease in dogs and cats, veterinarians can improve patient care. I would also hope that it poses some diagnostic and therapeutic problems that stimulate more research interest.

Louis N. Gotthelf
Montgomery, Alabama

Acknowledgments

It is important to recognize that I would not have the time to devote to the study of ear disease and to the preparation of a book manuscript if it were not for the support of my family, my staff at the Animal Hospital of Montgomery, and the clients who have the confidence in my abilities to allow me to treat their beloved companions.

But I would be remiss if I did not acknowledge the warm reception and constructive feedback that I have received as encouragement from my veterinarian colleagues all over the world. The letters and phone calls I receive thanking me for providing a book that helps them understand the mechanisms of ear disease and the logical approach to ear treatments have helped motivate me to write the second edition. Part of the reason for this second edition is that, through colleague comments and questions, I found that there is a thirst for new, useful information that needs to be quenched.

I would also like to again thank Ron Buck and Rodney Glass from MedRx, Inc. who have supported me since 1996. Their commitment to veterinary continuing education allows me to do 25 ear disease lectures and wet labs each year for veterinarians and technicians all over the United States and elsewhere. Their foresight in adapting their video otoscopic equipment to the needs of our profession makes it possible for me to show pictures of diseases of the ear in this book.

I have come to realize that writing the manuscript is the easy part of writing a book. Actually putting it all together into a meaningful end product is the hard part; from the language editing to the page layout, printing, marketing, and distribution, many people whom I do not even know had a part. So a big "thanks" to all of the people at Elsevier who worked as a team to get it into the final form.

Contents

1

Anatomy of the Canine and Feline Ear

A. Kumar, DVM, PhD

Margo Ruth Roman-Auerhahn, DVM

The basic anatomical components of the dog and cat ear are as follows:

- Auricle, or pinna
- Auditory canal, or external auditory meatus
- Middle ear
- Internal ear

Structure of the External Ear

The external ear is composed of three elastic cartilages: annular, scutiform, and auricular (Figure 1-1). The annular and auricular cartilages form the external ear canal, and the auricular cartilage expands to form the pinna. The scutiform cartilage lies

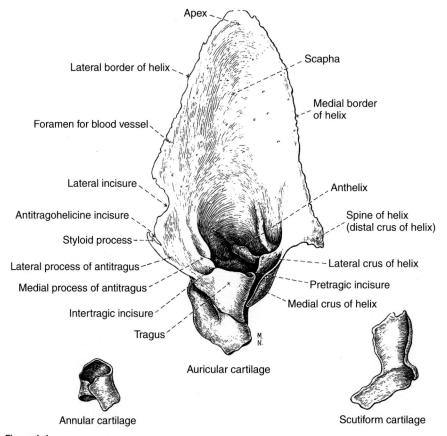

Figure 1-1

Cartilages of the right external ear. (From Evans HE, ed: *Miller's Anatomy of the dog,* ed 3, Philadelphia, 1993, WB Saunders.)

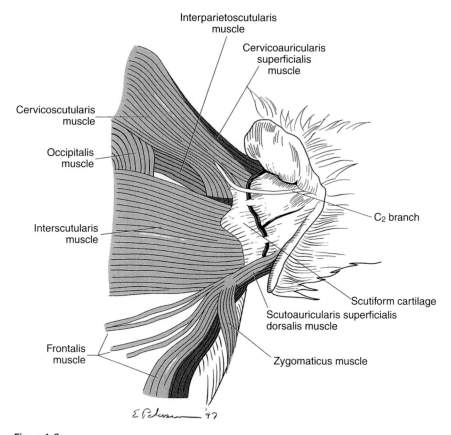

Interparietoscutularis
muscle

Cervicoauricularis
superficialis
muscle

Cervicoscutularis
muscle

Occipitalis
muscle

Interscutularis
muscle

C₂ branch

Scutiform cartilage

Scutoauricularis superficialis
dorsalis muscle

Frontalis
muscle

Zygomaticus muscle

Figure 1-2

Location of the scutiform cartilage in relation to some of the external ear muscles in the dog.

medial to the auricular cartilage within the auricular muscles that attach to the head (Figure 1-2).

Pinna, or Auricle

The pinna, or auricle, is a highly visible structure. Carriage of the pinna is breed-specific in the dog but mostly upright in the cat. It is designed to localize and collect sound waves and transmit them to the tympanic membrane (eardrum). The ear is moved by three sets of muscles (rostral, ventral, and caudal) that are innervated by branches of the facial nerve (cranial nerve VII).

The leaf-shaped pinna of the external ear is broad with medial (rostral) and lateral (caudal) margins. The caudal margin of the pinna exhibits a cutaneous pouch called the *marginal pouch* (Figure 1-3). This pouch has no obvious function. The skin on the concave surface of the pinna is very tightly connected to the underlying auricular cartilage, accentuating all the auricular prominences (see Figure 1-3). The skin covering the auricular cartilage may show breed-specific pigmentation. The shape and size of the external ear vary greatly among different breeds of dogs, mainly owing to the auricular cartilage that forms the skeleton of the pinna. It is the largest cartilage of the external ear. The broad auricular cartilage has numerous holes (see Figure 1-1), which are traversed by branches arising from the caudal auricular artery.

The auricular cartilage is broad dorsally and funnels to a narrow tubelike structure, the tubus auris, which fits around the annular cartilage ring. The parotid salivary gland occupies the base of the external ear, partially surrounding the tubus auris (Figures 1-4 and 1-5). The tubus auris encloses the vertical part of the external canal and, together

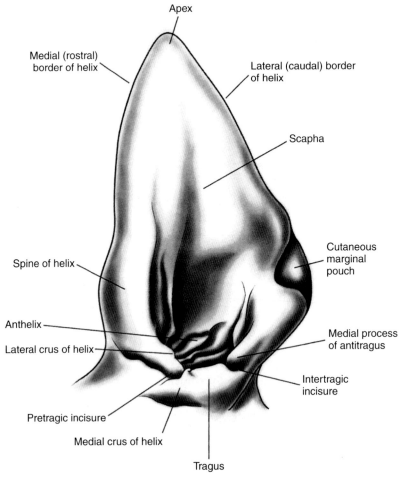

Figure 1-3

Anatomical features of the left external ear of the dog.

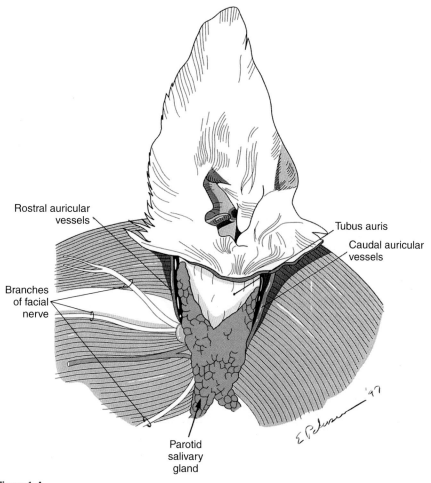

Rostral auricular
vessels

Tubus auris

Caudal auricular
vessels

Branches
of facial
nerve

Parotid
salivary
gland

Figure 1-4

Relationships of the tubus auris to the parotid salivary gland and auricular vessels. The facial nerve runs deep to the parotid salivary gland, immediately ventral to the annular cartilage, and gives off motor branches to the facial muscles.

with the tragal, antitragal, and antihelicene borders, forms the external acoustic meatus (see Figure 1-3).

Usually, the entrance to the external ear canal is guarded by a few fine hairs. Certain breeds, such as Airedales and Old English sheepdogs, exhibit hairy external ear canals. The external ear canal of the cat is devoid of hairs, and the ear canal is well ventilated. This may be a significant factor contributing to the lower incidence of external ear canal infections in cats. A hairy ear canal interferes with proper drainage and aeration of the canal in chronic otitis externa complicated by granulomatous lesions, leading to exacerbation of the condition.

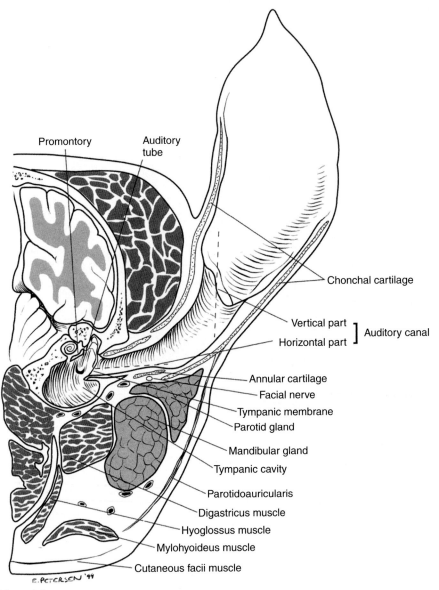

Figure 1-5

Structure of the ear canal. (Redrawn from Bojrab MJ: *Current techniques in small animal surgery I,* Philadelphia, 1975, Lea & Febiger.)

Annular Cartilage

The annular cartilage is part of the external ear canal. The pinna, formed by the cone-shaped auricular cartilage, articulates with the annular cartilage. The annular cartilage is a ring-shaped structure attached to the bony orbit of the external acoustic meatus of the temporal bone. A tubular cartilage piece, the annular cartilage surrounds the osseous external acoustic meatus (see Figure 1-7). It is attached to the bony rim of the external acoustic meatus by fibrous tissue that permits some degree of movement of the external ear. The annular cartilage encloses the horizontal part of the external ear canal.

Scutiform Cartilage

The scutiform cartilage is an L-shaped structure located over the temporalis muscle. It does not contribute to the formation of the external ear or its canal. The scutiform cartilage is attached to the midline raphe of the head and neck by numerous muscles (see Figure 1-2). Muscles also extend from the scutiform cartilage to the auricular cartilage. The scutiform cartilage functions like a fulcrum, providing for efficient movement of the auricle. It can be considered to function like a sesamoid cartilage. It lies over a fat cushion (corpus adiposum auriculae) on the dorsal surface of the temporalis muscle.

Structure of the Ear Canal

The external ear canal in the dog is 5 to 10 cm long and 4 to 5 mm wide (see Figure 1-5). The ear canal consists of an initial vertical part, which may extend an inch. The vertical canal runs ventrally and slightly rostrally before bending to a shorter horizontal canal that runs medially and forms the horizontal part of external ear canal. Because the external ear is elastic, the ear canal can be straightened enough to permit otoscopic examination.

The vertical part and most of the horizontal part of the canal are cartilaginous, but the deepest part is osseous. The ear canal is lined by skin containing sebaceous and ceruminous glands and hair follicles. The ceruminous glands are modified apocrine tubular sweat glands. The combined secretions of sebaceous and ceruminous glands constitute ear wax (cerumen). Cerumen (1) protects the external ear canal by immobilizing foreign objects and (2) keeps the tympanic membrane moist and pliable. The external ear canal is separated from the middle ear cavity by the semitransparent tympanic membrane.

Blood Supply to the External Ear

The external ear is generously vascularized by branches of the external carotid artery. A large caudal auricular artery arises from the external carotid artery at the base of the annular cartilage, medial to the parotid salivary gland and deep to the caudal

---

CLINICAL NOTE

Violent shaking of the head by the animal may contribute to fracture of the delicate auricular cartilage, resulting in severe hemorrhage within the cartilage. The blood clot (aural hematoma) may often fill the entire concave surface of the ear, requiring surgical removal of the clot.

---

auricular muscles. This artery gives off the lateral, intermediate, and medial auricular arteries, which pass along the convex surface of the pinna, wrapping around the helicene margins as well as penetrating the scapha and supplying the skin covering the cavum conchae. In addition to providing nourishment to the tissues of the external ear, the vascular supply to the pinna may also play a minor thermoregulatory role. Venous drainage occurs via the caudal auricular and superficial temporal veins into the maxillary vein.

Nerves of the External Ear

Sensory innervation of the pinna and external ear canal is provided by four nerves: the trigeminal, facial, vagus, and second cervical.

The auriculotemporal branch of the trigeminal nerve provides sensory innervation to the skin lining the horizontal part of the ear canal and to the tympanic membrane itself. This nerve also provides sensory innervation to the rostral margin of the pinna and the concave surface of the pinna close to the rostral margin and the skin over the tragus.

The facial nerve is related to the ventral surface of the annular cartilage, close to the osseous external acoustic meatus. The facial nerve provides substantial sensory innervation to the concave surface of the scapha and part of the cavum conchae via the rostral, middle, and caudal internal auricular branches (Figure 1-6). Most of the vertical along with part of the horizontal ear canal lining is supplied by the lateral internal auricular branch of the facial nerve, which may contain predominantly vagal fibers.

Communication between the facial nerve and the vagal nerve takes place as the facial nerve exits the stylomastoid foramen (see Figure 1-11). It is believed that these vagal branches are given off as the lateral internal auricular branch to the skin of the external ear canal. Reflex gastric vomiting may be triggered if the sensory endings of the vagus nerve are stimulated by mild ear canal irritation.

The convex surface of the pinna is provided with sensory innervation mainly by the second cervical nerve. All of the muscles of the external ear are innervated by the facial nerve.

Tympanic Membrane

The tympanic membrane (eardrum) is a thin, slightly opaque, membranous partition that separates the external ear from the middle ear. The tympanic membrane is

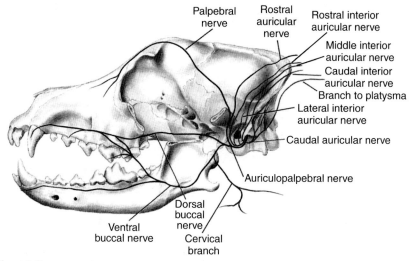

Palpebral nerve

Rostral auricular nerve

Rostral interior auricular nerve

Middle interior auricular nerve

Caudal interior auricular nerve

Branch to platysma

Lateral interior auricular nerve

Caudal auricular nerve

Auriculopalpebral nerve

Dorsal buccal nerve

Ventral buccal nerve

Cervical branch

Figure 1-6

Schematic drawing of sensory branches of the facial nerve that supply the external ear. Other important motor branches of the facial nerve are also shown.

located at a 45-degree angle in relation to the central axis of the horizontal part of the external ear canal (Figure 1-7; see also Figure 1-5). It is thin in the center and thicker near the periphery. The small upper portion is the pars flaccida, and the larger lower part is the pars tensa (Figure 1-8). With the exception of the pars flaccida, the membrane is tense, being firmly attached to the surrounding bone by a fibrocartilaginous ring, the annulus fibrocartilaginous. This ring is attached to the osseous ring of the external acoustic meatus by fibrous tissue.

The pars flaccida is a loose, opaque, pink triangular region forming the upper quadrant of the eardrum containing small branching blood vessels. Owing to its flaccid nature and rich blood supply, the pars flaccida heals rapidly if injured.

The pars tensa is thin, tough, and glistening, usually pearl-gray and translucent, although it may have opaque, radiating strands. The pars tensa, once broken, heals slowly. The external aspect of the tympanic membrane is concave because of traction on the medial surface by the manubrium of the malleus. The outline of the manubrium of the malleus is usually visible through the tympanic membrane as the stria mallearis (see Figure 1-8).

Opposite to the distal end of the manubrium, the depressed point on the external surface of the tympanic membrane is called the *umbo membrane tympani.*

Histologically, the tympanic membrane is made up of four layers: an external epidermal layer, an inner mucous layer, and two layers of intervening fibrous tissue. The epidermal layer is made up of a thin hairless skin consisting of a flat basal layer without any ridges, and a superficial layer only a few cells thick. This stratified squamous epithelium is continuous with the epithelial lining of the external ear canal. The thin dermis contains fibroblasts and a fine vascular supply. The thicker middle

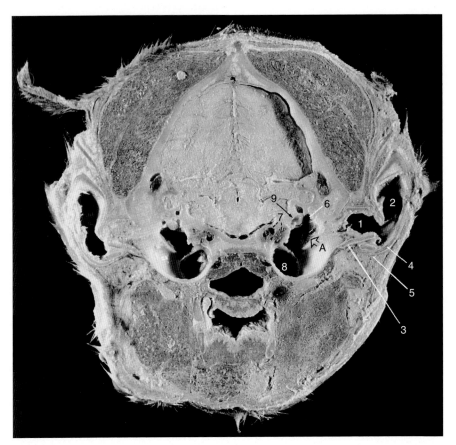

Figure 1-7

Transverse section through the head of the dog at the level of the tympanic bulla. *A,* Osseous external acoustic meatus covered by tympanic membrane. Note that the tympanic membrane is placed at an approximately 45-degree angle in relation to the central axis of the horizontal part of the ear canal. *1,* Horizontal part of the ear canal; *2,* vertical part of the ear canal; *3,* annular cartilage; *4,* auricular cartilage; *5,* parotid salivary gland; *6,* epitympanic recess; *7,* carotid canal accommodating the internal carotid artery, postganglionic sympathetic nerves, and the ventral petrosal venous sinus (the caudal continuation of cavernous venous sinus), which drains into the internal jugular and vertebral veins; *8,* cavity of the middle ear; *9,* osseous labyrinth accommodating the internal ear.

fibrous layer consists of an outer layer of fibers that radiate toward the annulus fibrocartilaginous from the center of the eardrum. A layer of inner fibers are circular and are found closer to the annulus. The manubrium of the malleus is buried in the fibrous layer intercalated between the two epithelial surfaces. The arrangement of fibers in the middle layer optimizes the vibratory faces. The arrangement of fibers in the middle layer optimizes the vibratory response of the tympanic membrane to incoming sound waves. The inner layer of the tympanic membrane is composed of

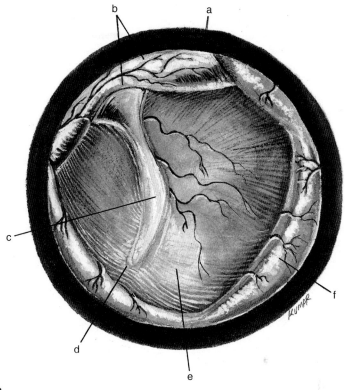

Figure 1-8

Tympanic membrane anatomy in the dog as observed through an otoscope. *a,* Rim of the otoscopic tube; *b,* flaccid part of the tympanic membrane; *c,* manubrium of malleus shining through the tympanic membrane; *d,* umbo of tympanic membrane; *e,* pars tensa of the tympanic membrane surrounding the manubrium; *f,* skin of the external acoustic meatus raised by the otoscopic tube. (Modified from DeLahunta A, Habel RE: *Applied veterinary anatomy,* Philadelphia, 1986, WB Saunders.)

a single layer of respiratory epithelium. The epithelium lining the inner surface of the tympanic membrane starts as columnar at the periphery, gradually becoming cuboidal and finally squamous at the center. This layer is continuous with the mucous membrane type of respiratory epithelium covering the middle ear cavity, auditory tube, and nasal cavity. The underlying lamina propria is thin, with a fine vascular supply.

Middle Ear

The middle ear consists of the space within the osseous tympanic bulla, the opening of the auditory tube, and the three ear ossicles with their associated muscles and ligaments.

Structure of the Osseous Tympanic Bulla

It is clinically relevant to appreciate the close relationships among the facial canal, which carries the facial nerve; the petrooccipital (or carotid) canal, which carries postganglionic sympathetic nerves to the eye; and the periorbital structures, structures of the inner ear, and the middle ear cavity. The tympanic bulla has approximately equal dimensions (8 to 10 mm) in width and depth. The wall of the bulla tympanica is very thin and easy to remove.

The roof of the tympanic cavity presents a barrel-shaped prominence called the *cochlear promontory* (Figures 1-9 and 1-10). The osseous bony cochlea is excavated within the cochlear promontory. At the caudolateral end of this promontory, a foramen called the *cochlear* (or round) *window* is located. The cochlear window is covered by a thin membrane that oscillates to dissipate the vibratory energy of the perilymph in the scala tympani. Immediately lateral to the barrel-shaped promontory, a narrow vestibular (or oval) window is present, which is covered by a thin diaphragm. The footplate of the stapes is attached to the diaphragm over the vestibular window. The bony facial canal is closely related to the middle ear cavity.

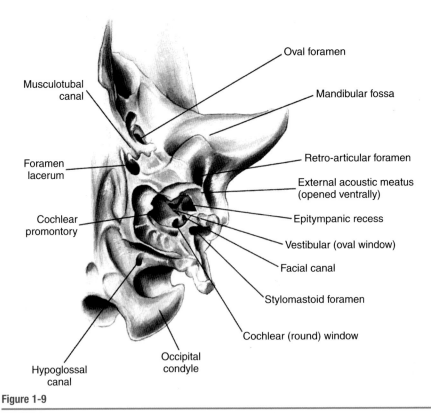

Figure 1-9

Internal anatomy of the left tympanic bulla, ventral view. The ventral wall of the bulla has been removed.

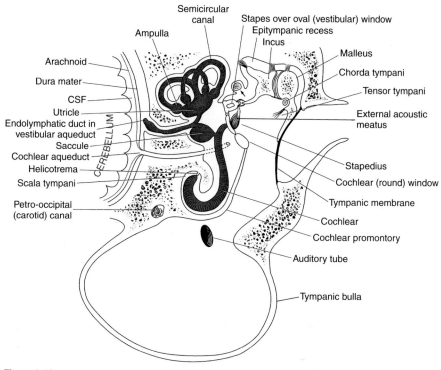

Figure 1-10

Schematic drawing of the internal and middle ear structures. The three ear ossicles form synovial joints with one another, supported by ligaments and two skeletal muscles. Note the location of the facial nerve in relation to the middle ear cavity *(arrow)*. Also shown are the relationships between subarachnoid space containing cerebrospinal fluid *(CSF)* and the inner ear via the cochlear aqueduct.

An open slit facing the vestibular window is present in the bony facial canal (see Figures 1-9 and 1-10). This slit is the open part of the facial canal, which is covered by mucous membrane lining the tympanic bulla. The other fossae close to the external acoustic meatus accommodate the tensor tympani and stapedius muscles. The small middle ear bones—the malleus, incus, and stapes—are accommodated in an epitympanic recess located dorsal to the oval and vestibular window, immediately medial to the opening of the external acoustic meatus.

At the caudal aspect of the tympanic bulla is a large fissure called the *tympanooccipital fissure,* which is also called the *petrobasilar* or *petro-occipital fissure.* A medial foramen in the tympanooccipital fissure that leads into a canal between the occipital and temporal bones is called the *caudal foramen lacerum.* The bony canal that extends rostrally from the caudal foramen lacerum is called the *carotid canal;* it transmits the internal carotid artery and postganglionic sympathetic plexus from the superior cervical ganglion (also called the *carotid plexus,* made up of the carotid nerves; Figure 1-11). The carotid canal in its caudal extent also accommodates the ventral petrosal venous sinus (the caudal continuation of the cavernous venous sinus), which drains into the internal jugular and vertebral veins.

Ear Ossicles

The auditory ossicles—the malleus, incus, and stapes—are small movable bones that extend like a chain from the tympanic membrane and functionally connect the tympanic membrane with the vestibular (oval) window (see Figure 1-10). The ossicles consist of compact bone formed by endochondral ossification. They form synovial joints with each other.

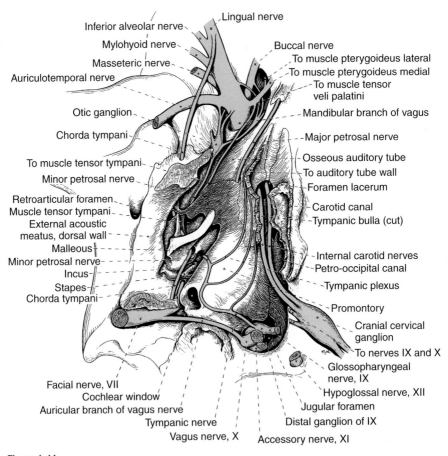

Figure 1-11

Nerves in relation to the middle ear cavity, ventral view, with most of the tympanic bulla removed. (From Evans HE, ed: *Miller's Anatomy of the dog,* ed 3, Philadelphia, 1993, WB Saunders.)

The malleus is the most lateral bone. It consists of a head that articulates with the incus, a thin neck, and a long manubrium, or handle. The lateral aspect of the handle is concave and is embedded in the tympanic membrane, as described earlier.

Articulating with the medial part of the incus is the stapes. It is in direct contact with the perilymph fluid through its footplate (base of stapes) attachment in the oval window.

Vibrations of the tympanic membrane are transmitted through the chain of these auditory ossicles to the perilymph fluid within the vestibule. The vestibular window is approximately 18 to 20 times smaller in area than the tympanic membrane, contributing significantly to the amplification of sound waves by the ear ossicles.

The middle ear ossicles are associated with two very small skeletal muscles (see Figure 1-10). The tensor tympani muscle is a spherical muscle that attaches to the malleus by a short tendon. It is supplied by a branch of the trigeminal nerve. The stapedius, the smallest skeletal muscle in the body, is closely related to the facial nerve at its origin. This muscle is supplied by the facial nerve. Reflex contraction of these two muscles in response to loud noises results in fixation of the ear ossicles, damping vibrations. This protective reflex is called the *tympanic reflex*. It takes approximately 40 to 160 milliseconds for the tympanic reflex to occur.

Tympanic Bulla

The osteum of the auditory tube lies in a rostrodorsomedial location in the tympanic bulla, coursing anteriorly. The auditory tube is lined by pseudostratified ciliated columnar epithelium containing goblet cells. The auditory tube opens into the nasopharynx and equalizes air pressure on either side of the tympanic membrane. On the medial wall of the tympanic cavity is the promontory, a bony shelf that houses the bony labyrinth (see Figure 1-10).

The central space of the labyrinth, called the *vestibule,* is continuous with the subarachnoid space via the cochlear aqueduct (see Figure 1-10). It is filled with peri-lymph, which is similar to cerebrospinal fluid. The vestibule connects to the three semicircular canals and the cochlea.

On the lateral side of the promontory is a thin bony plate containing two windows or fenestrations. The oval or vestibular window lies on the dorsolateral surface of the promontory immediately adjacent to the pars flaccida. It attaches to the base of the stapes and connects to the vestibule. Vibrations are transmitted to the endolymph contained within the cochlea from the tympanic membrane via the ear ossicle chain to the oval window. The round window, an opening in the bony shelf of the osseous cochlea, is covered by a secondary tympanic membrane. It is found in the anterior end of the vestibule, just ventral to the smaller oval window. This membrane permits vibrations that have already passed to sensory receptors to be dissipated into the air-filled tympanic bulla.

The middle ear cavity of the cat is divided by a septum into two separate tympanic cavities (Figure 1-12). In the small dorsolateral compartment lie the auditory ossicles, the osteum of the auditory tube, and the eardrum. The larger ventromedial compartment is an air-filled tympanic bulla. The two compartments of the tympanic

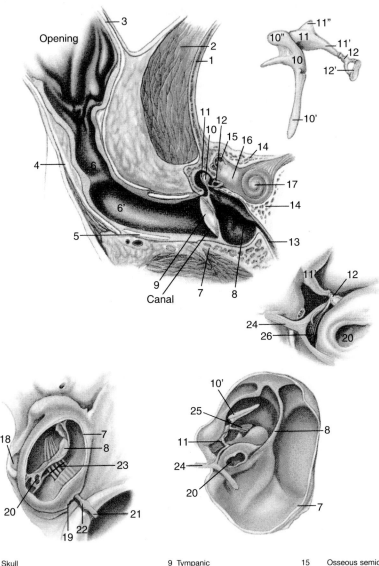

1	Skull		9	Tympanic		15	Osseous semicircular
2	M. temporalis			membrane			canals
3–6′	External ear		10–12	Ear ossicles		16	Vestibule
	3,4	Auricular cartilage		10	Malleus	17	Cochlea
	3	Scapha		10′	Manubrium	18	External acoustic meatus
	4	Concha		10″	Head	19	Tympano-occipital fissure
	5	Annular cartilage		11	Incus	20	Vestibular window
	6	External ear canal,		11′	Long crus	21	Cervical sympathetic trunk
		vertical part		11″	Short crus	22	Cranial cervical ganglion
		6′	External ear canal,	12	Stapes	23	Sympathetic rami
			horizontal part	12′	Base	24	Facial n.
7–12	Middle ear		13	Auditory tube		25	M. tensor tympani
	7	Tympanic bulla		14	Petrous temporal bone	26	M. Stapediurs
	8	Septum bullae		15–17	Osseous labyrinth		

Figure 1-12

Schematic views of the cat middle and internal ear. (From Hudson LC, Hamilton WP: *Atlas of feline anatomy for veterinarians,* Philadelphia, 1993, WB Saunders.)

bulla communicate via a small passage located dorsally near the cochlear window. This intervening bony septum should be perforated when necessary for proper drainage of the middle ear cavity. Rough handling of the bony septum may result in damage to the postganglionic sympathetic nerves. The nerves, which are visible submucosally as fine strands over the cochlear promontory, should be avoided during surgical removal of the septum in the cat.

Nerves

Two types of nerves should be considered in relation to the middle ear: (1) nerves in transit in close association with the middle ear but destined for a distant location and (2) nerves that play a role in normal function of the middle ear. All are susceptible to injury by disease of or trauma to the middle ear.

Those nerves that are in transit in relation to the middle ear are as follows:

- The sympathetic postganglionic nerves to the eye and orbit from nerve cell bodies located in the cranial cervical ganglion
- The facial nerve and a branch from it (chorda tympani)
- A branch of the glossopharyngeal nerve.

The sympathetic postganglionic nerve fibers are collectively called *internal carotid nerves* (see Figure 1-11), and they travel as a perivascular nerve plexus along with the internal carotid artery in the petrooccipital canal, which is separated from the middle ear cavity by a thin bony plate in the dog. Chronic infections in the middle ear cavity can erode the bone separating the carotid nerves from the middle ear cavity.

In the cat, the postganglionic sympathetic nerves run through the middle ear cavity submucosally below the septum of the tympanic bulla over the cochlear promontory. Damage to these nerves results in Horner's syndrome, consisting of miosis (constriction of the pupil) and enophthalmos (recession of the eyeball), which contributes to prolapse of the third eyelid. Ptosis (drooping of the upper eyelid) may also be present.

The facial nerve travels through the bony facial canal (Figure 1-13). As mentioned before, the facial canal is incomplete, exposing this nerve to the middle ear cavity. This can contribute to the involvement of the facial nerve in chronic middle ear infections. Early symptoms of facial nerve involvement may include blepharospasm. Other symptoms, such as drooping of the ear, paralysis of buccal muscles, and spasms of the platysma behind the ear on the affected side, may also be exhibited, depending on the degree of facial nerve involvement.

The chorda tympani, a branch of the facial nerve, runs through the middle ear cavity. It courses medial to the base of the malleus in the dorsal compartment of the middle ear (see Figures 1-10 and 1-13). The chorda tympani carries preganglionic parasympathetic nerves that synapse in the mandibular and sublingual ganglia to innervate the mandibular and sublingual salivary glands, respectively. This nerve also carries gustatory fibers from fungiform papillae in the rostral two thirds of the tongue. Because taste buds require neurotropic influences to remain functional, damage to the chorda tympani may result in atrophy of fungiform papillae on the affected side.

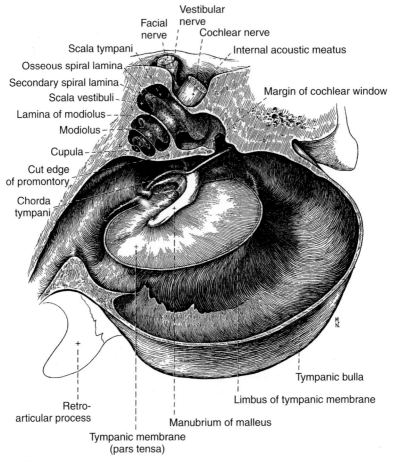

Vestibular
nerve
Facial
nerve
Cochlear nerve
Scala tympani
Internal acoustic meatus
Osseous spiral lamina
Secondary spiral lamina
Margin of cochlear window
Scala vestibuli
Lamina of modiolus
Modiolus
Cupula
Cut edge
of promontory
Chorda
tympani
Tympanic bulla
Limbus of tympanic membrane
Retro-
articular process
Manubrium of malleus
Tympanic membrane
(pars tensa)

Figure 1-13

Sculpted medial view of the right middle ear and cochlea. (From Evans HE, ed: *Miller's Anatomy of the dog,* ed 3, Philadelphia, 1993, WB Saunders.)

The tympanic nerve of the glossopharyngeal nerve supplies the mucous membrane lining of the tympanic bulla. The tympanic nerve gives off the tympanic plexus, which innervates the middle ear cavity (see Figure 1-11).

These nerves may be involved in sensing pressure changes across the tympanic membrane. They may also carry pain sensations from the middle ear cavity. The tympanic nerve itself runs through the middle ear cavity submucosally as the minor petrosal nerve, which mainly carries preganglionic parasympathetic nerve fibers to the otic ganglion. Postganglionic nerve fibers from the otic ganglion innervate the parotid and zygomatic salivary glands. Injury to the tympanic nerve may thus lead to partial loss of salivation on the affected side. The tensor tympani from the mandibular nerve of the trigeminal innervates the tensor tympani muscle. Stapedial nerves from the facial nerve provide motor innervation to the stapedius muscle. The tensor tympani and stapedial nerves are clinically not important.

Inner Ear

The main functions of the inner ear are receiving auditory signals and maintaining equilibrium. The inner ear is located within the osseous labyrinth of the petrous part of the temporal bone. The membranous labyrinth consists of three primary parts: the cochlea, vestibule, and semicircular canals. The vestibule is divided into an utricle and a saccule. The vestibulocochlear nerve (cranial nerve VIII) supplies the membranous cochlea, vestibule, and semicircular canals (Figure 1-14).

Osseous Anatomy

The petrosal part of the tympanic bone has an internal pyramid containing the internal acoustic meatus, the osseous and membranous labyrinths, and an external mastoid process. The pyramidal part of the petrous (meaning "rocklike") temporal bone is the hardest bone in the body. The rostrodorsal surface of the pyramid is in contact with the cerebrum and hence is called the *cerebral surface,* whereas the caudomedial surface contacts the cerebellum and is called the *cerebellar surface.* The mid-part of the cerebellar surface of the pyramid exhibits a foramen called the *internal acoustic meatus.* The internal acoustic meatus in turn presents two tiny foramina: (1) a dorsally located foramen that leads into the osseous facial canal for the seventh cranial nerve and vestibular component of the eighth cranial nerve, and (2) a ventrally located foramen for the cochlear component of the eighth cranial nerve (see Figure 1-13). Because of the close association of the facial and eighth cranial nerves within the petrous temporal bone, the two nerves may be affected simultaneously by the same lesion.

The excavation within the petrous temporal bone, called the *osseous labyrinth,* is approximately 15 mm long. It is divided into three compartments: the cochlea, vestibule, and semicircular canals. The osseous vestibule is continuous with the subarachnoid space via the cochlear aqueduct (see Figure 1-10). Via this duct, the perilymph is continuous with cerebrospinal fluid in the subarachnoid space surrounding the brain. Chronic middle ear infections can thus travel via the vestibular or cochlear window to affect the inner ear and eventually can spread via the cochlear aqueduct to the meninges. Within the osseous labyrinth, the membranous labyrinth is suspended in perilymph.

Cochlea

The membranous labyrinth within the osseous labyrinth is an interconnecting system of epithelium-lined tubules and spaces filled with a clear fluid called *endolymph.* As

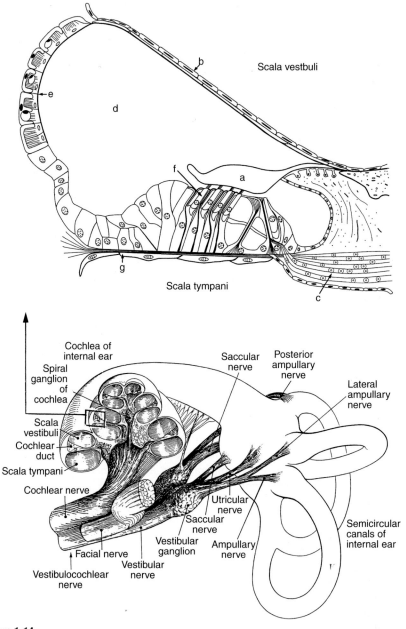

Scala vestbuli

Scala tympani

Cochlea of
internal ear

Spiral
ganglion
of
cochlea

Scala
vestibuli

Cochlear
duct

Scala tympani

Cochlear nerve

Saccular
nerve

Posterior
ampullary
nerve

Lateral
ampullary
nerve

Semicircular
canals of
internal ear

Utricular
nerve

Saccular
nerve

Facial nerve

Vestibular
ganglion

Vestibular
nerve

Ampullary
nerve

Vestibulocochlear
nerve

Figure 1-14

Schematic drawing of the inner ear. The membranous labyrinth is rotated 180 degrees ventrodorsally. *Top panel* shows the membranous cochlea in section and spiral organ (organ of Corti). *a,* Tectorial membrane; *b,* vestibular membrane; *c,* spiral ganglion of the cochlea; *d,* scala media; *e,* stria vascularis, which primarily produces endolymph; *f,* outer hair cells, which are sensory receptors for sound; *g,* basilar membrane. *Lower panel* shows innervation of the inner ear complex by branches of the eighth cranial nerve.

mentioned before, the vestibule consists of the utricle and the saccule. These sacs communicate directly with each other and also with the semicircular and cochlear ducts. The cochlea is receptive to vibrations in endolymph, and the rest of the membranous labyrinth is associated with the function of equilibrium. Problems within the membranous labyrinth lead to signs of deafness and vestibular disease, including vestibular ataxia, circling, head tilting, strabismus, and nystagmus.

The bony cochlea winds around a hollow central axis (modiolus) in a dorsoventral direction. The modiolus accommodates the cochlear nerve (see Figure 1-14). The osseous or bony spiral lamina is a bony shelf that projects from the modiolus into the interior of the canal. Like the cochlea, it makes three and one quarter turns to end at the apex, or cupula (see Figure 1-13). The bony spiral lamina reaches about halfway into the lumen of the bony cochlea, partially dividing its cavity into two parts, the dorsal scala vestibuli and the ventral scala tympani.

The membranous cochlear duct is an epithelium-lined and endolymph-filled structure that extends from the osseous spiral lamina to the outer bony wall, completely dividing the scala vestibuli and scala tympani. The scala vestibuli and scala tympani are continuous with each other at the apex of the modiolus through a small foramen called the *helicotrema.* The cavity of the membranous cochlea, called the *scala media,* is filled by endolymph.

A specialized thickened epithelium in the basilar membrane constitutes the spiral organ (organ of Corti), in which cochlear nerve endings innervate the sensory hair cells. The hair cells are exposed to a specialized leaflike structure, the tectorial membrane. Vibrations of perilymph are transmitted to endolymph by the intervening (vestibular) membrane between the scala vestibuli and the scala media. The tectorial membrane in turn vibrates, touching the hair cells and initiating nerve impulses that are carried by the cochlear nerve to the brain.

Damage to the hair cells leads to hearing deficits or loss. Congenital deafness may be either perceptive (inner ear defect) or central (lesion of the auditory brain center). Acquired deafness may be either central or peripheral, resulting from chronic disease, normal aging, or drug use. Aminoglycoside therapy can lead to ototoxicity, a leading cause of iatrogenic hearing loss. White cats with congenital deafness have numerous cochlear abnormalities, including lesions in the spiral ganglion of the cochlear nerve.

Suggested Readings

Blauch B, Strafuss AC: Histologic relationships of the facial (7th) and vestibulocochlear (8th) cranial nerves within the petrous temporal bone in the dog, *Am J Vet Res* 35:481, 1974.
Evans HE: *Miller's Anatomy of the dog,* ed 3, Philadelphia, 1993, WB Saunders.
Getty R: *Sisson and Grossman's The anatomy of the domestic animals,* ed 5, vol 2, Philadelphia, 1975, WB Saunders.
King AS, Riley VA: *A guide to the physiological and clinical anatomy of the head,* ed 4, Liverpool, UK, 1980, University of Liverpool.

2

Examination of the External Ear Canal

Louis N. Gotthelf, DVM

One of the most common ailments of dogs seen in a veterinary practice is ear disease. Approximately 15% to 20% of all canine patients and approximately 6% to 7% of all feline patients have some kind of ear disease, from mild erythema to severe otitis media. Many clients are unaware of their pets' otitis, and many pets do not show clinical signs of ear disease until it has become quite severe. Determining the cause of ear disease is often a difficult task.

Examination of the ear canals and tympanic membranes of dogs and cats can be extremely frustrating for the veterinarian presented with a patient suffering from ear disease. Simply manipulating the pinna or inserting the otoscope cone into the painful ear of a dog or cat can cause discomfort to the patient and may result in aggressive behavior toward the examiner. Looking through an otoscope in a patient that is shaking its head to relieve its discomfort gives the examiner a very quick, superficial look, at best. Painful ears prevent thorough examination, so sedation or anesthesia is required for a complete examination.

The Normal Ear

To become familiar with the appearance of the normal ear canal and eardrum, the veterinarian should perform a thorough ear examination on every patient anesthetized for any reason (such as ovariohysterectomy or a dental procedure). It is necessary to know (1) what the normal ear canal should look like, (2) where the eardrum should be located, if it is not readily visible, and (3) how to distinguish normal cerumen from otic exudates in order to determine whether the ear is affected by disease.

Ear Canal

The normal ear canal epithelium should be light pink with small superficial blood vessels visible (Figure 2-1). Small amounts of cerumen coating the epithelium give the surface a glistening appearance. Cerumen is a normal part of a healthy ear and should not be regarded as pathological unless it is excessive. Hairs are seen along the canal, being more numerous in the vertical canal (Figure 2-2).

The dog's ear canal gently bends approximately 75 degrees as it changes from the vertical to the horizontal (Figure 2-3). With the dog in the standing position, the examiner should gently place traction ventrally on the pinna; the ear canal will straighten out, because the normal underlying cartilage is soft and pliable. The otoscope cone should be advanced into the horizontal canal as the canal straightens. This technique enables the horizontal canal to be examined. In the anesthetized patient in lateral recumbency, the examiner can straighten out the canal by lifting the pinna vertically to the point of elevating the entire head.

Hairs are almost absent from the horizontal canal in most dogs. However, a clump of long, bristly hairs is often found at the distal end of the horizontal canal and may cause discomfort (Figure 2-4). An accumulation of wax may be seen along the

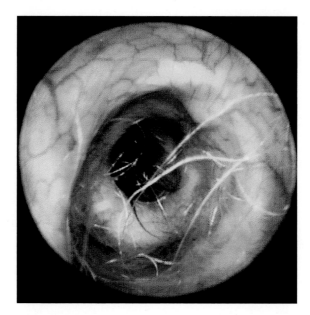

Figure 2-1

Normal ear canal of the dog.

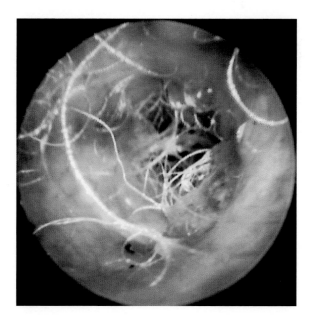

Figure 2-2

Numerous hairs and wax found in the vertical canal of a poodle.

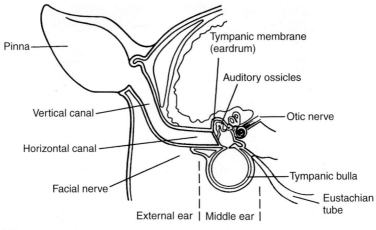

Figure 2-3

The anatomy of the dog's ear canal. The vertical canal bends at approximately 75 degrees to become the horizontal canal.

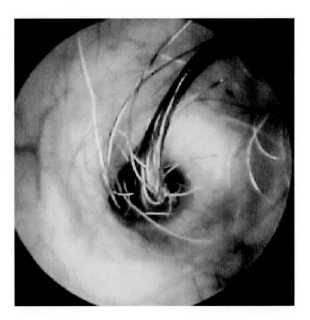

Figure 2-4

A tuft of long, thick, bristly hairs is sometimes found in the horizontal canal originating near the annulus of the eardrum. These hairs can be irritating and may become the matrix for wax plugs.

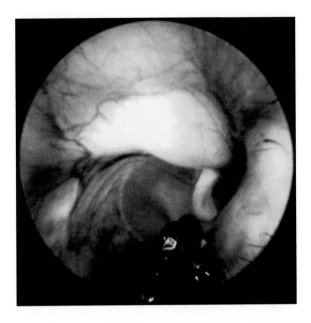

Figure 2-5

Accumulation of wax along the ventral floor of the horizontal canal. This wax is helpful for orienting the dorsoventral axis when examining the ear canals.

ventral floor of the horizontal canal (Figure 2-5). As the otoscope is advanced in the horizontal canal, the tympanic membrane, if present, should become visible.

Tympanic Membrane

The normal tympanic membrane in both the dog and the cat appears as a thin, transparent to translucent, reflective end of the horizontal ear canal (Figures 2-6 and 2-7). The normal eardrum has been described as having a pale, "rice paper" appearance. The outline of the footplate (manubrium) of the malleus is seen attached to the medial side of the tympanic membrane, frequently bulging outward (pars tensa). The malleus is seen as a thin rectangular white bone originating from the dorsal portion of the tympanic membrane and extending ventrally halfway across the membrane. The malleus is oriented dorsoventrally. The free distal end of the manubrium may have a gentle curve or a "hook" that points rostrally. This feature aids in distinguishing the right ear from the left ear on photographs of the eardrum.

Examination of the dorsal portion of the tympanic membrane (pars flaccida) reveals an opaque, pink or white, loose membrane often containing a network of small blood vessels that extend across the tympanic membrane (Figure 2-8). This "vascular strip" often has an edematous appearance, and this "pretympanic bleb" may obstruct visualization of dorsal portions of the eardrum. In many cases of otitis media, the vascular strip is destroyed, removing from the germinal epithelium of the

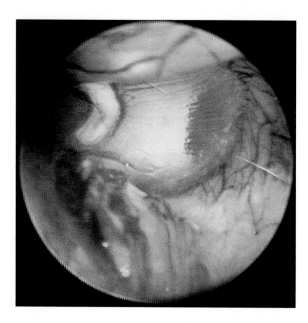

Figure 2-6

Normal canine left eardrum. The yellow wax is in the ventral portion of the horizontal canal. The footplate of the malleus can be clearly seen through the rice paper–thin *pars tensa*. The malleus has a "hook" that points rostrally. In the dorsal portion of the eardrum is the *pars flaccida* with the blood vessels that supply the epithelium over the malleus.

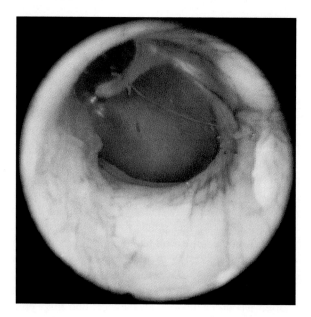

Figure 2-7

Normal feline eardrum.

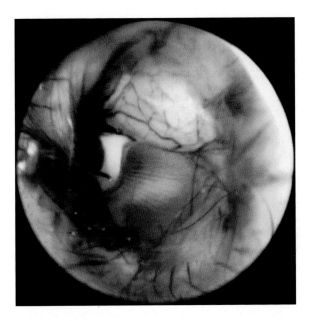

Figure 2-8

Prominent *pars flaccida* forming the "vascular strip." This provides the blood supply to the eardrum. Radial collagen fibers can be seen in the *pars tensa.*

eardrum the blood supply that is required for the eardrum to heal. If the vascular strip is unaffected by disease or trauma, the damaged eardrum has a much better chance of completely healing with time.

The tympanic membrane in dogs is oriented at an acute angle of as much as 45 degrees to the long axis of the horizontal canal, making visualization of the entire eardrum difficult.

Often, the lower portion of the eardrum's attachment to the horizontal canal is obscured from view due to a depression of the floor of the horizontal canal, forming a fornix. Some dogs may have negative pressure in the tympanic bulla, which causes retraction of the eardrum into the bulla and makes examination difficult. A condition known as a "false middle ear" has been described, in which the tympanic membrane is actually stretched inward into the bulla from exudates or negative pressure and becomes attached to the lining of the middle ear. In this condition, the entire middle ear cavity is obliterated. When such an ear is examined with the otoscope, no eardrum is visible, but a deep, dark hole can be seen.

In the anesthetized patient in lateral recumbency, the pinna is lifted vertically to straighten the curved ear canal, which makes advancing of the otoscope cone easier. The tip of the instrument can be advanced closer to the eardrum. The cat's tympanic membrane is easily visualized because the eardrum is oriented in a plane forming a 90-degree angle with the short ear canal.

Assessing the Ear Canals

With the otoscope, the examiner evaluates the ear canals for the following:
- Patency or stenosis
- Color changes
- Proliferative changes
- Ulcerations
- Exudates (Figure 2-9)
- Foreign bodies
- Parasites
- Tumors
- Excessive hair or waxy accumulation.

The location of the lesion along the canal should be noted. If visibility is impaired by hair or excessive cerumen or exudates, then either plucking the hair plug or flushing the external ear canal is mandatory. Cytological and culture specimens of any exudates or secretions should be collected with a small cotton-tipped swab, curette, or catheter prior to initiation of cleaning by any method.

In otitis externa, proteolytic enzymes are produced that have a depilatory effect, so hairs may be absent on examination. After therapy has resolved the ear disease, hair regrowth is a good indicator that the treatment was successful.

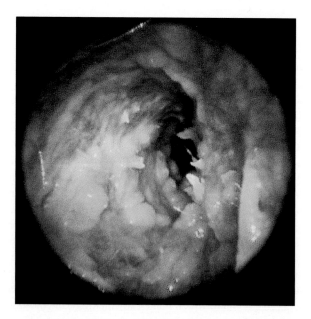

Figure 2-9

Otitis externa in a cocker spaniel. There is a yellow, creamy exudate present in the vertical canal. This cocker had a ceruminous otitis externa with large numbers of *Staphylococci*.

Flushing the Canals

Until a determination of the integrity of the eardrum is made, the choice of flushing solutions should be limited to nondetergent, nonfoaming types of flushing solutions. Tepid solutions (98° F) of saline or very dilute povidone-iodine solution are used to soften and loosen wax and debris. For gentle flushing, a bulb syringe should be used to irrigate the vertical canal, and a syringe and catheter should be used to irrigate the horizontal canal. This should be repeated until the ear canal is clean.

When ear disease is present, exudates accumulate along the ventral portion of the horizontal canal and remain in contact with the eardrum. Proteolytic enzymes elaborated as a result of inflammation break down the eardrum and weaken it. Therefore, even gentle flushing against a weakened membrane may cause it to rupture. Detergents and alcohols, along with many organic acids contained in ear cleaners, which are extremely irritating to the mucosa lining the bulla, may gain access to the middle ear in this manner. If this should happen, the tympanic bulla should be copiously irrigated with normal saline.

If the eardrum is visible and is normal, detergent ear cleaners are safe to use for flushing of the ceruminous ear canals. Various commercially available solutions designed to flush the ear canals are also safe for removing pus and serum from the ear canal where a detergent ceruminolytic is not required. Ear curettes of various sizes can be used to scrape large pieces of exudates off the ear canal.

Otoscopy

The conventional otoscope is configured to project a bright light through a conical tube. Objects in the ear canal reflect the light back to the examiner's eye. A large magnifying lens at the eyepiece focuses on the end of the otoscope cone and aids in enlarging the image. For procedures using an otoscope, an "operating" head is available with a very small lens at the eyepiece. This allows the examiner to place small instruments through the cone without having to move the lens. The disadvantages of this system are that (1) the light may not be strong enough to transilluminate the eardrum, and (2) when instruments are used, the view of the examiner is often obliterated.

The Video Otoscope

A video-based otoscope (MedRx Video Vetscope, MedRx, Inc., Largo, Florida) has been designed to overcome the shortcomings of the hand-held otoscope. This is a very useful instrument for examining, cleaning, and drying the ear canal because it gives the examiner a clear real-time image on a video monitor (Figure 2-10). The high-quality glass lens pack of the Video Vetscope probe begins with a 2-mm lens at the tip of the 4.75-mm diameter probe. This lens configuration provides a 110-degree angle of view and an infinite focus to the image ahead of the probe tip. Even in small patients in which the ear canal diameter is smaller than the tip of the probe, the wide

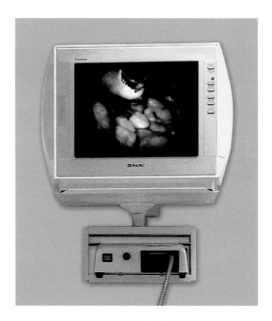

Figure 2-10

Video otoscopy allows the client and veterinarian to view the patient's ear canal on a video monitor. (Courtesy MedRx, Inc., Largo, Florida.)

viewing angle and the long focal length of this instrument allow examination of the ear canal. Light fibers within the tip of the probe are connected to a powerful halogen light source, providing excellent illumination. A 2-mm working channel is built into the Vetscope probe, separate from the lens system. Instruments can be placed through the working channel without obscuring the view of the procedure. The entire instrument is attached to a miniature color video camera (Figure 2-11), which is connected to a video monitor and a video printer.

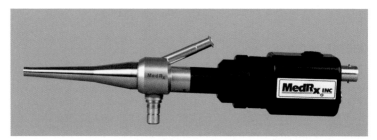

Figure 2-11

Video Vetscope probe attached to a miniature video camera. (Courtesy MedRx, Inc., Largo, Florida.)

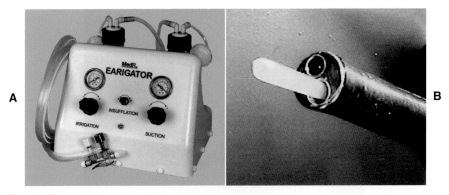

Figure 2-12

MedRx Earigator with independent flushing and suction. **A,** The free end of the trumpet valves connects to the flared end of a catheter. **B,** The catheter is extended through the 2-mm working channel. (Courtesy MedRx, Inc., Largo, Florida.)

For flushing and suctioning of the ear canals, a 5 Fr feeding tube or a polypropylene urethral catheter can be inserted through the video otoscope's working channel. Use of an irrigation/suction machine (Earigator, MedRx, Inc., Largo, Florida) (Figure 2-12) makes this procedure very efficient. The catheter is inserted into the working channel with the otoscope positioned in the ear canal. The catheter can be advanced into the ear canal with clear visualization (Figure 2-13). Small pieces of epithelium, wax, hairs, and pus can be flushed away from the ear canal epithelium and then suctioned out of the canal while the examiner views the procedure on the video monitor. In this manner, even the smallest pieces of detritus can be removed. The examiner can extract large pieces of debris and concretions of wax and medications from the ear canal under visualization with the Video Vetscope by using a grasping type of endoscopic forceps inserted through the 2-mm working channel or an ear curette (Figure 2-14).

The video otoscope also has documentation capability. When a lesion is encountered, the image on the video monitor can be "frozen" and then printed out as a 4- × 5-inch color glossy photograph with the use of a video printer. Thus, there is a photographic hard copy document of the ear disease to place in the medical record for comparison on rechecks. These photographs are also helpful in counseling owners and showing them the severity of the ear disease; they make the veterinarian's medical or surgical recommendations more valid. Documentation capability is very useful in a referral practice. The referring veterinarian can receive a color photograph of the ear canal in addition to the written report. The photographs can also be used to illustrate contributions to veterinary medical literature. The video otoscope can be coupled to a videocassette recorder so that the examination and surgical procedures can be videotaped and kept for documentation. A computer-based database system is also available to catalog and store video examination records as both digital photos and 30-second digital video clips (Figure 2-15).

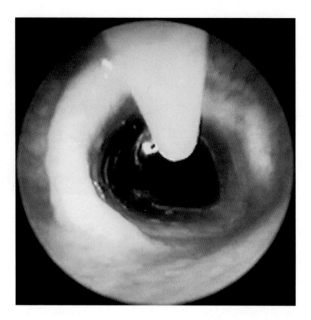

Figure 2-13

The open-ended tomcat catheter is advanced through the 2-mm channel of the Video Vetscope toward the flush solution. Advancing the catheter allows visualization of the suctioning process. Always keep the end of the catheter in view to prevent iatrogenic myringotomy.

After cleaning and examining the ear canal, the examiner can gain a better understanding of the ear disease and better formulate therapeutic protocols.

Assessing the Eardrum

In many cases of chronic canine otitis media, the eardrum is ruptured as a result of long-standing otitis externa. Examination of the ears of a patient with chronic otitis media often reveals the absence of the eardrum. The tympanic bulla may be filled with a dark material composed of epithelial cells, keratin, and cerumen (Figure 2-16). In acute suppurative otitis media, copious exudates resembling curdled milk are seen along the floor of the horizontal canal. Flecks of material are often seen floating in the liquid. After exudates and flush solution are suctioned from the external ear canal, the eardrum may not be visualized, but the bony tympanic bulla can be visualized beyond the annulus of the tympanic membrane. Many cases of otitis media are suspected due to the presence of an opaque eardrum or a bulging eardrum.

It is difficult to assess the integrity of the eardrum if this structure cannot be clearly seen. When stenosis or occlusion of the ear canal prevents visualization of the eardrum, a rigid tomcat catheter can be advanced through the stenosis carefully. As the catheter is slowly advanced, it encounters a spongy object, the eardrum. If the eardrum is not ruptured and pressure is applied to the catheter, there is resistance.

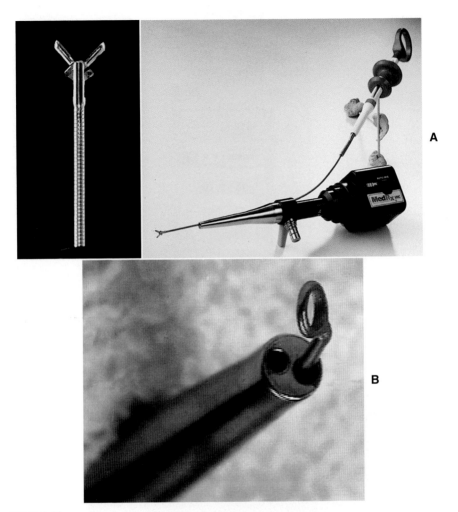

Figure 2-14

Using the working channel to work in the ear canal. **A,** An oval fenestrated endoscopic grasping forceps can be threaded through the Video Vetscope to remove foreign bodies, wax, polyps, and other material in the ear canal. **B,** Buck ear curette threaded retrograde into the 2-mm working channel of the Vetscope probe.

If the catheter advances, it will perforate the eardrum. If the catheter hits a hard object and does not advance, the object usually is the bone of the medial wall of the tympanic bulla, and the eardrum is not intact.

Sometimes when the eardrum is ruptured, using dilute povidone-iodine solution or fluorescein dye in the flushing solution will allow the colored solution to flush through the middle ear and out of the auditory tube. When this happens, the solution will come out of the nose or out of the back of the throat; the color indicates that there is a ruptured eardrum.

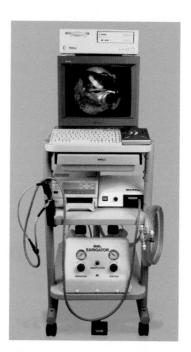

Figure 2-15

The Video Vetscope is assembled as a self-contained ear treatment station. (Courtesy MedRx, Inc., Largo, Florida.)

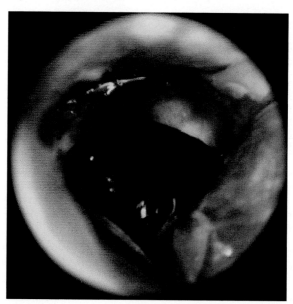

Figure 2-16

Appearance of otitis media. Otoscopic examination of this Toy Poodle revealed the absence of most of the eardrum. The *pars flaccida* can be seen in the dorsal portion of the annulus. The tympanic bulla is filled with a dark waxy material composed of squamous epithelium, keratin, and cerumen.

Alternatively, if there is a small hole in the eardrum, the ear canal can be filled with normal saline with the patient in lateral recumbency and the affected ear facing upward. The video otoscope is advanced through the saline toward the eardrum. Any rising air bubbles indicate that air from within the tympanic cavity is escaping through a hole in the tympanic membrane.

Pathological changes may be present in the bulla and eardrum as indicated by opacity or discoloration of the intact eardrum (Figure 2-17). These findings signify either an ascending otitis media, which is common in cats but rare in the dog, or an otitis media in which the eardrum has healed over, leaving material within the tympanic bulla. There may be tissue in the bulla indicating a tumor mass or polyp. The eardrum may be reddened in response to inflammation or from accumulation of blood in the bulla. Whitish opacity indicates pus or mucus in the bulla, and yellow fluid indicates a serous effusion. A bulging membrane signifies fluid pressure behind the eardrum. Retraction of the eardrum around the malleus indicates negative air pressure. To relieve pressure gradients and obtain specimens from the middle ear for cytological evaluation and culture, a myringotomy should be done (Figure 2-18). (See Chapter 14, Otitis Media.)

Cytological Evaluation

Cytological examination of specimens from every infected ear should be a routine part of every ear examination (see Chapter 3). Information gained from studying the cellular components of ear exudates becomes an integral part of the decision-making process in treatment of ear disease.

Cytological specimens are obtained from the proximal horizontal canal to minimize contaminants and are prepared as follows:

1. A small cotton-tipped swab is inserted into the ear without touching the ear canal. A plastic otoscope speculum to shroud the ear swab is helpful.
2. The sample is obtained by pressing the applicator tip against the ear canal as the swab is withdrawn. With this approach, packing of wax and exudates is minimal.
3. The swab is rolled onto a clean frosted-end microscope slide; the harvested material from the left ear is rolled onto the left side of the slide, and the material from the right ear onto the right side of the slide.
4. The slide is labeled with the patient's name and the date of the sample (Figure 2-18).
5. The slide is heat fixed and stained with a blood stain (Diff-Quik or Wright-Giemsa stain).
6. After the slide is dried, a drop of slide-mounting medium (Cytoseal60, Richard Allen Scientific, Kalamazoo, Michigan) is applied, and a coverslip is placed over the material.

In this manner, a permanent slide is made. A drop of mineral oil can be spread on the slide if permanent slides are not desired. This standardized approach to making slides allows uniform identification of organisms from each ear and allows comparison of cytological findings from visit to visit.

Evaluation of slides should begin with a low-power (100×) overview of the cell types. Look for clumps or clusters of cells. If there are large numbers of cornified

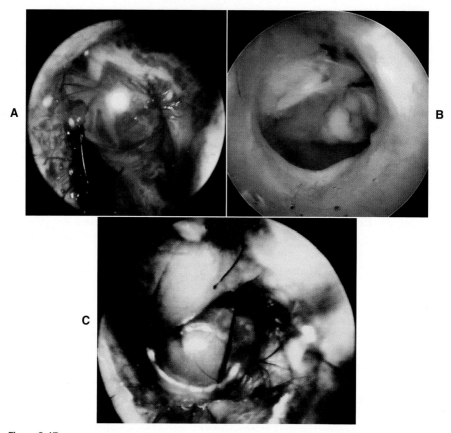

Figure 2-17

Examine for any change in shape and color of the eardrum. **A,** Bulging eardrum in a Golden Retriever puppy with purulent exudate behind the eardrum. **B,** Granulomatous exudate behind the eardrum of a cat. **C,** Bulging eardrum in a 6-year-old German Shepherd with otitis media.

epithelial cells or nonstaining sebaceous cells and few microorganisms, noninfectious causes of otitis such as seborrheic conditions should be considered. High-power (400×) examination is needed to characterize bacteria and yeasts. Large numbers of bacteria or yeast represent secondary invaders. When neutrophils are seen in addition to bacteria or yeasts, infection and inflammation of subcutaneous tissues must be considered. Ear mites are not often seen on stained ear swabs, but the eggs may be found. Clumps and clusters of vacuolated epithelial cells may indicate neoplasia. Inflammatory cells and acantholytic cells may also signify autoimmune disease.

To look for ear mites under the microscope, the examiner rolls swabs onto a slide containing a drop of mineral oil and applies a coverslip. Low-power examination reveals mites scurrying around on the slide, along with typical long oval eggs in the field.

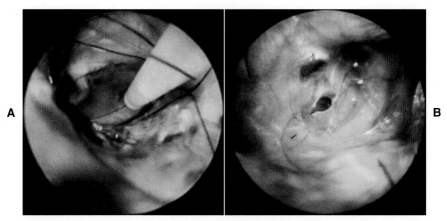

Figure 2-18

Using a 5 Fr polypropylene catheter to perform a myringotomy. **A,** The catheter is positioned under visualization at the 5 o'clock position. A gentle push on the catheter will make a small perforation in the eardrum. The malleus and vascular strip are visible to the left of the catheter in the dorsum of the eardrum. **B,** A small hole in the eardrum remains to allow exudates to drain and give access to the bulla so that it can be flushed and suctioned.

Skin Diseases Affecting the Ear

Pets with itchy ears may not have ear disease at all but may be responding to a localized pruritus associated with an underlying pruritic skin disease. Because many diseases found in the ear arise as a result of an underlying skin disease, the veterinarian should also carefully evaluate the pet's skin to determine the underlying cause if possible. Often, treatment for atopy, food allergy, or hypothyroidism diminishes the severity of the ear disease.

Suggested Readings

August JR: Evaluation of the patient with otitis externa, *Dermatology Reports, Solvay Veterinary* 5(2), 1986.

Kwochka KW: Mites and related disease, *Vet Clin North Am Small Anim Pract* 17:1263-1284, 1987.

Little CJL, Lane JG: An evaluation of tympanometry, otoscopy, and palpation for assessment of the canine tympanic membrane, *Vet Rec* 124:5-8, 1989.

Reedy LM, Miller WH: *Allergic skin diseases of dogs and cats,* Philadelphia, 1989, WB Saunders.

Simpson D: Atresia of the external acoustic meatus in a dog, *Austr Vet J* 75:18-20, 1997.

Sirigu P, Perra MT, Ferelli C: Local immune response in the skin of the external auditory meatus: an immunohistochemical study, *Microsc Res Tech* 38:329-334, 1997.

Stout-Graham M, Kainer RA, Whalen LR, et al: Morphologic measurements of the external horizontal ear canal of dogs, *Am J Vet Res* 51:990-994, 1990.

3

Cytology and Histopathology of the Ear in Health and Disease

John C. Angus, DVM

Cytology

Otitis externa is a multifactorial disorder affecting the quality of life of 10% to 20% of dogs and 2% to 6% of cats presenting to veterinarians.[1-3] Although a common problem, management of otitis externa is frequently challenging. Seemingly simple cases can become complicated by treatment failure, recurrence, and progressively worsening physical changes. Successful management of otitis requires accurate identification and management of both the primary cause (e.g., atopy, adverse food reaction, parasites, neoplasia) and concurrent perpetuating factors (e.g., bacterial or yeast infection, edema, glandular hyperplasia, loss of epithelial migration, otitis media).

In addition to a detailed history and physical examination, otic cytology should be considered part of the minimum database for all patients with clinical signs of ear disease. Cytology is a simple, practical, and inexpensive diagnostic test that provides rapid results indicating the presence and numbers of bacteria and yeast. Preparation of a diagnostic-quality slide does not require any special skills or equipment, and the slide can be quickly and easily evaluated during a standard office examination. The immediate result allows for rational decision making at the time of the initial consultation, prior to return of culture and sensitivity results 48 to 72 hours later.

The value of cytology exceeds simple identification of organisms. Cytology can characterize the severity of overgrowth or infection; also, in cases of mixed infection, cytology assists in evaluating the relative significance of each organism, strengthening interpretation of culture and sensitivity data. When performed routinely on each subsequent visit, cytology provides an accurate method for monitoring the patient's response to therapy.

Observation of quality and odor of exudates found during physical examination provides practitioners with a rough guide regarding potential organisms present in the external canal. Classically, dry, grainy, black discharge is most often associated with *Otodectes cynotis* infestations; waxy, brown exudates indicate *Malassezia*[4]; and yellow discharge indicates bacterial infection. Unfortunately these observations are not consistent or reliable.[5,6] Veterinarians should not make a diagnosis or select therapy based on past experience, physical character of discharge, or odor. Instead, decision making should be based on cytologic evidence established by careful microscopic evaluation. Failure to do so may result in misidentification of the most relevant pathogen and inappropriate selection of antimicrobial therapy. The consequence is often poor case management, prolongation of treatment, or even treatment failure and progression of disease. Cytology should be viewed as a routine diagnostic test for every patient with clinically significant ear disease.

Technique

In order to obtain the best diagnostic slide, be prepared to collect the sample prior to introduction of any cleaning agent or other therapy. In most cases, material obtained from the deeper horizontal canal is more clinically relevant than material obtained from the superficial vertical canal.[5,7] In well-behaved or anesthetized dogs, the ideal sample is obtained by inserting a cotton-tipped applicator through a disinfected otoscopic cone positioned beyond the junction of the vertical and horizontal canals. The cone shields the swab from contents of the vertical canal, which may contain numerous, irrelevant commensal organisms. Once in position, the swab is extended beyond the cone and pressure is applied laterally against the epithelium, collecting the exudates; the swab is then pulled back into the cone and removed from the canal. Unfortunately, with an awake patient, safely inserting a swab into a painful deep horizontal canal can be challenging at best. The presence of stenosis, inflammation, and voluminous exudate makes the exercise difficult and potentially dangerous if the patient moves suddenly or unpredictably. Overaggressive insertion of the swab into the patient's ear canal in an effort to obtain the deepest possible sample may result in further damage to irritated epithelium, or worse, in accidental perforation of the tympanic membrane. To obtain consistent samples in awake or painful patients, veterinarians should aim for the junction of the vertical and horizontal canals, where the cartilage bends at a 75-degree angle. If the veterinarian avoids straightening the canal, the bend should prevent the swab from advancing too deeply and damaging the tympanic membrane. Veterinarians who are gentle, cautious, and quick can safely obtain a diagnostic sample from the majority of patients. In patients anesthetized for ear flush, otoscopy, or other procedures, time should be taken to collect an ideal specimen properly from the deep horizontal canal or in some cases the tympanic cavity.

Although cotton-tipped applicators appear to be soft and gentle, when applied with pressure to inflamed epithelium, the surface of the swab is actually quite abrasive and can traumatize fragile tissue. An alternative to the swab is a rounded ear curette. The curette can be placed within the disinfected otoscopic cone positioned in the deep horizontal canal; the curette is advanced beyond the cone and gently scraped along the epithelium, collecting the exudate within the curette head. However, if a neoplasia is suspected, exfoliative cytology is preferred. The best sample for cytologic evaluation of a mass or polyp can be obtained by using a more traumatic surgical curette, using the same method described previously.

A separate cytologic specimen should always be prepared from both the right and the left ear canals, even if the patient presents for unilateral disease. Separate evaluation allows for comparison between the diseased ear and the normal ear, as well as early recognition of bacterial or yeast overgrowth in the less obviously affected ear. In patients with bilateral disease, clinically relevant differences in bacteria and yeast are common when comparing the two sides.[8,9] Without independent evaluation, documentation, or monitoring of each ear separately, veterinarians may fail to make appropriate management decisions.

In the case of otitis media, systemic therapy and bulla infusions of antibiotics should be directed at organisms colonizing the middle ear rather than the external canal. In one study, isolates from the tympanic cavity differed from isolates from the horizontal canal in 89.5% of cases.[8] In the same study, the tympanic membrane appeared to be intact in 71.1% of the ears with proven otitis media. If otitis media is suspected and the tympanum appears to be intact, sample collection should be performed by myringotomy—the intentional perforation of the tympanic membrane with a sterile swab, needle, or catheter. Because organisms from the middle ear may be coated in mucus, which prevents adequate uptake of stain, cytology from the middle ear should always be accompanied by a sample for culture and sensitivity obtained at the same time. In the external canal, cytology has been shown to be more sensitive than culture and sensitivity[5,10]; but this is not always the case in samples collected from the tympanic cavity.[8]

Once the sample is collected, roll the swab or curette onto a clean glass slide, evenly distributing a thin layer of material (Figure 3-1). Label each slide to identify correctly which ear was sampled. Alternatively, using one slide with a frosted end, holding the frosted end toward oneself, roll the sample from the left ear on the left part of the slide and the sample from the right ear on the right part of the slide. The precise method for marking slides is less important than consistency. Because cerumen has high lipid content, briefly heat the slide with an open flame to fix the material to the glass. This precaution will prevent loss of valuable information into the stain solvent. Avoid overheating the slide; excess heat will distort cells and organisms. Stain selection is a matter of personal preference; however, the same stain should be used for all samples in order to gain familiarity and produce consistent and reliable results. A modified Wright's stain, such as Diff-Quik (Baxter Scientific Products, McGraw Park, Illinois) is recommended. Modified Wright's stains are designed for evaluation of peripheral blood smears; therefore, leukocytes will retain easily recognized characteristics. Both gram-positive and gram-negative bacteria, as well as yeast, will appear blue or purple. Performing a gram stain is necessary to obtain this additional information, but extra staining is often an unnecessary and time-consuming task. In general, morphologically coccoid bacteria found in the ear canal are gram-positive organisms (e.g., *Staphylococcus, Streptococcus,* and *Enterococcus*) and the majority of rod bacteria are gram-negative (e.g., *Pseudomonas* spp., *Proteus* spp., coliforms). Only *Corynebacterium,* a gram-positive coccobacillus, and less common organisms such as *Actinomyces* and *Nocardia* spp. and filamentous gram-positive rod bacteria do not follow this rule.

Following staining, allow the specimen to air dry prior to microscopic examination. If desired, the slide can be permanently preserved by placing a drop of slide-mounting medium onto the stained material, applying a coverslip, then allowing the glue to set. Archiving of otic cytology is not always necessary if a detailed description is written into the medical record.

Scan the slide at low magnification to locate an area of interest. Cerumen and ointment-based medications do not take up stain and are of little interest. Avoid areas of thick, deeply stained debris, as the confluence will make characterization of individual organisms and cells difficult. Select a field containing thinly spread cellular or keratin debris for closer evaluation. Because different areas of the slide may yield different results, evaluate several fields to be sure all clinically relevant findings are discovered.

The high-dry, 40× objective (400× magnification) is adequate for identification of leukocytes, red blood cells, cornified epithelium, and neoplastic cells. Infectious organisms such as yeast and larger bacteria are also easily recognized. After examining several fields with the high-dry objective, switch to the high-magnification,

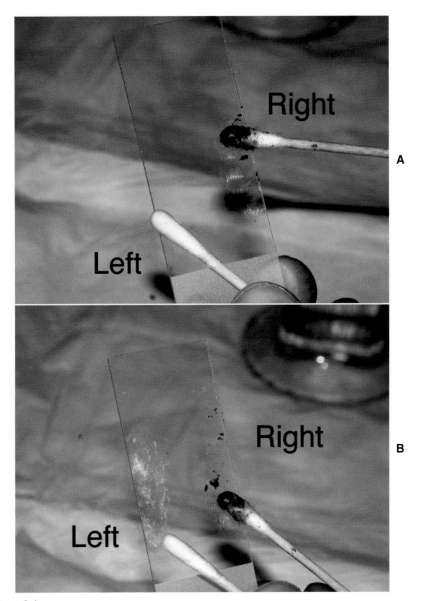

Figure 3-1

Technique for staining a cytologic specimen from the ear. **A,** Roll swab along glass slide. Swab with brown debris came from the right ear. Swab with purulent debris came from the left ear. **B,** Both specimens applied to the same slide, the right ear on the right side of the slide, the left ear on the left.

Continued

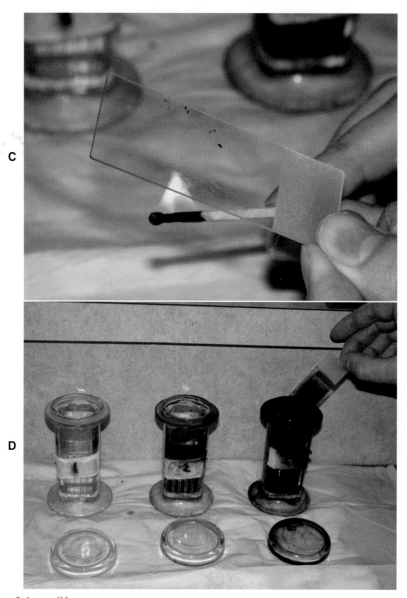

Figure 3-1—cont'd

C, Briefly heat-fix specimen to the slide. **D,** Stain with modified Wright's stain according to label instructions (Diff-Quik) shown.

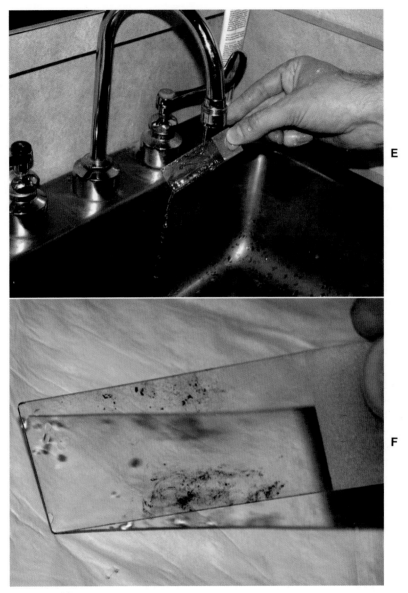

Figure 3-1—cont'd

E, Rinse slide by placing unstained side of slide under gentle water stream; this permits laminar flow of water to remove excess stain. **F,** Allow to air dry.

oil-immersion lens (100× objective, 1000× magnification) for detailed evaluation. The higher magnification is necessary to identify smaller or lightly stained bacteria that may be easily missed with the high-dry objective. The high-oil magnification also permits detailed evaluation of the cytoplasm of neutrophils and macrophages for phagocytized bacteria—another important indicator of that particular organism's acting as a pathogen rather than a commensal.

In order to maintain consistency in cytologic evaluation, each specimen should be specifically evaluated for the presence, estimated number, and morphologic characteristics of three specific features: yeast, bacteria, and leukocytes. To estimate the numbers, evaluate five to 10 areas, and record the average count per high-powered field (Figure 3-2). A complete record of all three cytologic features is necessary to monitor progression of disease or response to therapy. Recording "bacterial otitis" alone does not supply sufficient information for later comparison. Each cytologic description should contain information regarding the morphologic characteristic of bacteria (cocci or rod), the presence or absence of *Malassezia* and leukocytes, whether bacteria were phagocytized by leukocytes, and a semiquantitative estimation of the relative numbers of each type of organism seen. This level of detail permits either the primary clinician or any colleague following the case to determine accurately whether the "bacterial otitis" is resolving, changing, or worsening.

In addition to bacteria, yeast, and leukocytes, veterinarians occasionally identify parasites such as *Demodex* or *Otodectes cynotis* on stained specimens prepared in this manner; however, this technique is unreliable for purposeful diagnostic evaluation for parasites. Instead, prepare a separate slide using a direct mineral-oil technique. Apply several drops of mineral oil to a clean glass slide. Collect a large quantity of otic exudate from any level of the canal with a clean cotton swab and transfer the debris to the mineral oil on the glass slide. Unlike stained cytology, debris from both ears can be pooled onto the same slide. Place a coverslip directly onto the mineral oil and examine the specimen with low magnification (4× or 10× objective). Examine the entire area defined by the margins of the coverslip, using a consistent back-and-forth sweep, similar to the technique used for fecal flotation specimens.

Patient name _____			Date _____
Left ear cytology			
• Yeast	No [ ]	Yes [ ]	Estimated _____ per [40x / 100x] field
• Cocci	No [ ]	Yes [ ]	Estimated _____ per [40x / 100x] field
• Rod	No [ ]	Yes [ ]	Estimated _____ per [40x / 100x] field
• WBC	No [ ]	Yes [ ]	Phagocytosis: No [ ] Yes [ ]
Right ear cytology			
• Yeast	No [ ]	Yes [ ]	Estimated _____ per [40x / 100x] field
• Cocci	No [ ]	Yes [ ]	Estimated _____ per [40x / 100x] field
• Rod	No [ ]	Yes [ ]	Estimated _____ per [40x / 100x] field
• WBC	No [ ]	Yes [ ]	Phagocytosis: No [ ] Yes [ ]

Figure 3-2

Suggested medical record insert for documenting cytologic findings.

Normal Cytology

Cytology is not performed to identify the disorder otitis externa; this diagnosis is based on history and clinical signs. Instead, cytology is used to characterize the nature of otic exudate in order to identify potential primary causes and clinically significant perpetuating factors. Thus, cytology is rarely performed on normal asymptomatic ear canals. However, since determining the relative significance of cytologic findings requires a thorough understanding of what is and is not normally found in the external ear canals of dogs and cats, a discussion of normal cytology is appropriate.

The epithelial lining of the normal ear canal is coated with a thin layer of cerumen, the combined product of secretions by modified apocrine glands (ceruminous glands) and sebaceous glands. Cerumen forms a protective barrier, which traps debris, organisms, hair, and desquamated corneocytes. A sample taken from a normal ear canal should yield minimal material consisting mostly of waxy, yellow cerumen, exfoliated epithelium, resident microorganisms, and little else.

Because cerumen is predominantly lipid, the sample does not take up much stain; on gross examination a stained slide from a normal ear should be nearly colorless. Normal cornified squamous epithelial cells are seen on microscopic examination as sheets of lightly stained, basophilic keratin. The cells may roll up on themselves during smear preparation, resulting in a deeper staining, shardlike appearance. Desquamated keratinocytes may also contain melanin granules, which appear as tiny yellow to brown ovoid or round structures. Recognition of these melanin granules as a normal finding is important; otherwise, the structures may easily be misidentified as cocci or small rods colonizing the surface of the keratinocyte. Melanin granules do not take up stain; therefore, granules can be differentiated from purple-stained bacteria by focusing up and down through the cell until the true color of the structure is recognized.

The external ear canals of dogs and cats contain small numbers of normal resident bacteria. Coagulase-negative *Staphylococcus* spp., coagulase-positive *Staphylococcus* spp., and *Streptococcus* spp. are the most frequently isolated bacteria from normal ear canals. With the exception of *Corynebacterium,* rod-shaped bacteria are rarely found in normal ear canals.[4,6,11] Any bacteria found in the presence of leukocytes should be considered abnormal.[5-7] Because stain precipitate can resemble coccoid bacteria, high-oil magnification is necessary to visualize morphologic characteristics of bacteria. Clinically significant organisms should be symmetrical, have a distinct smooth edge, and be uniformly stained; they are typically present in pairs or chains of bacteria equal in size (Figure 3-3). In contrast, debris and precipitate vary in size and may be asymmetrical, irregular, and granular in appearance.

Another common finding on otic cytology is basophilic staining yeast, ranging in size from 2.0 μm × 4.0 μm up to 6.0 μm × 7.0 μm.[12] For comparison, canine red blood cells are approximately 7.0 μm in diameter; feline red blood cells are 5 μm. The most commonly encountered yeast exhibits unipolar budding, which creates the commonly described "peanut," "snowman," or "footprint" shape, easily recognizable as *Malassezia* (Figure 3-4). Although these organisms are normal residents of the canine and feline ear canal, under the appropriate circumstances *Malassezia* can

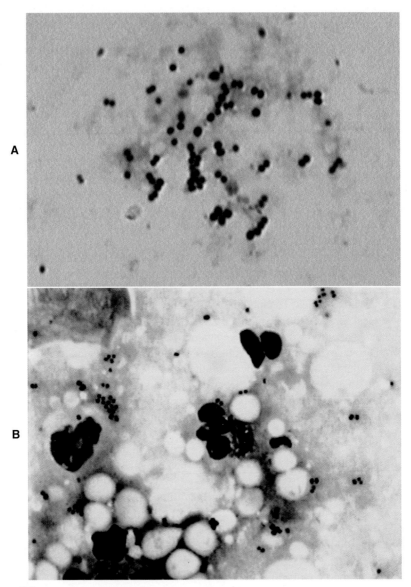

Figure 3-3

A, Cluster of paired coccoid bacteria photographed under high-oil immersion lens (100×
objective). **B,** Paired coccoid bacteria with neutrophils and an eosinophil (400× objective).

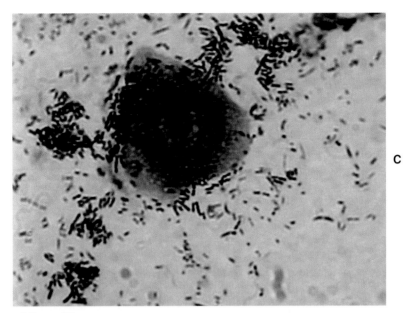

C

Figure 3-3—cont'd

C, Numerous rods and a keratinized epithelial cell (1000× objective).

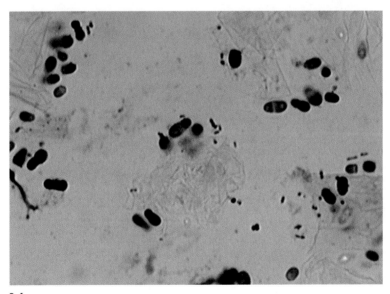

Figure 3-4

Malassezia pachydermatis with occasional paired coccoid bacteria in background. Note the oval shape of nonbudding yeast and unipolar budding of actively replicating organisms.

become important opportunistic pathogens, contributing directly to the severity of clinical signs, as well as to the progression and perpetuation of disease.

Because bacteria and yeast are considered normal inhabitants of the external ear canal, veterinarians need to determine whether the bacteria present cytologically are clinically relevant. In contrast, any finding of leukocytes on cytology is considered abnormal. The finding of bacteria that have been engulfed by phagocytic neutrophils and macrophages is one clear indication of relevance (Figure 3-5). The absence of leukocytes does not rule out the role of bacteria or yeast as pathogens. In general, heavy colonization of the canal by opportunistic pathogens is reflected in the number of bacteria seen per high-powered field. This semiquantitative method for determining clinical significance is discussed in detail in the sections on abnormal cytology.

Abnormal Cytology

Malassezia

Malassezia spp. can be found on cytology from up to 96% of dogs and 83% of cats with normal ear canals.[10] *Malassezia pachydermatis* is widely recognized as the predominant commensal yeast of dogs.[12-15] However, the genus actually consists of eight species, including seven distinct lipid-dependent species: *M. furfur, M. sympodialis, M. globosa, M. obtusa, M. restricta, M. sloofiae,* and *M. equi.*[12,13] In dogs with otitis externa, *Malassezia pachydermatis* is present 83% of the time.[16-18]

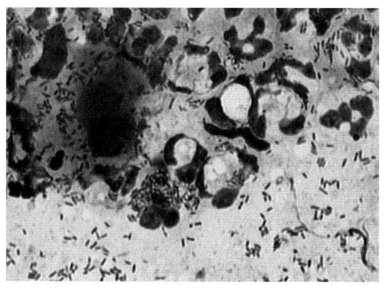

Figure 3-5

Cytology from severe bacterial otitis with *Pseudomonas aeruginosa*. Numerous polymorphonuclear neutrophils are present. Rod bacteria can be seen intracellularly (phagocytosis) and extracellularly.

Recent studies have demonstrated *M. furfur* and *M. obtusa* in 4.5% of cases of canine otitis externa, whereas *M. sympodialis* and *M. furfur* were present in 8.9% of diseased ear canals of cats.[18,19] *M. sympodialis,*[20,21] *M. globosa,*[21] and *M. furfur*[18,21] can be recovered from normal-haired skin, ear canals, and mucosa of healthy cats. Of these, *M. sympodialis* is believed to be a normal resident of the feline ear canal.[15]

Because the different species may have variable morphologic features and staining characteristics, veterinarians may notice unusually shaped yeast bodies on cytologic preparations. Most likely these variations represent multiple species of *Malassezia*. Current research demonstrates that different species have variable pathogenicity, virulence factors, and host responses; however, the clinical relevance of these differences has not been demonstrated.[13] Unless there is a compelling reason to differentiate between *Malassezia* species using laboratory techniques, cytologic recognition of any member of the genus is sufficient for management of clinical cases.

Because *Malassezia* can be found in normal patients or mixed in with predominantly bacterial infections, veterinarians need to determine the clinical significance of *Malassezia* for each patient. Cytology is the most useful tool for differentiating between normal resident colonization and overgrowth. Unlike bacterial infections, suppurative inflammation is not a common feature of *Malassezia* otitis[5] and therefore cannot be used to determine a pathologic state.

At what threshold does yeast become a contributing factor to disease rather than an incidental finding? Precise breakpoints for maximum acceptable number of yeast vary from patient to patient. Cytologic estimation of numbers can provide a guideline for the clinician; in the end, however, the decision to treat *Malassezia* depends on a combination of cytologic findings, severity of clinical signs, past history of yeast otitis, and response to previous therapy in that individual patient. A recent comparison of cytologic specimens from normal and diseased ears demonstrated that up to an average of two yeast per high-dry field (40× objective, 400× magnification) in the dog and cat should be considered normal.[22] Mean counts greater than 5 yeast per field in dogs, and 12 yeast per field in cats are abnormal. Intermediate values are considered a gray zone (Table 3-1). These criteria had a specificity of 95% in dogs and 100% in cats. However, because the study included bacterial otitis, not all cases of otitis externa had yeast as a component; as a result, sensitivity was only 50% for

TABLE 3-1 Recommended Breakpoints for Numbers of Organisms Identified Cytologically. Reported as Mean Number of Organisms per High-Dry Field (40× Objective)

	NORMAL	INTERMEDIATE	ABNORMAL
Malassezia			
Dog	≤2	3-4	≥5
Cat	≤2	3-11	≥12
Bacteria			
Dog	≤5	6-24	≥25
Cat	≤4	5-14	≥15

dogs and 63% for cats. A study by Tater et al[10] evaluated otic cytology from 50 normal dogs and 52 normal cats; it found a range of 0 to 2.6 yeast per high-dry field in dogs and 0 to 3.3 per high-dry field in cats. Diseased dogs were not included for comparison, but these findings would be consistent with previously reported normal breakpoints. The authors also demonstrated that ear conformation did not result in differences in normal yeast numbers when comparing dogs with pendulous pinna with dogs with erect ear carriage. Therefore, ear conformation should not influence interpretation of cytologic findings.

Malassezia may also colonize the tympanic cavity, causing or contributing to otitis media. In one study, *Malassezia* was recovered from 65.8% of external ear canals and 34.2% of middle ears of dogs with chronic otitis.[8] Yeast can be found mixed with bacteria; however, in the study by Cole et al,[8] 23.7% of dogs had otitis media associated with *Malassezia* infection alone. *Malassezia* is not a normal resident of the tympanic cavity; therefore, any finding on cytology from this space is considered abnormal, and systemic antifungal therapy is indicated.

Candida

Candida albicans is a normal resident of the skin and gastrointestinal (GI) tract of dogs and cats. Under appropriate circumstances, *Candida* can become an opportunistic pathogen. Compared with *Malassezia, Candida* spp. are not common pathogens in cases of otitis externa. In a study by Ginel et al,[22] three of 24 dogs (12.5%), and two of 22 cats (9.1%) with clinical signs of otitis externa had cytologic and culture evidence of *Candida* spp. Cytologically, *Candida* are thin-walled, round to oval, and approximately 2 to 6 μm in diameter.[23] A thin, clear capsule displaces stain and sediment, giving the appearance of a halo around the yeast body. The organism exhibits narrow-based budding and can form short, tubular, septate pseudohyphae. In contrast, *Malassezia* is unencapsulated, has broad-based budding, and never forms pseudohyphae or hyphae.

Bacteria

One of the primary uses of otic cytology is detection of the presence of bacteria. Unlike yeast, which can be readily identified using the 40× objective, proper evaluation for bacteria requires high magnification with an oil-immersion lens (100× objective, 1000× magnification). The diameter of most coccoid bacteria is typically 0.3 μm; coliform, rod bacteria are typically less than 1.5 μm in length.[24] In spite of this small size, and given quality equipment and practiced skill and ability, cytology can actually be more sensitive than culture for detecting bacteria.[5,10] In one study of normal ear cytology, gram-positive cocci were identified in 42% of dogs by cytology but only 25% by culture. The actual percentage of normal patients with cytologic or culture evidence of bacteria may vary significantly based on geographic location and humidity. Ear conformation has not been shown to influence cytologic findings.[10]

Determining the significance of bacteria seen on cytology depends on several factors: morphology, numbers, and concurrent leukocytes. After bacteria have been identified, the clinician should determine whether there is a monoculture of a single morphologic type or whether a mixed infection is present, and then describe the morphology of bacteria seen. The presence of larger cocci arranged in pairs or tetrads is typical morphology for *Staphylococcus* spp; small cocci in short chains are characteristic of *Streptococcus* and *Enterococcus* spp. Even with these guidelines, laboratory culture is necessary to make a definitive speciation; clinicians should record findings as pairs of cocci or chains of cocci rather than attempt to make a specific diagnosis based on cytology. *Corynebacterium* is a large plump rod that may be found in normal or diseased ears. The most common rod-shaped pathogens associated with otitis externa are *Pseudomonas* spp. and *Proteus* spp. In tropical climates, coliform bacteria may be considered a normal finding. In more arid regions, only gram-positive cocci are commonly observed in normal patients.

In addition to morphology, the number of bacteria present should be estimated for each case. A semiquantitative cytologic criteria, similar to that proposed for *Malassezia,* can be used for bacteria (see Table 3-1). Based on the results reported by Ginel et al,[22] fewer than five bacteria per high-powered dry field (40× objective) should be considered normal; more than 25 bacteria per field supports the diagnosis of an abnormally increased population. Using higher magnification, fewer than two bacteria per high-oil field (100× objective) is normal, and more than 10 bacteria per field is abnormal. For cats, fewer than four bacteria per 40× field (1.6 per 100× field) was consistent with normal conditions, and more than 15 bacteria per 40× field (6 per 100× field) was abnormal. Intermediate numbers in a gray zone are subject to interpretation. Using these mean-count breakpoints to differentiate normal from diseased ears yielded 95% specificity and 50% sensitivity in dogs, and 100% specificity and 63% sensitivity for cats.

An important concept in determining the clinical significance of bacteria seen on cytology is the distinction between bacterial "overgrowth" and bacterial "infection." In general, *overgrowth* refers to increased numbers of resident bacteria in the debris and on the epithelial surface of the external canal. Overgrowth may contribute to disease through the production of exotoxins that perpetuate inflammation; however, overgrowth does not typically warrant culture and susceptibility testing or expensive systemic therapy. In these cases, systemic therapy may be less effective than topical medications because the concentration of antibiotic achieved by topical medications can far exceed that achievable by systemic routes. Overgrowth can usually be managed effectively by frequent flushing, antiinflammatory therapy, and topical antibiotics directed at the specific organism(s). *Bacterial infections* typically describe cases with purulent response to bacteria, ulceration of epithelial lining, or colonization of the tympanic cavity. These cases often require high-dose, long-term systemic antibiotic therapy for successful resolution.

The most direct evidence supporting a diagnosis of infection instead of overgrowth is the presence of neutrophils on cytology. Leukocytes are not found in the normal ear canal. Bacterial overgrowth on surface debris rarely elicits the same neutrophilic response as bacterial infection of the external canal or tympanic cavity. The finding of bacteria within neutrophils (phagocytosis) strongly supports a diagnosis of infection with a significant bacterium.

Cytology, however, is not the only test that should be performed when evaluating bacterial otitis externa. Although cytology can demonstrate the presence, number, and relative significance of cocci or rods, it cannot be used to determine the species of bacteria. Bacterial culture is performed to identify species and determine the antimicrobial susceptibility of clinically relevant bacteria. Because culture does not differentiate between normal resident bacteria, bacterial overgrowth, and bacterial infection, cytology is the best tool to determine the relative significance of bacteria present in the external canal. Similarly, because culture does not accurately evaluate changes in numbers or the presence or absence of neutrophils, sequential bacterial cultures are not useful for monitoring response to therapy. Cytology is necessary to determine whether numbers of organisms are decreasing, if there is a change in the predominant organism, or if there is a change in the presence or absence of neutrophils. Bacterial culture in the absence of cytology is an inaccurate tool (Table 3-2).

When evaluating otitis media, a separate cytology should be performed from the tympanic cavity. Veterinarians should not assume that the same organism contaminates both sites. In a study comparing isolates from the horizontal canal and the tympanic cavity of dogs with chronic otitis externa and media, differences were noted in the species or antimicrobial susceptibility of bacteria isolated in 89.5% of the cases.[8] Therefore, samples for cytology and culture should be obtained from the tympanic cavity rather than the external canal.

Leukocytes

Unlike bacteria and yeast, which may be found in the normal ear canal, white blood cells are only present in cytologic specimens from abnormal ears. Leukocytes enter the ear canal as the result of exocytosis across severely inflamed epithelial lining, through ulceration of epithelial lining, or by extension from the tympanic cavity during otitis media. Therefore, practitioners should always examine slides carefully for white blood cells, in addition to bacteria and yeast, and document the findings in the medical record.

TABLE 3-2 **Comparison of Cytology and Culture for Evaluation of Otitis Externa**

ATTRIBUTE	CYTOLOGY	CULTURE
Time to available results	Immediate	48-72 hours
Sensitivity for yeast	High	Low
Sensitivity for bacteria	High	Moderate to high
Sensitivity for leukocytes	High	None
Estimation of numbers	Semiquantitative	Categorical data
Rank significance in mixed infection	Yes	No
Monitor response to therapy	Yes	No
Detection of antimicrobial resistance	No	Yes

Because neutrophils rarely respond to bacterial overgrowth in debris, the presence or absence of neutrophils is a reliable tool for differentiating overgrowth from true infection. Phagocytosis of bacteria is also worth noting, particularly in mixed infections; the organism being targeted is more likely the significant pathogen compared with bacteria free in the background. Extension of purulent exudate from the middle ear to the external canal may be the only evidence readily available to clinicians that a concurrent otitis media is present in a dog presenting for otitis externa. Because otitis media is present in 16% of dogs with acute otitis externa and up to 82% of dogs with chronic disease,[6,8] any cytologic evidence of leukocytes in the external canal should increase the clinician's suspicion for concurrent otitis media, warranting specific diagnostic evaluation. As a general rule, if the patient's body is responding to an infection with suppurative or pyogranulomatous inflammation, systemic antibiotic therapy is almost always indicated. Whenever appropriate, a culture and susceptibility should be obtained to modify empirical antibiotic selection; in the case of otitis media the sample should be obtained directly from the tympanic cavity.

The presence or absence of leukocytes on cytology is a useful tool for monitoring the progression of disease or response to therapy. Progression from otitis externa to otitis media, or progression from *Malassezia* otitis or bacterial overgrowth to bacterial infection should not be missed due to failure to perform and document otic cytology. When monitoring therapy in a difficult case of *Pseudomonas* otitis, the disappearance of leukocytes during the first recheck is a strong indication of improvement even if small numbers of bacteria remain; in contrast, bacterial culture would simply identify *Pseudomonas* on both visits, leading the veterinarian to believe the case was not responding adequately. A serial cytologic record from each episode helps veterinarians avoid inappropriate therapeutic decisions.

Parasites

Heat-fixed, stained cytologic specimens from otic debris will occasionally contain evidence of parasites, but direct mineral-oil preparation is a more reliable method for specific parasite evaluation. Low-magnification (4× objective) microscopic examination of a mineral-oil preparation is sufficient for identifying ear mites. In all cases the presence of any insect or mite in the external ear canal is considered abnormal and should be pursued accordingly.

In both dogs and cats the most common parasite associated with otitis externa is *Otodectes cynotis*.[6,7,25] When large numbers of mites are present in the external ear canal, the diagnosis can be easily confirmed by direct visualization of the mites with a magnified operating-head otoscope or video otoscope. *O. cynotis* has a psoroptiform body type, similar to *Sarcoptes*, but is larger and has short, unjointed pedicles extending from the legs. The larger adult female mite is approximately 280 μm wide and 450 μm long[26]; the rudimentary fourth pair of legs does not extend beyond the body. The slightly smaller adult males (250 × 320 μm) are frequently observed attached to eight-legged deutonymphs (220 × 320 μm). Other life stages include the protonymph (160 × 240 μm) and six-legged larva (115 × 240 μm). Numerous large eggs (100×210 μm) are commonly found lodged in the keratin debris. Identification of a single egg or mite of any life stage provides a definitive diagnosis. However, ear mites cannot be ruled out by the absence of *O. cynotis* on microscopic evaluation. A treatment trial with appropriate miticidal therapy is strongly recommended for all cases of chronic otitis externa.

Other mites occasionally found on cytologic preparations include *Demodex* spp., *Sarcoptes scabiei, Notoedres cati, Eutrombicula alfreddugesi,* and *Neotrombicula autumnalis.*

Demodex, the follicular mange mites of dogs and cats, can colonize any hair follicle, including those of the external ear canal. In normal dogs, *Demodex* rarely causes any significant problems; however, in patients with juvenile-onset or adult-onset demodicosis, overpopulation and colonization of hair follicles of the ear canal may cause secondary bacterial infections, folliculitis, furunculosis, inflammation, and edema, resulting in clinical otitis externa. Although *Demodex* is considered a normal resident organism, these mites are very rarely found in ear cytology from normal dogs. Therefore, if *Demodex* mites are found on microscopic evaluation of otic exudate, demodicosis should be suspected, and a thorough examination and skin scrapings of multiple regions of haired skin are indicated.

Sarcoptes scabiei and *Notoedres cati,* the sarcoptic mange mites of cats, most commonly affect the host's pinna, rarely causing inflammation of the external canal. Chiggers, or harvest mites, *Eutrombicula alfreddugesi,* and *Neotrombicula autumnalis* cause pruritus, papules, erythema, and crusting where they attach to the skin. Occasionally the parasitic larval stage is found tightly adhered to the skin around the entrance to the external ear canal. The large (500 μm), six-legged larvae are easily distinguished from *Otodectes cynotis* by their different body type and bright red-orange color.

Neoplasia

Although not common, the external ear canal can be a site for development of many different types of neoplastic and non-neoplastic masses. Symptoms of masses in the ear canal such as otorrhea, head shaking, and malodor are similar to presenting signs for other causes of otitis. The presence of secondary bacterial or yeast infections and subsequent debris may also obscure the actual cause of disease. Not all tumors exfoliate on normal cytology, but the finding of large sheets of epithelial cells is one cytologic finding that should always prompt further investigation for neoplasia.

Any nodule found in the external canal should be evaluated for neoplastic potential. Under sedation, cytologic samples can be obtained by fine-needle aspirate or curettage. Fine-needle aspirate is most useful for masses easily visible in the vertical canal. For nodules in the horizontal canal, curettage can be performed through an otoscopic cone, with one hand holding the otoscope and the other manipulating a sharp-edged curette. The curette is positioned over or just beyond the tumor and then angled and dragged back across the surface. The cells collected are spread gently across two or three glass slides and allowed to air dry prior to staining; heat fixing is not recommended because this will distort cellular features. Occasionally small tumors may be removed and submitted for histopathology by this method; for larger tumors the goal is to differentiate inflammatory hyperplasia, benign neoplasia, and malignant neoplasia.

If the predominant cell type is inflammatory, appropriate antiinflammatory therapy can be prescribed, followed by reevaluation. Sheets or clusters of large round cells may be indicative of an epithelial tumor such as ceruminous gland adenoma or adenocarcinoma, squamous cell carcinoma, basal cell tumor, lymphoma, histiocytoma, or plasmacytoma. Spindle-shaped cells may represent fibrosis of the canal, fibrosarcoma, or other nonepithelial tumor. Mast cells are more easily recognizable. Cytology from nasopharyngeal polyps may be characterized by epithelial cells with visible respiratory cilia at one margin. If cytologic evaluation is uncertain or the cytologist is concerned about either epithelial or nonepithelial tumors, specimens should be submitted for laboratory evaluation by a clinical pathologist and an incisional biopsy for histopathology should be obtained to confirm the diagnosis.

Conclusion

Cytology is a simple, rapid, and practical diagnostic test that should be performed routinely for every patient with clinical signs of otitis externa. Cytologic specimens should be evaluated for the presence, numbers, and characteristics of three key features: yeast, bacteria, and leukocytes. More than five yeast or 25 bacteria per high-powered field is suggestive of significant microbial activity, warranting therapeutic intervention. The presence of white blood cells on cytology indicates true infection, warranting systemic therapy, as opposed to bacterial overgrowth in debris, which can often be managed successfully with topical therapy. Cytology improves all aspects of case management, including diagnosis of secondary infections, monitoring progression of disease, and evaluating response to therapy.

Histopathology

Despite the frequency with which otitis externa occurs in veterinary patients, minimal attention has been paid in the veterinary literature to the histologic features of normal and abnormal ear canals. Most of what is known is derived from a sparse collection of early anatomic studies from the 1950s,[27] 1960s,[28-30] and a few more recent publications. Indeed, only four articles addressing this topic have appeared in peer-reviewed journals since 1980.[31-34] In the available literature, the majority of work is focused on the canine ear, with remarkably little scientific investigation of the histopathology of the feline ear. Familiarity with the normal histoanatomy and abnormal pathologic changes associated with otitis is useful for veterinarians seeking better understanding of the causes of otitis, progression of disease, and therapeutic intervention.

Normal Histoanatomy

External Canal

The external ear canal consists of two telescoping tubes of cartilage lined by normal squamous epithelium (analogous to epidermis) and normal subepithelium (analogous to dermis). The epithelial lining transitions with normally haired skin at the opening to the pinna. This tissue continues along the entire length of the vertical and horizontal canal, where it intersects with the tympanic membrane, forming a closed-ended tube. Similar to normal haired skin, the lining of the ear canal contains hair follicles, sebaceous glands, modified apocrine glands, vessels, lymphatics, nerves, collagen fibers, elastin fibers, and other cellular components common to dermis and epidermis. Several important variations from normal skin are worth noting.

The epithelium is stratified squamous epithelium (like normal skin) but is much thinner than that found on most areas on the body, consisting of only two to three cell layers (Figure 3-6).[28] In normal epidermis the terminally differentiated keratinocytes are shed directly into the environment. If this occurred in the blind-ended tube of the external canal, the lumen would fill with dead cells and debris. Because the ear canal does not contain cilia to evacuate the accumulated debris, living epithelial cells

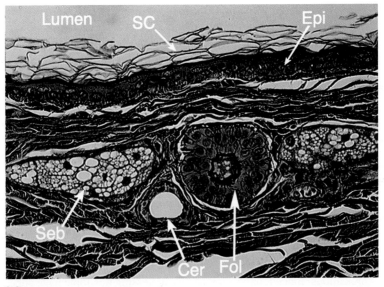

Figure 3-6

Photomicrograph of normal vertical ear canal. Lumen of the ear canal is visible at the top. *SC,* Stratum corneum, normal "basket-weave" appearance of healthy end-differentiated epithelial cells; *Epi,* epithelium, one to two cell-layer thick normal epithelial layer; *Seb,* sebaceous glands, small normal cluster of sebaceous gland cells associated with every hair follicular unit; *Cer,* ceruminous gland, single cross-section of modified apocrine gland associated with every hair follicular unit, *Fol,* follicle, cross-section of hair follicle with actively growing hair shaft visible in center.

migrate centripetally from a point of origin on the tympanum, up and out of the ear canal, depositing debris, cerumen, and desquamated corneocytes onto the pinnae.[35] In the normal ear, this process of epithelial migration keeps the tympanum and ear canal free of debris.

Hair follicles are sparsely distributed throughout the entire length of the ear canal. Most breeds have simple follicles with single hair shafts, compared with compound primary and secondary follicles found elsewhere in haired skin.[28,32] In addition to being sparse and simple, hair follicles in the ear canal are also miniaturized relative to haired skin (Figure 3-7). Cocker spaniels are the exception; this breed has been shown to have in the ear canal predominantly compound follicles that occupy a larger cross-section of tissue than non-spaniel breeds.[32]

Each hair follicle is associated with two types of adnexal glands: (1) sebaceous glands and (2) ceruminous glands. Sebaceous glands are similar in appearance to those found in haired skin. These glands supply neutral lipids to the lumen of the ear canal via a duct that opens in the hair follicle. The lipids coat the hair shaft, spread to the surface, and diffuse into the stratum corneum, contributing to the normal barrier function of the epithelium. On histopathologic specimens, sebaceous glands are easily recognized by the characteristic clustering of round to polygonal cells with pale foamy cytoplasm and a small, centrally located nucleus (Figure 3-8). Variation in sebaceous gland concentration occurs along the length of the canal. In general, sebaceous glands are most prominent in the tissue toward the opening of the ear

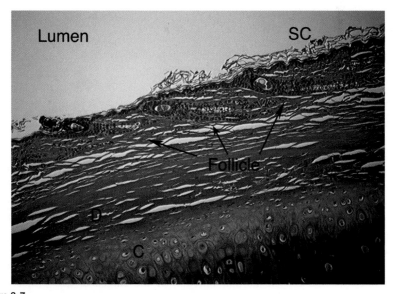

Figure 3-7

Photomicrograph demonstrating multiple small hair follicles that line the length of the external ear canal. Note how thin the section of tissue is between the lumen of the canal and the cartilage boundary. *SC,* Stratum corneum; *D,* dermis; *C,* cartilage.

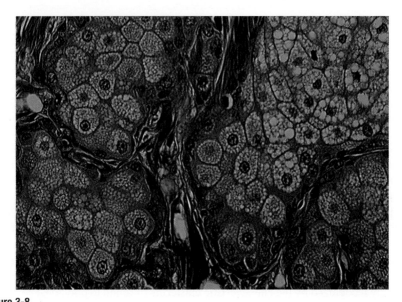

Figure 3-8

Photomicrograph close-up of sebaceous gland tissue.

canal and become less concentrated in proximal tissues closer to the tympanic membrane.[32]

Ceruminous glands are modified apocrine, or sweat, glands that also have ducts opening into the hair follicle. Typically they are positioned deeper in the dermis than sebaceous glands.[32] In contrast to sebaceous glands, ceruminous glands are most abundant near the tympanum, decreasing in size toward the opening onto the pinna.[32] Ceruminous glands are easily recognized as a single layer of cuboidal to columnar glandular epithelium surrounding a large central lumen. Ceruminous glands are actually coiled, so on cross-section a single gland may appear to be multiple adjacent glands as the slide transects the same lumen multiple times (Figure 3-9).

In the normal ear canal the ratio of sebaceous glands to ceruminous glands varies depending on location. As one moves farther away from the tympanic membrane, the ratio transitions from predominantly ceruminous glands in the horizontal canal to predominantly sebaceous glands in the vertical canal.[32] On the epithelial surface, sebaceous secretions mix with apocrine secretions to form a thin, tenacious layer of cerumen. Since sebaceous secretions are thicker and contain primarily neutral lipids, while ceruminous glands produce a thinner secretion containing phospholipids and acid mucopolysaccharides, the variation in gland ratios may influence cerumen composition in the horizontal canal compared with the vertical canal.[34]

Cerumen is vital for the normal function of the ear canal and protection of the tympanic membrane. Cerumen traps debris and pathogenic organisms, contains immunoglobulins and antimicrobial peptides that provide local protection, and forms a barrier to transepithelial water loss, maintaining a moist, pliable tympanic membrane and epithelium.

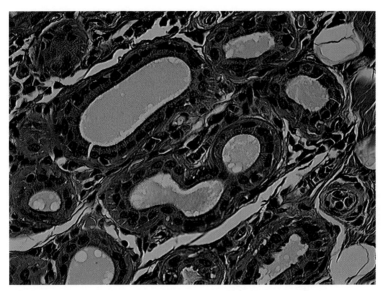

Figure 3-9

Photomicrograph close-up of ceruminous gland tissue. Note the multiple cross-sections of a single, coiled gland give the appearance of multiple adjacent glands.

Beneath the cerumen and epithelium and between follicles, the tissue of the ear canal is quite similar to the interfollicular dermis of the skin. This area contains numerous large collagen bundles, elastin fibers, blood vessels, capillaries, fibroblasts, mast cells, and other cells of the immune system. Below this layer are the auricular and annular cartilage tubes that define the boundaries of the ear canal.

Tympanic Membrane

The tympanic membrane consists of two sections: the pars tensa and pars flaccida. The pars tensa is a tough, semitransparent, multilayered tissue stretched taut across a fibrocartilaginous ring. The ring is in turn attached to the skull. Histopathologically, the pars tensa consists of four distinct layers. The first layer is continuous and equivalent to the epithelial surface of the external canal. The stratified squamous epithelium is only a few layers thick. Epithelial migration originates from a germinal center in this layer. The second stratum is roughly equivalent to the dermis, containing a thin layer of fibroblasts, fine nerves, and blood vessels. Hair follicles and glandular tissue are totally absent from this layer. Next is a fibrous intermediate layer, which connects to the fibrocartilaginous ring. This is the thickest layer of the pars tensa. The first of the auditory ossicles, the malleus, is embedded in this layer. The arrangement of fibers is orderly, to maintain strength and maximize transmission of vibrations. The fourth layer consists of a single sheet of respiratory epithelial cells overlying a thin lamina propria. Centrally, the cells of squamous morphology become more cuboidal toward the margins and finally columnar as the layer becomes continuous with the lining of the tympanic cavity. Unlike normal respiratory epithelium, this layer contains no cilia or goblet cells.[27,28,36,37]

The pars flaccida is a soft, pliable portion of the tympanum located dorsal to the pars tensa. This tissue contains a loose arrangement of collagen fibers covered by a thin layer of epithelium. Unlike the pars tensa, the pars flaccida is highly vascular and gives rise to the capillary branches that supply the germinal epithelium of the pars tensa. With acute inflammation, such as that associated with atopy, the pars flaccida may become severely erythematous and edematous.

Cocker Spaniels

American Cocker Spaniels differ substantially from other breeds in normal histoanatomy. In the study by Stout-Graham et al, Cocker Spaniels with normal ear canals were found to exhibit increased ceruminous gland tissue relative to non-spaniel breeds (Greyhounds, mixed).[32] In the same study, Cocker Spaniels were found to have compound hair follicles rather than simple follicles seen in other breeds; furthermore, Cocker Spaniel hair follicles were more densely packed.

Chronic Inflammatory Otitis

Nearly all of the pathologic changes that occur in ear disease are associated with alteration in form and function of one or more of these structures: cerumen, epithelium, sebaceous glands, ceruminous glands, fibroblasts, or cells of the immune system.

Without repeating a detailed analysis of the pathogenesis of otitis externa, the primary causes of disease can be summarized as chronic inflammatory diseases (atopy, adverse food reaction, parasitism), transient inflammatory diseases (parasitism, viral, contact hypersensitivity), obstructive diseases (neoplasia, foreign objects), and hyperkeratotic diseases (hypothyroidism, primary keratinization defects). Secondary bacterial and yeast infections can be associated with any of these causes, contributing to inflammation, worsened clinical signs, and perpetuation of the disease state. This section focuses on the histopathologic changes associated with chronic inflammatory diseases such as atopy and adverse food reactions.

In response to acute inflammatory stimulus, three principal changes occur: (1) dilation of blood vessels and increased vascular permeability, resulting in dermal edema; (2) alteration of epidermal barrier function; and (3) changes in cerumen composition. Grossly, edema and vascular dilation are seen as erythema and stenosis of the canal with inflamed but still pliable tissue. Loss of barrier function increases penetration of microorganism antigens and exotoxins, exacerbating local inflammation. Cerumen production tends to increase as the result of inflammation. Alterations in composition may also affect antimicrobial function, but the precise changes and effects are not well understood.[29,32,38] Narrowing of the canal and occlusion with ceruminous debris provide a better environment for microorganism overgrowth. This cycle amplifies both primary inflammatory disease and secondary infection, resulting in progressive worsening of clinical otitis externa. Early ceruminous gland dilation or hyperplasia may be seen at this stage. This can be observed grossly as dilated ceruminous glands throughout the ear canal appear slightly raised over the surrounding epidermis, contributing to what is described as a "cobblestone" appearance of the ear canal.

With continued inflammation the epithelium changes from a thin layer of migrating cells to hyperplastic stratified squamous epithelium, characterized by multiple layers of cells, increased cellular turnover, and orthokeratotic hyperkeratosis.[30-32] Normal epithelial migration is disrupted, resulting in greater accumulation of debris and shedding of keratin sheets directly into the lumen. If bacteria colonization or infection is a significant component of otitis, neutrophils may infiltrate the dermis, migrate through the epidermis, and form a purulent exudate in the lumen. The combination of bacterial exotoxins and neutrophil proteases can result in significant damage to the epithelium, causing erosion and ulceration. This is particularly true of infections by *Pseudomonas aeruginosa*.

Ongoing inflammatory stimuli from hypersensitivity to environmental allergens, dietary antigens, and bacterial or yeast products, result in hyperplasia of the three prominent cell types in the dermis: sebaceous glands, ceruminous glands, and fibroblasts. The precise mechanism for hyperplasia of these tissues is not well described but likely involves cytokines and growth factors associated with inflammation. With glandular hyperplasia there is a dramatic change in the volume of tissue occupying the limited diameter of the cartilage boundaries.[28,30,32] As glandular tissue increases, the lumen of the ear canal decreases, leading to severe stenosis of the canal. Frequently, large hyperplastic folds of tissue are visible on gross and otoscopic examination; occasionally folds completely fill the canal, and no obvious opening can be found.

In one study comparing histopathologic specimens from the horizontal ear canal of dogs undergoing total ear canal ablation surgery for end-stage otitis externa, three primary tissue reaction patterns were observed: (1) predominantly sebaceous glandular hyperplasia, (2) predominantly ceruminous glandular hyperplasia, and (3) fibrosis.[33] Interestingly there is substantial variation in the predominant tissue response pattern, depending on the breed of dog affected. Cocker Spaniels were found to have predominantly ceruminous gland response, while non–Cocker Spaniels exhibited fibrosis most often. Less commonly observed tissue reactions included lichenoid interface dermatitis, eosinophilic infiltration, and ulcerative otitis.

A separate study reported similar findings. The area covered by sebaceous glands was not significantly different in a comparison of spaniel dogs with or without otitis externa.[32] However, the area covered by ceruminous glands was markedly increased with otitis externa. Increases in glandular tissue occurred by both hyperplasia and marked dilation of the central lumens (ectasia). Grossly, this may be seen as hyperplastic folds with a cobblestone surface or in some cases dilated purple, blue, or clear cystic structures.

Hyperplasia and dilation of ceruminous glands is frequently accompanied by inflammation, resulting in ceruminous gland adenitis (Figure 3-10). The resultant destruction of glandular epithelium and leakage of glandular contents into the interstitial space results in large amounts of lipid. Macrophages filled with lipofuscin, a wear-and-tear pigment associated with oxidative stress, were observed around inflamed ceruminous glands (Figure 3-11). The presence of lipofuscin-laden macrophages is positively correlated with breed, ceruminous gland tissue response

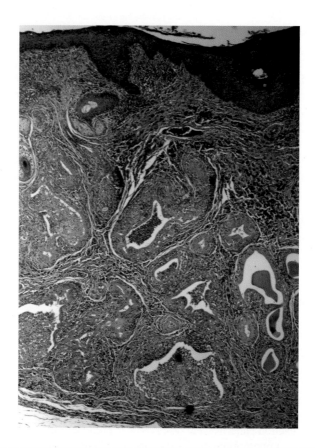

Figure 3-10

Severe ceruminous gland hyperplasia, ectasia, and inflammation. Large numbers of neutrophils are present both around the glands, in the gland walls, and in the dilated gland lumens. Note the tremendous thickening of the epithelial layer from one to two cells thick to 20 to 30 cells thick.

pattern, and osseous metaplasia (unpublished data). Lipofuscin cannot be broken down by the body; as a result, the large amounts of lipofuscin-laden macrophages may create a chronic granulomatous inflammation that cannot be resolved. Continued cytokine and growth factor production from these macrophages may contribute to perpetuation of glandular hyperplasia, fibrosis, osseous metaplasia and other changes observed in end-stage otitis externa.

In addition to macrophages, ear canal tissue may be infiltrated with large numbers of neutrophils, T-lymphocytes, and plasma cells. With chronicity, lymphoid nodules may develop in the deep dermis.

One of the most clinically significant histopathologic changes associated with chronic inflammatory otitis is calcification. A common misconception of this process is that the cartilage tube transforms to calcified tissue. In fact, the majority of calcification occurs in the soft tissue outside the cartilage boundaries (Figure 3-12). The process is true osseous metaplasia, where the resident fibroblasts transform to

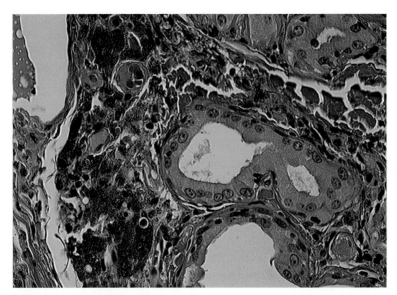

Figure 3-11

Photomicrograph of lipofuscin-laden macrophages. Lipofuscin is the yellow-brown granular pigment in the tissue adjacent to the ceruminous gland.

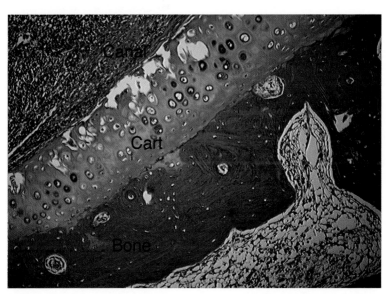

Figure 3-12

Osseous metaplasia. Figure shows a cross-section of vertical ear canal from a dog with end-stage otitis externa. The ear canal tissue is filled with large numbers of white blood cells. The cartilage border separates the ear canal tissue from the new bone being formed outside of the ear canal.

produce bonelike tissues in an inappropriate location. Palpation of the para-aural space reveals rigid calcification, usually surrounding the dorsal, lateral, and ventral canal in a semicircular formation. The new bone is easily visible on computed tomography (CT) scans or radiographs of the skull (Figure 3-13). This change is irreversible and represents progression toward an end-stage canal, which is less likely to respond to medical therapy.

Progression from edema to epidermal hyperplasia, glandular hyperplasia and ectasia, deposition of lipofuscin, lymphoid nodules, fibrosis, and osseous metaplasia represents a spectrum of histopathologic changes associated with otitis externa. Understanding these changes and the mechanisms driving them can assist in diagnosis, prognosis, and appropriate therapeutic decision making in the management of chronic inflammatory otitis.

Cocker Spaniels

In a review of 80 dogs undergoing total ear canal ablation for end-stage inflammatory otitis externa, 48 of the dogs were Cocker Spaniels (60%).[33] Over the same time period, Cocker Spaniels represented only 4.2% of the general hospital population. The next most commonly represented breeds were six mixed-breed dogs (7.5%). No other pure breed was represented by more than two dogs (2.5%). Cocker Spaniels do not have a higher incidence of atopy, food allergy, or ear mites, which would have

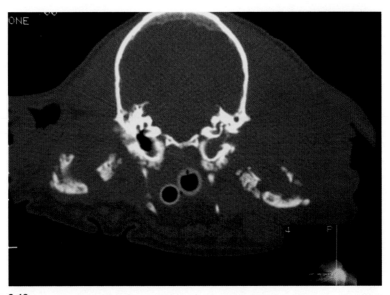

Figure 3-13

CT scan of a Cocker Spaniel with osseous metaplasia. The skull is visible centrally. Both tympanic bullae can be seen. Contrast the air-filled bulla on the left with the fluid-filled bulla on the right. Bone lining the bulla is thickened and irregular. New bone is visible in the soft tissue on both sides of the skull.

explained the 24-fold increase in incidence of end-stage otitis over the next most represented pure breed or a 14-fold increase over the incidence predicted by breed popularity. The most likely explanation for the observed overrepresentation is that Cocker Spaniels have a different pathologic response to primary conditions causing otitis externa. This hypothesis was supported by substantial differences in histopathologic findings from the horizontal ear canal. Most notably, 72.9% of Cocker Spaniels had changes dominated by ceruminous gland hyperplasia and ectasia (Figures 3-14 and 3-15). By comparison, only 28.1% of all other breeds demonstrated this tissue response pattern. The most common pattern observed in other breeds was fibrosis, seen in 40.6% of other breeds and 8.3% of Cocker Spaniels (Figure 3-16).[33]

Cocker Spaniels were also found to have a higher incidence of lipofuscin-laden macrophages infiltrating the tissue than other breeds of dogs; this feature was observed in 70.8% of the Cocker Spaniels, compared with 25% of other breeds. Osseous metaplasia in the soft tissue surrounding the horizontal canal was observed in 60.4% of the Cocker Spaniels but only 21.9% of non–Cocker Spaniel breeds.[33]

Overall, these differences in histopathologic changes in end-stage otitis externa suggest that American Cocker Spaniels have different physiologic responses to inflammatory stimuli. The differences in tissue response result in more severe expression of disease, confirming previous observations that Cocker Spaniels have more frequent and more severe otitis externa than other breeds.

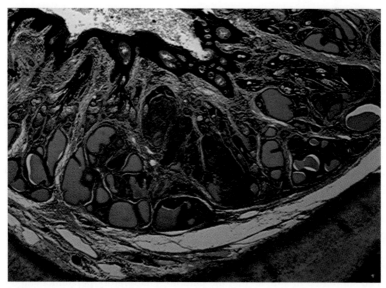

Figure 3-14

Cocker Spaniel with ceruminous gland tissue response, characterized by hyperplasia of ceruminous glands, dilation of glands, and inflammation.

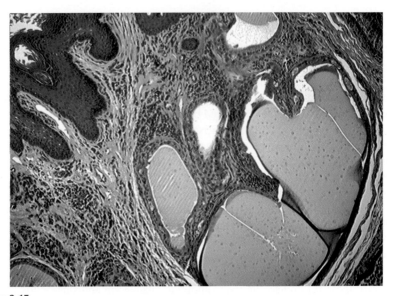

Figure 3-15

Close-up of single-hair follicular unit from same dog as in Figure 3-14.

Neoplasia

In general the ear canal is an uncommon site for tumor development. The true incidence of ear canal tumors in dogs and cats is not known, but based on surveys of total submissions to pathology laboratories, less than 1% of all tumors in dogs and less than 2% of all tumors in cats occur in the ear canal.[39] Tumors can arise from epithelium, ceruminous glands, sebaceous glands, fibroblasts, mast cells, and virtually any other cell type found in the lining of the external canal.

Any nodule, mass, or polyp found in the ear canal should be biopsied for histopathologic diagnosis. Biopsy of nodules deep in the canal can be difficult due to the limited confines of the canal and diminished visualization due to debris. Care should be taken not to crush the tissue with hemostats, alligator forceps, or other blunt, grasping instruments. A diagnostic sample can best be obtained using biopsy forceps (Figure 3-17). If available, video-otoscopic guided CO_2 laser can be a practical alternative to grasping and pulling.

Because neoplasia can occur due to transformation of chronically inflamed tissue, histopathology should also be obtained of any tissue removed during lateral ear canal resection or total ear canal ablation, even if the patient has a history of long-standing disease. Do not section the ear canal prior to submission; the entire canal should be submitted in situ, so that the pathology laboratory personnel can trim ear canals using a standard method.

The most common tumors of the ear canal in both cats and dogs are ceruminous gland adenoma and adenocarcinoma. Contrary to early reports indicating that tumors

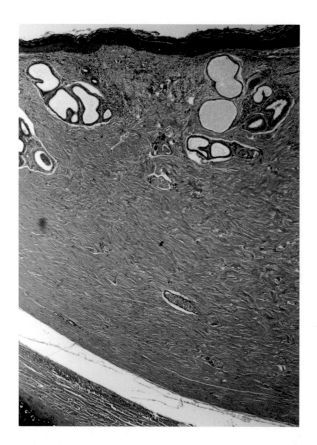

Figure 3-16

Example of fibrosis tissue response pattern. Note the absence of inflammation and sparse follicular units in the deep dermis, which is replaced by large amounts of collagen tissue.

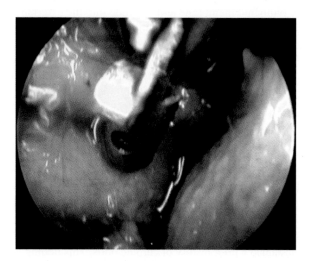

Figure 3-17

Video-endoscopic biopsy forceps obtaining sample from nodule in the vertical canal.

of ceruminous gland origin were more frequently benign in dogs and malignant in cats, this distinction may not be entirely accurate or reliable. In a large review of 124 ceruminous tumors, 61% of dogs and 69% of cats had adenocarcinoma.[39] The frequency of malignancy is high enough that any tumor of the ear canal should be treated suspiciously until proven otherwise by histopathologic diagnosis.

Typical histopathologic findings of adenoma are well-differentiated proliferation of polypoid cuboidal-to-columnar epithelium. The neoplastic tissue forms acini and secretory ducts. Mitotic figures are rare. Individually cells have minimal atypia, ovoid-to-round nuclei, and a single prominent nucleolus. Glands tend to retain normal myoepithelial basement membrane boundaries and do not invade connective tissue parenchyma.[39]

In contrast, adenocarcinoma is characterized by moderate or marked nuclear atypia and common mitotic figures. Neoplastic tissue fails to form normal-appearing secretory gland patterns. Orientation of the apical surface to the myoepithelial basement membrane is absent. Squamous differentiation, characterized by individual necrotic keratinocytes, dyskeratosis, and keratin pearl formation, can be seen. As tumors outgrow effective blood supply, central necrosis can be observed. Most significantly, adenocarcinoma frequently invades connective tissue parenchyma, occasionally penetrating the auricular or annular cartilage.[39]

Other tumors diagnosed by histopathology include squamous cell carcinoma, mast cell tumor, malignant melanoma, hemangiosarcoma, fibrosarcoma, lymphoma, and basal cell carcinoma.

Nasopharyngeal polyps are a common tumorlike disease in cats. Polyps are fleshy, nodular masses of fibrous connective tissue that develop from respiratory epithelial tissue of the nasopharynx, eustachian tube, or tympanic cavity. Some patients present with respiratory signs such as nasal discharge, sneezing, and stertor or with dysphagia and recurrent gagging. If the polyp fills the tympanic cavity, it may rupture the tympanic membrane and protrude into the external canal, resulting in obstructive otitis. Biopsy should be taken to rule out neoplasia. Histopathologically, polyps are characterized by an irregular mass of fibrous connective tissue covered by a layer of respiratory epithelium. The pathognomonic finding is respiratory cilia on the surface of the mass. Less commonly, dogs can also develop benign fibrous polyps arising from the external ear canal, tympanic membrane, or respiratory epithelium.

Cocker Spaniels

Not only are Cocker Spaniels more likely to have more severe histopathologic changes associated with chronic inflammation, but American Cocker Spaniels are also over-represented in studies of ear canal tumors.[31,40] In a large review of 81 dogs with ear canal tumors, Cocker Spaniels were found to represent 17% of all cases of malignant tumors, and 27% of the benign tumors.[41] In the same review, 35% of dogs with malignant neoplasia had a prior history of chronic otitis. This finding is not surprising, since chronic inflammation and ceruminous gland hyperplasia are suspected risk factors for neoplastic transformation.[42]

Conclusion

The external ear canal of a dog is lined with tissue that in many ways is very similar to normal epidermis and dermis elsewhere on the body. However, tissue response to inflammatory stimuli is unique to the ear canal. Familiarity with the changes that occur in cerumen volume and content, epithelial migration, glandular activity, fibrosis, and osseous metaplasia contributes to a better understanding of the progression of chronic inflammatory otitis from acute edema to irreversible end-stage disease. Findings such as ceruminous gland adenitis and lipofuscin-laden macrophages may provide clues to further understanding of the transformation of hyperplastic glands to cerumen gland adenocarcinoma.

Important breed differences in histopathology support clinical observations that American Cocker Spaniels have more severe otic disease than any other breed. Although Cocker Spaniels are less likely than other breeds to exhibit severe fibrosis of the ear canal, they have a demonstrated predisposition for ceruminous gland ectasia, proliferative ceruminous gland hyperplasia, osseous metaplasia, and lipofuscin-containing macrophages. These changes result in increased risk for end-stage otitis externa requiring total ear canal ablation surgery. In fact, Cocker Spaniels are 24 times more likely to require this surgery than any other breed and 14 times more likely than would be predicted based on breed popularity.

References

1. Baba E, Fukata T, Saito M: Incidence of otitis externa in dogs and cats in Japan, *Vet Rec* 108: 393-395, 1981.
2. Griffin CE, Song M: Otitis workshop. In Kwochka K, Willemse T, von Tscharner C, eds: *Advances in veterinary dermatology,* vol 3, Boston, 1996, Butterworth-Heinemann.
3. Rosychuk RA, Luttgen P. Diseases of the ear. In Ettinger SJ, Feldman EC, eds: *Textbook of veterinary internal medicine: diseases of the dog and cat,* ed 5, Philadelphia, 2000, WB Saunders.
4. Kowalski JJ: The microbial environment of the ear canal in health and disease, *Vet Clin North Am Sm Anim Pract* 18:743-754, 1988.
5. Harvey RG, Harari J, Delauche AJ: Diagnostic procedures. In Harvey RG, Harari J, Delauche AJ, eds: *Ear diseases of the dog and cat,* Ames, Iowa, 2001, Iowa State University Press.
6. Scott DW, Miller WH, Griffin CE: Diseases of eyelids, claws, anal sacs, and ears. In Scott DW, Miller WH, Griffin CE, eds: *Muller and Kirk's Small animal dermatology,* ed 6, Philadelphia, 2000, WB Saunders.
7. Chickering WR: Cytologic evaluation of otic exudates, *Vet Clin North Am Sm Anim Pract* 18: 773-782, 1988.
8. Cole LK, Kwochka KW, Kowalski JJ, et al: Microbial flora and antimicrobial susceptibility patterns of isolated pathogens from the horizontal ear canal and middle ear in dogs with otitis media, *J Am Vet Med Assoc* 212:534-538, 1998.
9. Colombini S, Merchant SR, Hosgood G: Microbial flora and antimicrobial susceptibility patterns of dogs with otitis media, *Vet Dermatol 2000* 11:235-239, 2000.
10. Tater KC, Scott DW, Miller WH, et al: The cytology of the external ear canal in the normal dog and cat, *J Vet Med A* 50:370-374, 2003.
11. Harvey RG, Harari J, Delauche AJ: The normal ear. In Harvey RG, Harari J, Delauche AJ, eds: *Ear diseases of the dog and cat,* Ames, Iowa, 2001, Iowa State University Press.

12. Guillot J, Bond R: *Malassezia pachydermatis:* a review, *Med Mycol* 37:295-306, 1999.

13. Bond R: Pathogenesis of *Malassezia* dermatitis. In Thoday KL, Foil CS, Bond R, eds: *Advances in veterinary dermatology,* vol 4, Oxford, UK, 2002, Blackwell Science.

14. Morris DO: *Malassezia* dermatitis and otitis, *Vet Clin North Am Sm Anim Pract* 29(6):1303-1310, 1999.

15. Scott DW, Miller WH, Griffin CE: Fungal skin diseases. In Scott DW, Miller WH, Griffin CE, eds: *Muller and Kirk's Small animal dermatology,* ed 6, Philadelphia, 2000, WB Saunders.

16. Bond R, Saijonmaa-Koulumies LE, Lloyd DH: Population sizes and frequency of *Malassezia pachydermatis* at skin and mucosal sites on healthy dogs, *J Small Anim Pract* 36(4):147-150, 1995.

17. Greene CE: Otitis externa. In *Infectious diseases of the dog and cat,* ed 2, Philadelphia, 1998, WB Saunders.

18. Crespo MJ, Abarca ML, Cabanes FJ: Occurrence of *Malassezia* spp. in the external ear canals of dogs and cats with and without otitis externa, *Med Mycol* 40:115-121, 2002.

19. Crespo MJ, Abarca ML, Cabanes FJ: Otitis externa associated with *Malassezia sympodialis* in two cats, *J Clin Microbiol* 38:1263-1266, 2000.

20. Bond R, Anthony RM, Dodd M, et al: Isolation of *Malassezia sympodialis* from feline skin, *J Med Vet Mycol* 34:145-147, 1996.

21. Bond R, Howell SA, Haywood PJ, et al: Isolation of *Malassezia sympodialis* and *Malassezia globosa* from healthy pet cats, *Vet Rec* 141:200-201, 1997.

22. Ginel PJ, Lucena R, Rodriquez JC, et al: A semiquantitative cytological evaluation of normal and pathological samples from the external ear canal of dogs and cats, *Vet Dermatol* 13:151-156, 2002.

23. Baker R, Lumsden JH: The head and neck. In Baker R, Lumsden JH, eds: *Color atlas of cytology of the dog and cat,* St Louis, 2003, Mosby.

24. Clinkenbeard KD, Cowell RL, Morton RJ, et al: Diagnostic cytology: bacterial infections, *Compend Cont Ed* 17(1):71-85, 1995.

25. Harvey RG, Harari J, Delauche AJ: Etiopathogenesis and classification of otitis externa. In Harvey RG, Harari J, Delauche AJ, eds: *Ear diseases of the dog and cat,* Ames, Iowa, 2001, Iowa State University Press.

26. Loshe J, Rinder H, Gothe R, et al: Validity of species status of the parasitic mite *Otodectes cynotis,* *Med Vet Entomol* 16:133-138, 2002.

27. Getty R, Foust HL, Presley ET, et al: Macroscopic anatomy of the ear of the dog, *Am J Vet Res* 17:364-375, 1956.

28. Fraser G: The histopathology of the external auditory meatus of the dog, *J Comp Pathol* 71:253-258, 1961.

29. Fernando SDA: A histological and histochemical study of the glands of the external auditory canal of the dog, *Res Vet Sci* 7:116-119, 1966.

30. Fernando SDA: Certain histopathologic features of the external auditory meatus of the cat and dog with otitis externa, *Am J Vet Res* 28:278-282, 1966.

31. van der Gaag I: The pathology of the external ear canal in dogs and cats, *Vet Q* 8:307-317.

32. Stout-Graham M, Kainer RA, Whalen LR, et al: Morphologic measurements of the external ear canal of dogs, *Am J Vet Res* 51:990-994, 1990.

33. Angus JC, Lichtensteiger C, Campbell KL, et al: Breed variations in histopathologic features of chronic severe otitis externa in dogs: 80 cases (1995-2001), *J Am Vet Med Assoc* 221(7):1000-1006, 2002.

34. Chaudhary M, Mirakhur KK, Roy KS: Histopathologic and histochemical studies on chronic otitis in dogs, *Indian J Anim Sci* 72(2):128-129, 2002.

35. Gotthelf LN: Failure of epithelial migration: ceruminoliths. In Gotthelf LN, ed: *Small animal ear diseases: an illustrated guide,* Philadelphia, 2000, WB Saunders.

36. Kumar A, Roman-Auerhahn MR: Anatomy of the canine and feline ear. In Gotthelf LN, ed: *Small animal ear diseases: an illustrated guide,* Philadelphia, 2000, WB Saunders.

37. Harvey RG, Harari J, Delauche AJ: The normal ear. In Harvey RG, Harari J, Delauche AJ, eds: *Ear diseases of the dog and cat,* Ames, Iowa, 2001, Iowa State University Press.

38. Masuda A, Sukegawa T, Mizumoto N, et al: Study of lipid in the ear canal in canine otitis externa with *Malassezia pachydermatis, J Vet Med Sci* 62(11):1177-1182, 2000.

39. Moisan PG, Watson GL: Ceruminous gland tumors in dogs and cats: a review of 124 cases, *J Am Anim Hosp Assoc* 32:449-453, 1996.
40. Kirpensteijn J: Aural neoplasms, *Sem Vet Med Surg (Sm Anim)* 8:17-23, 1993.
41. London CA, Dubilzeig RR, Vail DM, et al: Evaluation of dogs and cats with tumors of the ear canal: 145 cases (1978-1992), *J Am Vet Med Assoc* 208:1413-1418, 1996.
42. Rogers KS: Tumors of the ear canal, *Vet Clin North Am Sm Anim Pract* 18(4):859-868, 1988.

4

Diagnostic Imaging of the Ear

Mauricio Solano, MV, DACVR

Selecting the appropriate imaging method, correctly applying the technique selected, and accurately interpreting the examination are the key steps in imaging ear disorders in dogs and cats. Conventional screen-film radiography (including positive contrast canalography), computed tomography (CT), and magnetic resonance imaging (MRI) should be considered complementary techniques, since no single imaging modality perfectly depicts the complex anatomy of the ear. The physics and instrumentation that form the basis of these diagnostic procedures will not be discussed. This chapter provides an overview of the indications for and limitations of different modalities, emphasizing the key points in selecting and performing the appropriate studies and interpreting the images. Readers will find the information needed to decide which modality will be most effective in a specific clinical setting. One guideline applies to all imaging described here—general anesthesia is required for a full assessment of the middle and inner ear. Attempting to evaluate these areas with sedation alone or without chemical restraint is an exercise in futility.

Conventional Radiography

The five radiographic projections needed to visualize the soft tissue of the external acoustic canal and the bone of the tympanic bullae and petrous temporal bones are referred to collectively as a *bulla series*. These views are: lateral, two opposite obliques (left 20-degree ventral–right dorsal oblique and right 20-degree ventral–left dorsal oblique), open-mouth (rostral 30-degree ventral–caudodorsal open-mouth oblique), and a ventrodorsal (VD) or dorsoventral (DV).

Technique and Normal Radiographic Findings

High-detail film screen combinations (Kodak Lanex fine screens with Ektascan M film or 3M SE plus film with Assymetrix detail screens) are required to provide the contrast and spatial resolution needed to recognize the typical abnormalities seen in the canine and feline ear.

Lateral View

The animal is placed in lateral recumbency with the nasal septum parallel and the hard palate perpendicular to the tabletop cassette (Figure 4-1, *A* and *B*). The primary beam is centered on the external acoustic canal. A foam wedge or gauze roll placed beneath the rostral third of the nose is needed to maintain proper alignment. The head should be slightly extended to avoid superimposition of the bullae on the pharynx. Portions of the larynx and pharynx should be included in this view (Figure 4-1, *C*) to assess the temporomandibular joints and the nasopharynx because as some diseases, such as nasopharyngeal polyps and craniomandibular osteopathy, can also affect the middle ear. This author prefers a subtle rostral offset of one bulla from the other to compare them. To achieve this, the primary beam can be centered just rostral to the external acoustic meatus, or the rostral third of the nose can be elevated slightly from

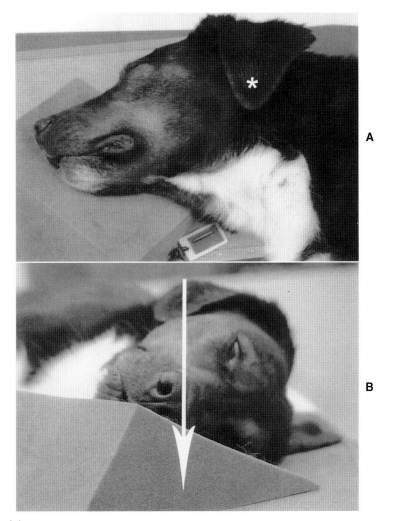

Figure 4-1

A, Patient positioning to obtain a lateral view of the middle ear. The *asterisk* indicates the point where the primary x-ray beam enters the patient. A foam wedge under the maxillary bones ensures the nasal septum is parallel to the table. **B,** The *arrow* indicates the trajectory of the primary beam. The skull should be positioned with the hard palate parallel to the primary beam.

Continued

parallel to the cassette (Figure 4-1, *D*). In animals with a large pinna covering the acoustic canal, such as hound or spaniel breeds, the pinna should be unfolded and placed dorsal to the skull to avoid allowing skin artifacts to obscure the area of interest. The endotracheal tube can be left in place. The external acoustic meatus is a circular to oval, gas-filled structure with well-defined inner borders. The tympanic bullae have smooth, thin-walled bone margins and a gas-filled lumen (see Figure 4-1, *C*

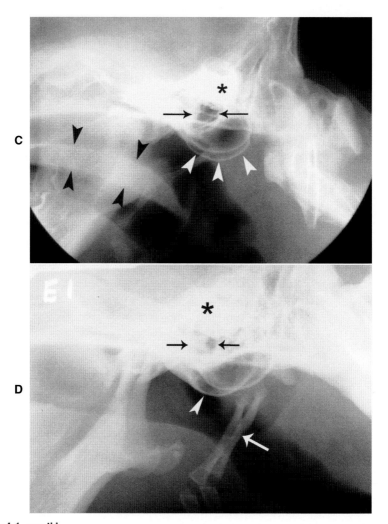

Figure 4-1—cont'd

C, Lateral radiograph of the middle ear. The left and right tympanic bullae are superimposed *(white arrowheads).* The petrosal portions of the temporal bones *(asterisk)* are located dorsal to the bullae. The soft palate is indicated with *black arrowheads.* The external acoustic meatus *(arrows)* is dorsal to the tympanic bullae. **D,** Lateral radiograph of the middle ear with one bulla rostrally positioned *(arrowhead).* The petrosal portions of the temporal bones *(asterisk)* are located dorsal to the bullae. The stylohyoid bones *(white arrow)* overlie the caudal aspect of the nasopharynx. The external acoustic meatus *(black arrows)* is also visible.

and *D*). Thickness of the wall varies between breeds. There is less variation in the thickness of the bullae walls between breeds in cats. The petrosal portions of the temporal bones are highly radiopaque and superimposed on each other in this view; therefore, they cannot be fully assessed. In cats the bullae appear larger in proportion to the head than in dogs.

Oblique Views

Two opposite oblique views are taken. With the animal in lateral recumbency, the bulla to be imaged is placed closer to the cassette. The thoracic limbs, sternum, nasal cavity, and mandible are rotated 20 degrees from the horizontal plane and are held in position with foam wedges (Figure 4-2, *A* and *B*). The mouth is closed to avoid superimposition of the mandible on the area of interest. The primary beam is centered at the base of the ear, ventral to the tragus. The primary beam travels through the patient in a lateral 20-degree ventral–left dorsal oblique direction. The tympanic bulla to be assessed is projected ventrally, while the contralateral bulla is superimposed over the caudal third of the calvarium and therefore cannot be assessed fully (Figure 4-2, *C*). Portions of the stylohyoid bone may be superimposed over the bulla of interest. The tympanic bullae have smooth, thin-walled bone margins and a gas-filled lumen. The external acoustic meatus is projected on the bulla as a circular to oval, gas-filled structure with well-defined inner borders.

VD and DV Projections

Choosing between a DV and VD projection is more a function of hospital protocol or personal preference than clinical need. To obtain the VD view, the animal is placed in dorsal recumbency. The primary beam enters the patient in a VD orientation at the

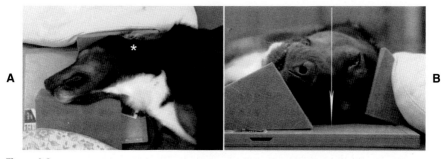

A   B

Figure 4-2

A, Patient positioning to obtain an oblique view of the middle ear. The resultant radiograph is named the *left 20-degree ventral–right dorsal oblique view,* which describes the entrance and exit points of the primary beam. The *asterisk* indicates the point where the primary x-ray beam enters the patient. **B,** Patient positioning to obtain a right 20-degree ventral–left dorsal oblique radiograph. The *arrow* indicates the trajectory of the primary beam.

Continued

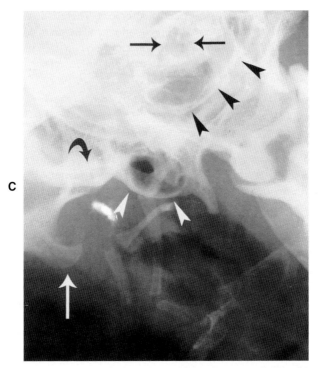

Figure 4-2—cont'd

C, Left 20-degree ventral–right dorsal oblique radiograph of the middle ear. The right bulla is displaced ventrally *(white arrowheads)*. Only a faint outline of the wall of the left bulla can be seen *(black arrowheads)* with the left external acoustic meatus located dorsally *(black arrows)*. There is superimposition of the right stylohyoid bone over the right tympanic bulla. The angular process of the right hemimandible *(white arrow)* is visible ventral to the right temporomandibular joint *(curved arrow)*.

midline halfway between the external acoustic meatuses (Figure 4-3, *A*). The animal is placed in sternal recumbency to obtain a DV view. The primary beam is directed vertically centered at a point where an imaginary line connecting the bullae intersects with the midsagittal plane. The body of the mandible should be parallel to the cassette, to avoid distortion. The tongue should be pulled forward and maintained on the midline. These views are used to assess the ear canals and to compare symmetry of the bullae and the petrosal portion of the temporal bones. The tympanic bullae cannot be evaluated fully in this view because they are superimposed over the petrosal portions of the temporal bones (Figure 4-3, *B*). There is no specific bone pattern associated with the petrous temporal bones, however; they should exhibit a symmetrical shape, size, and opacity on these projections. Reducing the milliamp seconds (mAs) by half to highlight the soft tissues allows visualization of the

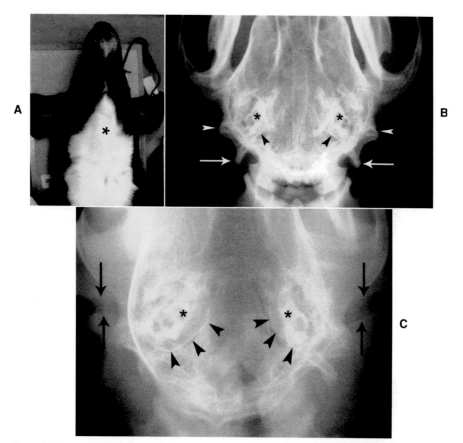

Figure 4-3

A, Patient positioning to obtain a VD view of the middle ear. The *asterisk* indicates the entrance point of the primary x-ray beam. Choosing between a VD and a DV view is more a function of hospital protocol or personal preference than clinical need. **B,** VD radiograph of the middle ear. The most caudal walls of the tympanic bullae *(black arrowheads)* are noted caudal to the more radiopaque petrosal portions of the temporal bones *(asterisks).* Rostral to the mastoid process *(white arrowheads)* lies the external acoustic meatus. The paracondylar process *(white arrows)* projects caudally. **C,** DV radiograph of the middle ear. The soft tissue exposure technique allows visualization of the external ear canals *(arrows).* The walls of the tympanic bullae *(arrowheads)* surround the petrosal portions of the temporal bones *(asterisks).*

horizontal portion of the external acoustic canals (Figure 4-3, *C*), which are noted as well-defined lucent structures. The canals tend to be wider laterally as the auricular cartilage expands to form the pinna. The average diameter of the proximal end of the annular cartilage is 4.1 ± 0.7 mm in dogs in which the tympanic membrane is visible otoscopically.[1]

Open-Mouth View

A commercially available U-shaped acrylic head rack can be used to facilitate positioning (Figure 4-4, *A*). Without a positioning device, medical-grade adhesive tape can be used to separate the mandible from the maxilla (Figure 4-4, *B*). With the animal in dorsal recumbency, the head is acutely flexed toward the thoracic inlet. The vertical primary beam is directed rostroventral to caudodorsal and centered immediately ventral to the hard palate. The hard palate and mandible are 30 degrees from the vertical plane. This will highlight both tympanic bullae with minimal superimposition from the surrounding structures. The endotracheal tube should be removed or secured against the mandible. To avoid increased bullae opacity due to superimposition, the tongue should be pulled rostrally and secured to the mandible on the midline. The normal bullae are noted as thin-walled structures with a lucent center ventral to the base of the skull (Figure 4-4, *C*). Increasing the angle of the hard palate relative to the primary beam can be used as an alternative to the open-mouth projection (Figure 4-4, *D*). This projection is easier to perform because it is a closed-mouth view that highlights the most caudal surface of the tympanic bullae. Caution should be taken in assessing abnormal findings on this projection because its clinical value has not been studied as extensively as the open-mouth view.[2] Normal bullae are thin-walled

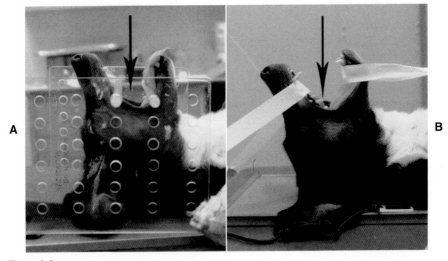

Figure 4-4

A, Patient positioning to obtain a rostral 30-degree ventral–caudodorsal open-mouth oblique projection. The *arrow* indicates the trajectory of the primary beam. The positional device is known as an *acrylic head rack,* which is radiolucent on radiographs. **B,** Patient positioning to obtain a rostral 30-degree ventral–caudodorsal open-mouth oblique projection without the aid of a positional device. Medical-grade adhesive tape is used to keep the mouth open. The *arrow* indicates the trajectory of the primary beam.

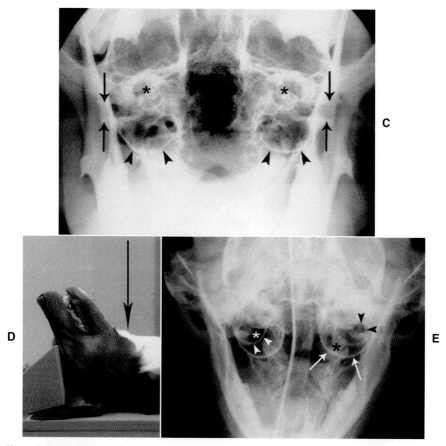

Figure 4-4—cont'd

C, Rostral 30-degree ventral–caudodorsal open-mouth oblique radiograph of a normal dog. The tympanic bullae *(arrowheads)* are located ventral to the petrosal portions of the temporal bones *(asterisks)*. The external acoustic meatus *(arrows)* is partially obscured by the overlying coronoid process of the mandible. **D,** Patient positioning to obtain a rostroventral-caudodorsal closed-mouth oblique radiograph. There is an increased angle of the hard palate in relationship to the primary beam represented by the *arrow*. This projection is technically easier to perform, but its clinical value has not been studied as extensively as the open-mouth projection. It highlights the caudal aspect of the tympanic bullae. **E,** Rostral 30-degree ventral–caudodorsal open-mouth oblique radiograph of a normal cat. An osseous septum *(white arrowheads)* separates the dorsolateral compartment *(white asterisk)* from the larger ventromedial compartment *(black asterisk)*. The *white arrows* indicate the walls of the medioventral compartment. The external acoustic meatus *(black arrowheads)* is visualized overlying the dorsolateral compartment.

structures with a lucent center ventral to the base of the skull (see Figure 4-4, *C*). Their walls are of uniform thickness. They are symmetrical in size, shape, and opacity when compared with one another.

In cats an osseous septum divides the bullae into two separate but communicating tympanic cavities—a smaller dorsolateral compartment and a larger ventromedial compartment (Figure 4-4, *E*). There is less variation in the thickness of the bulla walls between breeds in cats. The external acoustic meatus is sometimes superimposed on the dorsolateral compartment.

Abnormal Radiographic Findings

Otoscopic evaluation is the method of choice to evaluate the external ear canal. However, radiographs can reveal narrowing of its lumen by soft-tissue proliferation from extraluminal masses in cases of neoplasia or by inflammatory tissue, exudates, or debris in cases of otitis externa or trauma (Figure 4-5, *A*). Dystrophic calcification can be seen associated with chronic otitis externa (Figure 4-5, *B*).

Diseases affecting the middle ear, such as otitis media, neoplasia, and craniomandibular osteopathy, as well as polyps can be evaluated with a bullae series. Radiographic findings are nonspecific; therefore the list of differential diagnoses

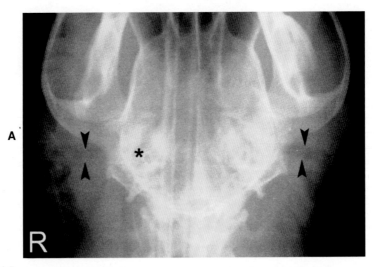

Figure 4-5

A, VD radiograph of a 4-year-old Doberman diagnosed with chronic bilateral ear infections. Both external acoustic canals *(arrowheads)* are narrowed and somewhat tortuous. The right canal is smaller and less defined than the left. There is an increased opacity associated with the right tympanic bulla and petrosal portion of the temporal bone *(asterisk)*. Compare the canals with the normal external acoustic canals depicted in Figure 4-3,*C*.

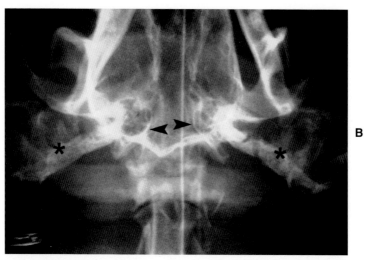

Figure 4-5—cont'd

B, VD radiograph of a 2-year-old Bulldog diagnosed with chronic bilateral otitis. Radiographs were taken prior to a total ear canal ablation. There is exuberant bilateral dystrophic calcification of the external acoustic canals *(asterisks)*. The visible walls of the tympanic bullae *(arrowheads)* appear normal.

should be generated in light of the clinical history and not radiographic findings alone.

Common findings in otitis media include thickening of the wall of the bullae, increased soft tissue opacity within the bullae, and increased size of the bullae (Figure 4-6). In the large majority of cases it is not possible to differentiate a fluid-filled bulla from one with a thickened wall. If the process is chronic, the increased opacity is likely the result of both thickening and fluid accumulation. Rare mineral concretions within the bullae, also known as *middle ear otoliths,* have been reported in four dogs.[3,4] Middle-ear otolithiasis may be associated with nonactive or active cases of otitis media. If the otitis media is secondary to otitis externa, narrowing and mineralization of the external acoustic canal can also be seen.

Common findings associated with neoplasia affecting the middle ear include soft-tissue swelling, which may or may not obliterate the external acoustic canal; lysis of the wall of the bullae; and increased opacity of the bullae without lysis (Figure 4-7). Less commonly, ill-defined periosteal reactions arising from the bullae and surrounding bones can be seen. Neoplasia of ceruminous glands, squamous cell carcinomas, and anaplastic carcinomas have been diagnosed among others.[5,6]

Increased opacity of the bulla as the result of thickening of the walls can also occur in cases of invading nasal polyps[7] and craniomandibular osteopathy (Figure 4-8).

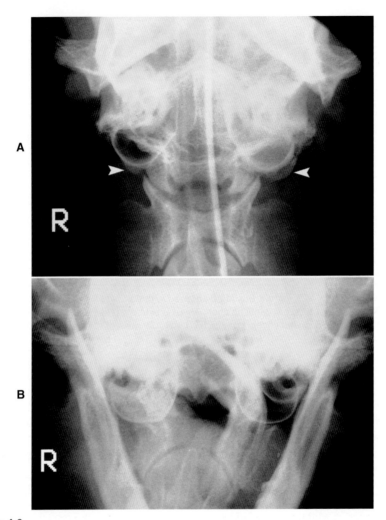

Figure 4-6

A, Rostroventral–caudodorsal closed-mouth oblique radiograph of a 14-year-old cat diagnosed with a nasopharyngeal polyp. There is bilateral thickening of the caudal aspect of the walls of the bullae *(arrowheads)*. The left bulla is increased in opacity, which can be the result of fluid or a mass within the bulla or the result of the sclerosis and thickness of the wall. **B,** Rostroventral–caudodorsal open-mouth oblique radiograph of an 11-year-old cat diagnosed with otitis media, which presented with right-sided head tilt and circling. The right bulla is mildly enlarged with a generalized increase in opacity, which is compatible with a diagnosis of otitis media. However, radiographically it is not possible to determine whether the increased opacity is the result of fluid or a mass within the bulla. Otoscopic examination reveals generalized thickening of the external and middle ear.

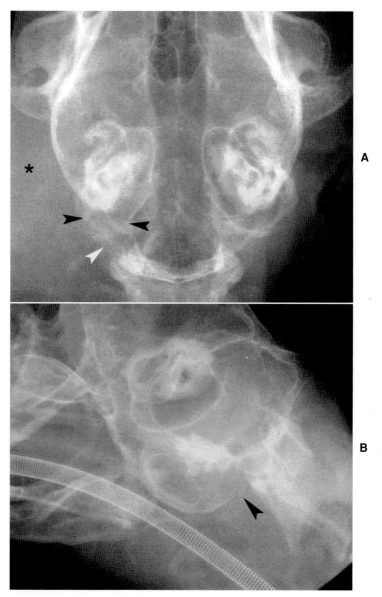

Figure 4-7

A, Ventrodorsal radiograph of a 10-year-old cat diagnosed with a ceruminous gland carcinoma. There is lysis of the caudal aspect of the occipital bone *(white arrowhead)*, thinning and lysis of the caudal aspect of the wall of the bulla *(black arrowheads)*, and an increased soft tissue opacity obliterating the external acoustic canal *(asterisk)*. **B,** Oblique radiograph of a 10-year-old cat diagnosed with a ceruminous gland carcinoma. There is lysis of the most caudal aspect of the tympanic bullae *(black arrowhead)*.

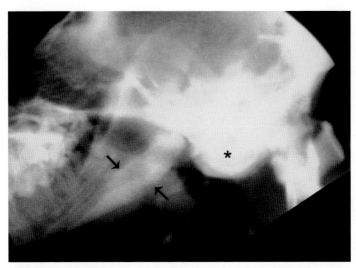

Figure 4-8

Lateral radiograph of the middle ear of a 1-year-old Scottish Terrier diagnosed with cranio-mandibular osteopathy. There is marked increased opacity associated with the tympanic bullae *(asterisk),* which is the result of thickening of the walls. The visible cortex of the mandibular body *(arrows)* is also thickened. VD radiographs (not shown) confirmed bilateral bullae thickening. Compare the bullae with the normal bullae in Figure 4-1, *C.*

Positive Contrast Canalography

This technique uses nonionic iodine-based contrast material to assess the integrity of the tympanic membrane as well as the anatomy of the external acoustic canal.[1,8] The technique is more accurate than otoscopy for detecting iatrogenic rupture of the tympanic membrane in normal dogs and can be used to assess stenosis of the external acoustic canal. Its usefulness in cases of otitis media remains uncertain, as inflammatory secretions may block the flow of contrast material and prevent it from filling the canal completely.[8]

Technique and Normal Radiographic Findings

The canals should be gently cleaned before the study. The animal is placed in sternal recumbency, and 1 cc of iohexol (300 mg iodine per cc) is placed within the lumen of the canal. After a massage of its vertical and horizontal portions, the canal is slowly filled with contrast until it reaches the level of the tragus. A final massage is then performed to ensure adequate distribution of the contrast in the canal. To avoid leakage of contrast, a cotton swab is placed to plug the vertical portion of the ear canal. A DV view is taken, followed by the rostrocaudal open-mouth projection. The resultant radiographs (Figure 4-9) are compared with the precontrast survey study.

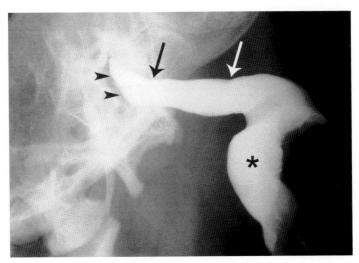

Figure 4-9

DV radiograph of a normal canalogram in a 5-year-old mixed-breed hound dog. There is complete filling of the canal by contrast material. The proximal *(black arrow)* and distal borders *(white arrow)* of the annular ligament are noted as slight indentations in the diameter of the canal. The slightly concave border that abruptly stops the flow of contrast into the tympanic bulla represents the tympanic membrane *(arrowheads)*. It is oriented at an oblique angle to the axis of the canal. The vertical portion of the ear canal *(asterisk)* is also noted.

After the study is completed, the ear is flushed with saline solution and dried. No side effects have been reported as the result of the procedure.[1,8]

The diameter of the proximal end of the annular cartilage tends to be smaller than the distal end of the annular cartilage. On the DV view these ends can be noted as minor indentations in the wall of the canal (see Figure 4-9). The tympanic membrane is a straight or slightly concave border overlying the tympanic bullae. It is oriented at an oblique angle in relationship to the longitudinal axis of the horizontal ear canal.

Abnormal Radiographic Findings

An intact tympanic membrane should prevent the flow of contrast material into the tympanic bullae; therefore, any leakage of contrast into the middle ear is considered diagnostic of a ruptured tympanic membrane. Stenosis of the ear canal has been documented in Shar-Peis and in Pugs.[1] Although canalography can effectively determine the degree of ear canal stenosis, additional studies are needed to establish fully stenosis as a predictor of chronic inflammatory ear disease. The average diameter of the proximal end of the annular cartilage in stenotic canals is 2.6 ± 0.8 mm. In dogs in which the tympanic membrane is visible otoscopically, the range is 4.1 ± 0.7 mm.[1]

Computed Tomography (CT)

CT provides cross-sectional imaging of the ear. By eliminating superimposition of surrounding bone, CT can clearly depict the anatomy of the inner, middle, and external ear. The CT anatomy of the middle and inner ear has been described by comparing transverse CT images in reference to a standard anatomy textbook.[9] CT is slightly more sensitive than radiography in the diagnosis of otitis media.[10] CT can detect subtle soft tissue changes before they are apparent on radiographs, due to its higher soft-tissue contrast resolution. However, CT is more expensive and less available to general practices than radiography. It requires a higher degree of technical expertise to operate a CT unit than a routine x-ray room, as well as a complete knowledge of the acquisition protocols and associated image post-processing software to generate diagnostic images.

Technique and Normal CT Findings

As with conventional radiography, assessment of the images relies on symmetry; therefore, careful positioning of the patient under anesthesia in the CT gantry is crucial. Most new units have laser-positioning guides to ensure that the longitudinal axis of the head enters the gantry at a 90-degree angle to the primary beam. Head-positioning devices can also facilitate positioning the hard palate parallel to the CT table (Figure 4-10). Higher kilovolt potential (kVp) and mA settings than conventional radiographs are used to reduce artifacts and noise. In dogs, a kVp of 120 and an mA of 200 are used with a full field of view and a 512 matrix. In cats, an mA of 150 with a half field of view and a 512 matrix are used. Contiguous or overlapping transverse slices 1 to 3 mm thick extending from the middle third of the nasal cavity to the foramen magnum are generated. Either the helical or axial mode of scanning can be used. A cursory look at adequately positioned images should reveal symmetry between contralateral anatomical landmarks in the head (Figure 4-11). Both frontal sinuses, temporomandibular joints, zygomatic portions of the temporal bones, occipital brain lobes, and atlantooccipital joints should appear similar in size and shape when they are being imaged in a slice (see Figure 4-11). Two different window settings, which determine the range of tissues that will appear gray on the image, are used to depict fully the anatomy of the middle and inner ear. Wide window-width settings are used to highlight bone, whereas narrow window widths centered at a soft tissue level are used to highlight soft tissues (Figure 4-12).[11] A typical window for bullae is 3200 at a level of 500, whereas a soft-tissue window width is 375 with a level of 40. Subtle changes commonly noted in cases of otitis media such as sclerosis and thickening of the bulla could be missed if a wide window width is not used. On the other hand, small amounts of fluid within the bulla can be missed if a narrow window width centered at soft-tissue settings is not used. Intravenous injection of iodinated contrast material, such as meglumine diatrizoate, should be performed to enhance inflammatory and neoplastic lesions, at a dose of 1 cc per pound of body weight (375 mg iodine per cc).

    Like conventional radiography, CT can identify the major anatomical landmarks of the external and middle ear. A major advantage of CT over conventional radiography

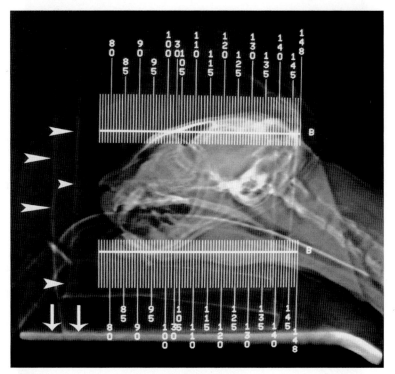

Figure 4-10

Scout image generated by the CT unit. The head of the cat is positioned in a U-shaped head holder *(arrowheads)* that facilitates positioning. The holder elevates the head over the CT table *(arrows),* maintaining the area of interest in the center of the unit's gantry. Each numbered line represents a single transverse slice. In this patient, approximately 20 slices are required to cover the ear anatomy. The tracheal tube does not need to be removed.

is the detailed visualization of the structures of the middle and inner ear, such as the tympanic membrane, the auditory ossicles, the cochlea, the vestibular aqueduct, and the semicircular canals (Figure 4-12, *C*). An artifact known as *beam hardening,* however, often obscures the area of the pons. This artifact can be identified as streak-like black bands generated by the petrosal portions of the temporal bones. Beam hardening is the result of absorption of low-energy x-ray photons by the highly dense bone. Visualization of the middle and inner ear structures requires careful patient positioning, generation of thin slices, wide window settings, and reconstruction of images using bone algorithms.[9]

Abnormal CT Findings

Evaluation of CT images follows criteria similar to those of conventional radiography; both techniques use x-ray absorption in tissues to generate images.

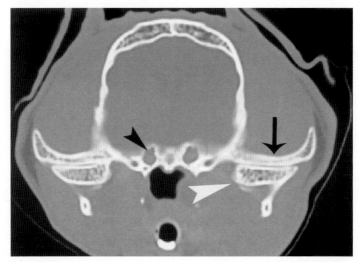

Figure 4-11

Transverse CT image at the level of the temporomandibular junction. A well-positioned patient should show symmetry between the right and left halves of the skull. Both temporomandibular joints show simultaneously in the image. The zygomatic portions of the temporal bone *(arrow)* and condyles of the mandible *(white arrowhead)* are similar in size and shape. The oval foramina *(black arrowhead)* are also symmetric.

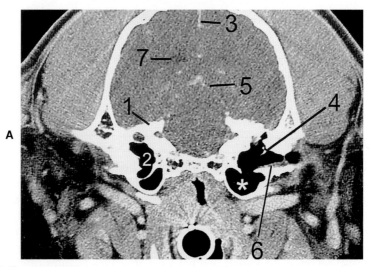

Figure 4-12

A, Post-contrast transverse CT image of a normal cat at the level of the bullae using a soft-tissue window. The septum bulla divides the bulla into a smaller dorsolateral *(2)* and a larger ventromedial *(asterisk)* compartment. The anatomical detail of the petrosal portion of the temporal bone and its contents *(1)* is obscured when compared with image 4-12, *B*. Only a faintly visible malleus *(4)* is seen. However, cerebral landmarks such as the falx cerebri *(3)*, contrast enhanced meninges *(5)*, and portions of the lateral ventricles can be identified. There is a small amount of cerumen overlying the horizontal portion of the external acoustic canal *(6)*.

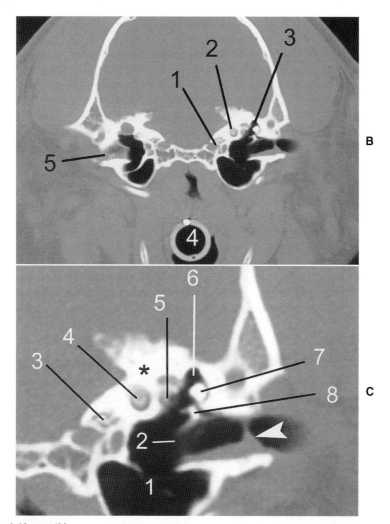

Figure 4-12—cont'd

B, Transverse CT image depicted in 4-12, *A,* with a bone-tissue window. Compare the detail of the middle ear with image 4-12, *A.* The epitympanic recess *(3),* cochlea *(2),* and carotid canal *(1)* are now visualized. By using the proper window, structures such as the external acoustic meatus *(5),* noted here with a small amount of cerumen, become apparent. The endotracheal tube is indicated with the number *4.* **C,** Transverse CT image at the level of the inner ear in the patient depicted in images 4-12, *A* and *B.* There is a small amount of cerumen overlying the horizontal portion of the external acoustic canal *(arrowhead).* The septum bullae *(1)* and tympanic membrane *(2)* are faintly visible as linear areas of increased density. The carotid canal *(3)* is medial and ventral to the cochlea *(4).* The vestibular window *(5)* is medial to the incus *(7)* and malleus *(8),* which are located within the epitympanic recess *(6).* The petrosal portion of the temporal bone *(asterisk)* also contains the vestibular aqueduct and semicircular canals (not pictured).

Diseases such as otitis,[10] neoplasia,[12] nasopharyngeal polyps,[13] and craniomandibular osteopathy can be assessed with CT.

Common findings in otitis include thickening of the external acoustic canal, with or without mineralization (Figure 4-13). Also, enlargement, thickening, and sclerosis of the walls of the bulla (Figure 4-14), as well as sclerosis of the petrosal portion of the temporal bone, can be seen (Figure 4-15). Unlike radiography, CT can differentiate fluid within the bullae from thickening of the walls (Figure 4-16). An exception to the latter arises when the bullae are completely obliterated by soft-tissue density. Use of contrast can help differentiate whether the density is fluid or mass because masses tend to enhance with intravenous injection of contrast material. However, this author has seen inflammatory exudates associated with otitis externa and media that have enhanced after contrast medium administration. An inflamed external acoustic canal can be seen as a contrast-enhancing tubular structure (see Figure 4-13). If the enhancement is limited to the canal, it is possible to be more confident in a diagnosis of otitis than when the enhancement extends out of the canal, such as in cases of neoplasia.

Abnormalities noted in otitis can also be seen associated with neoplasia or osteomyelitis. Therefore, findings should be interpreted in light of the clinical history. However, neoplasia can be placed at the top of the list of differential diagnoses when

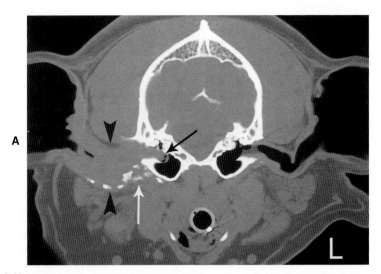

Figure 4-13

A, Transverse view of the bullae of a 5-year-old male Beagle diagnosed with chronic otitis externa imaged with a bone-tissue window. Otoscopic examination of the middle ear was not possible. The diameter of the right external acoustic canal *(arrowheads)* is increased. A soft-tissue density has completely replaced the air in the canal. Scattered foci of dystrophic mineralization are also noted *(white arrow)*. The tympanic bullae are considered normal. However, there is a bulge at the level of the right tympanic membrane *(black arrow)*, which suggests a compromise of its integrity.

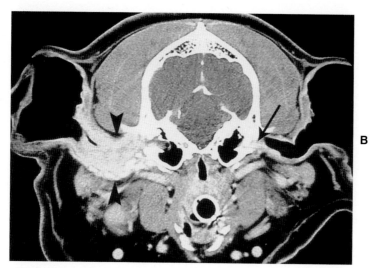

B

Figure 4-13—cont'd

B, Soft tissue window after injection of contrast material of the dog imaged in image 4-13, *A*. The obliteration of the lumen is the result of severe thickening of the walls, which exhibit well-defined contrast enhancement, likely the result of the chronic inflammatory changes *(arrowheads)*. Cerumen or inflammatory exudates are also noted lateral to the left tympanic membrane *(arrow)*.

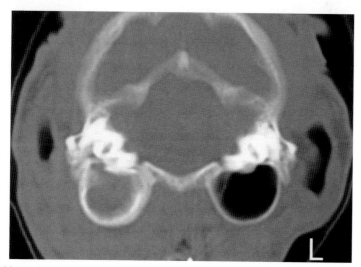

Figure 4-14

CT image of a 6-month-old cat diagnosed with otitis media. There is generalized thickening of the walls of the right bulla. The bulla is filled with dense material, which represents fluid. The affected bulla is mildly enlarged compared with the contralateral one, which is considered normal. The petrosal portions of the temporal bones are symmetrical.

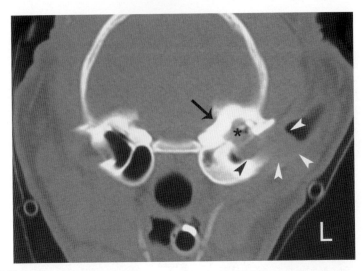

Figure 4-15

CT image at the level of the bullae of an 18-month-old-male cat diagnosed with a polypoid mass. The mass *(arrowheads)* is noted as a homogeneous space-occupying dense structure at the level of the external acoustic meatus and extending into the middle ear. The petrosal portions of the left temporal bone *(arrow)* as well as the bulla wall are thicker and sclerotic when compared with the contralateral normal right. The left septum bulla is no longer present and the epitympanic recess *(asterisk)* is wider, likely the result of pressure bone atrophy caused by the mass.

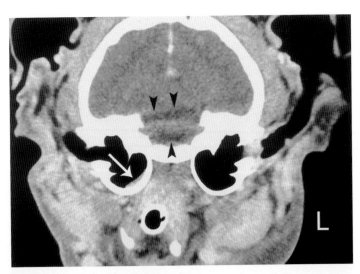

Figure 4-16

CT image at the level of the bullae of a castrated male cat diagnosed with otitis and a fibrosarcoma of the most rostral third of the mandible. There is a minimal volume of dense fluid *(arrow)* on the dependent portion of the right bulla. The corresponding radiographs of the bullae were considered within normal limits. The black streaks *(arrowheads)* are known as *beam hardening*, which is a common CT artifact generated by the petrosal portions of the temporal bones. The artifact hampers full visualization of the pons.

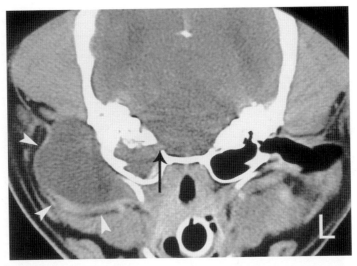

Figure 4-17

Transverse CT image of a 7-year-old Chihuahua. There is a large homogeneously dense mass lateral to the right bulla *(arrowheads)*. Lysis of the medial aspect of the petrosal portion of the temporal bone is also noted *(arrow)*.

there is a space-occupying lesion (Figure 4-17) of variable enhancement character-istics, extension of the lesion into the caudal fossa, and lysis of the tympanic bullae (Figure 14-18).

Magnetic Resonance Imaging (MRI)

The reader is referred elsewhere[11] for an overview of the basic concepts of MRI tech-nology. MRI does not use ionizing radiation (x-rays); therefore, it is considered a noninvasive imaging modality. MRI manipulates the spinning behavior of hydrogen protons within a strong magnetic field to produce an image. Changes in this behav-ior are achieved by sending radio-frequency pulses to the hydrogen protons. The hydrogen protons in turn send radio frequencies back to a receiver antenna. A computer uses the signal from the hydrogen protons to form a gray-scale image. MRI provides cross-sectional imaging of the ear. By eliminating superimposition, the structures medial to the external acoustic canal can be seen clearly. Unlike CT, the area of interest can be imaged in an infinite number of planes without relying on slice reconstruction and without changing the position of the animal in the gantry. The image quality of the CT reconstructions is less desirable (Figure 4-19, *A*) than the equivalent MRI plane. MRI offers better soft-tissue contrast resolution than CT or conventional radiographs.[14] Assessment of the pons is not hampered by the pres-ence of beam-hardening artifacts commonly noted on CT (Figure 4-19, *B*). On the other hand, tissues with minimal hydrogen protons such as bone, air, or areas of

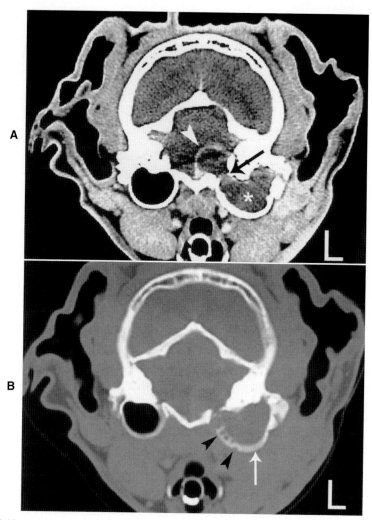

Figure 4-18

A, Transverse CT image of a 10-year-old spayed female cat presented with a unilateral persistent drainage from the ear. There is a space-occupying mass of heterogeneous enhancement *(asterisk)* causing enlargement of the left bulla. There is ringlike enhancement associated with the left half of the pons *(arrowhead)* and lysis of the medial aspect of the petrosal portion of the temporal bone *(arrow)*. The beam-hardening artifact overlying the caudal fossa lesion precludes full assessment of the pons. **B,** CT of the cat depicted in Figure 4-18, *A,* imaged with a bone-tissue window. Permeative lysis *(arrowheads)* of the medial wall of the left bulla as well as thickening of the ventral wall *(arrow)* become apparent. The aggressive process not only extends into the caudal fossa but also medial to the affected bulla. No further diagnostics were performed due to the poor prognosis.

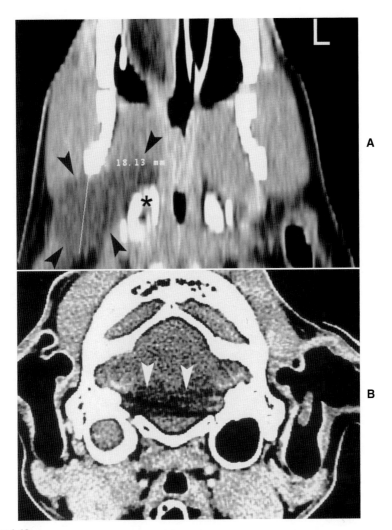

Figure 4-19

A, CT dorsal plane reconstruction of the dog depicted in Figure 4-17. There is a hypodense mass *(arrowheads)* located lateral and rostral to the right bulla *(asterisk).* The mass extends laterally to the right hemimandible. The spatial resolution of this image is poor compared with the MRI image of another dog in Figure 4-23, *A.* **B,** Transverse CT image at the level of the bullae. The beam hardening artifact *(arrowheads),* generated by the dense petrosal portion of the temporal bones, hampers full visualization of the intracranial structures. The right bulla is fluid filled. MRI images offer a better view of the area due to the lack of artifacts as well as to higher soft-tissue contrast resolution.

calcification will have little signal on MRI and are represented as a signal void or black on the resultant image. Therefore the normal petrosal portion of the temporal bone, the bulla wall, and the air within the bulla will appear black on MRI images and cannot be assessed with the same degree of detail as with CT (Figure 4-20). Ferromagnetic foreign material such as gun pellets, hemoclips, and identification

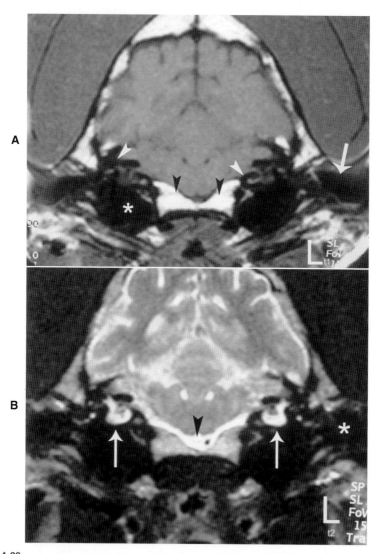

Figure 4-20

A, T1-weighted transverse image of the normal bulla of a dog. There is a large signal void, which represents the air and the walls of the bullae *(asterisk)*. The petrosal portions of the temporal bone are also represented as irregular structures without signal *(white arrowheads)*. Portions of the external acoustic canal *(arrow)* and the basisphenoid bone *(black arrowheads)* are also included. **B,** T2-weighted transverse image of the normal bullae of a dog. The hyperintense signal of the intralabyrinthine fluid associated with the cochlea and semicircular canals is noted *(arrows)*. Low cellular fluid such as the cerebrospinal fluid is hyperintense on this sequence *(arrowhead)*. The *arrows* are overlying the bullae.

chips close to the areas of interest may render the study nondiagnostic due to abrupt changes in the magnetic field, which distort and degrade the image.[14] Finally, MRI is less available and significantly more expensive than CT or conventional radiography. Obviously, a higher degree of expertise and training is required to run an MRI unit than an x-ray room.

Technique and Normal Findings

Patient motion causes severe degradation of the MRI signals; therefore, general anesthesia is required.[14] All equipment brought inside the MRI room should be approved MRI-compliant equipment because metal objects attracted to the strong magnetic field may cause injury to the patient.[15] Generation of a complete MRI study takes longer than the equivalent CT examination because several different sequences are produced to highlight tissues of different characteristics. A typical examination may last between 60 to 90 minutes, depending on the number of sequences and the number of planes generated. Transverse sequences known as *T1-weighted spin-echo, T2-weighted spin-echo, fluid-attenuation inversion recovery (FLAIR),* and *fluid-attenuation spoiled gradient echo (FLASH)* can be performed for the examination of the middle ear. Additionally, T1-weighted sequences after injection of contrast material in transverse, sagittal, and dorsal planes are also generated. The contrast material used is gadopentetate dimeglumine, a paramagnetic agent that appears hyperintense (white) on the T1-weighted sequence. Obtaining 5-mm transverse slices, as commonly performed for the brain, may obscure the fine structures of the membranous labyrinth due to partial volume averaging with surrounding bone.[7] Thin slices of 1 to 2 mm thickness, generated by volume acquisition protocols, have been used to detect the intralabyrinthine fluid.[16]

On T1- and T2-weighted images the air and walls of the bullae and the petrosal portion of the temporal bone are represented as black areas (signal void) and cannot be evaluated[17] (see Figure 4-20, *A*). The intralabyrinthine fluid is isointense tissue (to brain) on the T1-weighted sequence and hyperintense on the T2-weighted sequence (see Figure 4-20, *B*). The signal resembles the lateral silhouette of a duct[18] and represents the fluid (endolymph) associated with the semicircular canals and cochlea. The appearance of the fluid has not been studied with the FLASH and FLAIR protocols. This author has noted a hyperintense (white) signal on the FLASH sequence and speculates that a low-intensity signal exists on the FLAIR protocol.

Abnormal Findings

Hyperintense thickening of the epithelium and a hypointense thick external ear canal have been reported in a dog with chronic otitis externa on both T1- and T2-weighted sequences.[19] The two most commonly reported abnormalities in otitis media are the presence of hyperintense material within the bullae on T2-weighted sequences[17,19] (Figure 4-21, *A*), which is compatible with accumulation of fluid, and enhancement of the inner surface of the bulla, likely due to inflammation, on T1-weighted sequences after injection of contrast material[7] (Figure 4-21, *B*). MRI is the first imaging modality

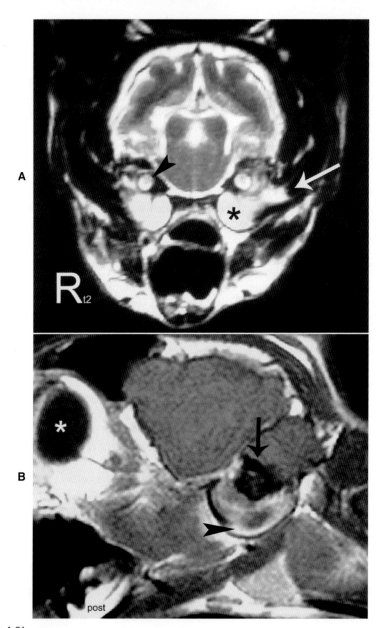

Figure 4-21

A, T2-weighted transverse image of a 13-year-old spayed female cat with a diagnosis of bilateral otitis. There is bilateral hyperintense volume of fluid associated with the tympanic bullae *(asterisk)*. The fluid also fills the horizontal portion of the left external acoustic canal *(arrow)*. The hyperintense signal of the intralabyrinthine fluid *(arrowhead)* is well visualized. **B,** T1-weighted sagittal image of a bulla of the cat depicted in Figure 4-21, *A,* obtained after injection of contrast material. There is a well-defined rim of enhancement *(arrowhead)* associated with the inner surface of the wall of the bulla. The curvilinear thin black signal void representative of the wall of the bulla is better defined because the air in the bulla has been replaced by isointense fluid. The globe *(asterisk)* and the petrosal portion of the temporal bone *(arrow)* are also noted.

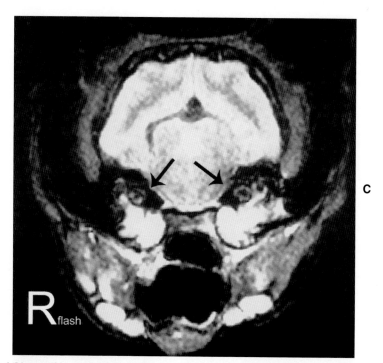

Figure 4-21—cont'd

C, Corresponding FLASH transverse image of the cat depicted in Figure 4-21, *A.* The fluid within the bullae is again noted. This sequence provides finer detail between the petrosal portion of the temporal bone and the intralabyrinthine fluid *(arrows).*

available to veterinarians that has the potential to diagnose otitis interna based on the detection of the intralabyrinthine fluid surrounding the semicircular canals. Preliminary studies suggest that MRI findings in otitis interna include absence of the hyperintense signal on T2-weighted spin-echo images of the intralabyrinthine fluid.[16] The appearance of the intralabyrinthine fluid on additional sequences other than T1- and T2-weighted protocols needs further study before this sign can be used as a predictor of otitis interna in small animals.

MRI excels in depicting changes in the soft tissues surrounding the middle ear as well as in the caudal fossa because no artifacts hampering evaluation of the pons are produced. MRI has proven to be valuable in the diagnosis of dogs with vestibular disorders.[16] By generating multiple sequences with different acquisition parameters, it is possible to further characterize the diseased tissue (Figures 4-22 and 4-23). Low-cellularity fluids, such as cerebrospinal fluid or true cystic lesions, appear hypointense (dark) on FLAIR sequences. Highly cellular or proteinaceous fluids, such as those present in inflammatory exudates in otitis, are hyperintense (white) on T2-weighted and FLAIR sequences. Blood and mineral appear as a signal void (black) on FLASH sequences.

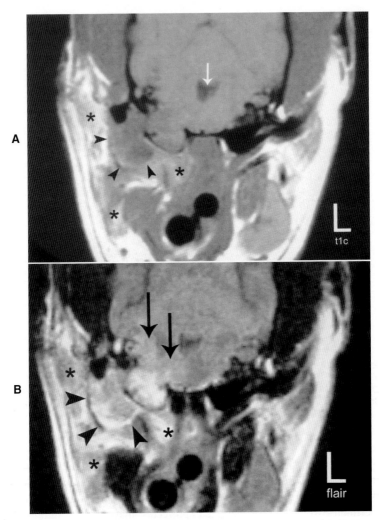

Figure 4-22

A, Transverse T1-weighted spin-echo image obtained after injection of gadolinium of a 7-year-old spayed female Chihuahua depicted in Figure 4-17 after an attempt to perform an ear canal ablation was aborted due to uncontrollable bleeding. The nonenhancing hypointense mass *(arrowheads)* is surrounded by heterogeneous enhancing tissue *(asterisks)* representative of inflamed muscle. The right bulla is completely obliterated by isointense tissue, and most of the petrosal portion of the temporal bone is absent. The mesencephalic aqueduct *(arrow)* is mildly distended. **B,** Corresponding transverse FLAIR image of the dog in Figure 4-22, *A.* There is ill-defined perilesional edema associated with the right half of the pons *(arrows).* The mass *(arrowheads)* is a combination of fluid at the periphery and a more solid content in the center. Extensive inflammatory changes associated with the surrounding musculature *(asterisks)* are also noted.

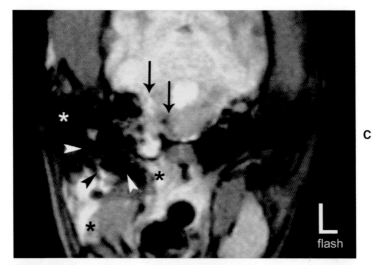

C

Figure 4-22—cont'd

C, Corresponding transverse FLASH image of dog depicted in Figure 4-22, *A.* The mass *(arrowheads)* is mostly blood, as indicated by the large signal void surrounded by a rim of fluid. The mass within the right bulla is also a combination of blood, solid tissue, and inflammatory fluid. The caudal fossa lesions *(arrows)* are representative of hemorrhage and inflammatory fluid. Inflamed surrounding musculature is again detected *(black asterisks),* with a more hemorrhagic component noted dorsolaterally *(white asterisk).*

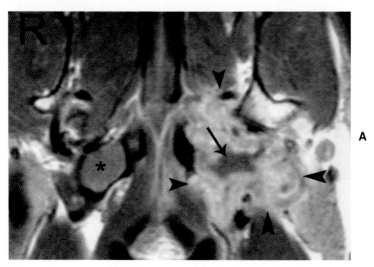

A

Figure 4-23

A, T1-weighted dorsal image at the level of the bullae of a Labrador-Golden Retriever mixed breed after injection of contrast material. There is a large mass of heterogeneous enhancement effacing the left tympanic bulla *(arrowheads)* and extending rostrally medial to the mandibular condyle. Nonenhancing areas within the mass suggest lack of blood supply to the center of the mass *(arrow).* There is a moderate volume of homogeneous fluid in the contralateral bulla *(asterisk).* The spatial and contrast tissue resolution of this image is higher than a similar CT dorsal plane reconstruction depicted in another dog in Figure 4-19, *A.*

Continued

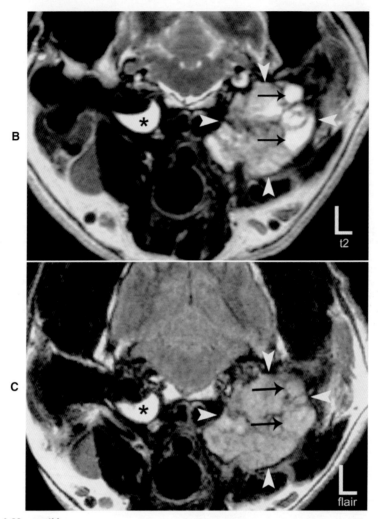

Figure 4-23—cont'd

B, Transverse T2-weighted image of the dog depicted in Figure 4-23, *A.* The increased inten-sity in the right bulla *(asterisk)* is fluid, which is considered the result of otitis media. Within the mass *(arrowheads)* several foci of increased intensity *(arrows)* may also represent fluid or tissue. **C,** Transverse FLAIR image of the dog depicted in Figure 4-23, *A.* The fluid within the bulla *(asterisk)* remains hyperintense, which suggests fluid with a high cellular content. The mass *(arrowheads)* is of more homogeneous intensity than the corresponding T2-weighted image, as the intense foci noted on Figure 4-23, *B,* are now isointense *(arrows).* These foci are likely made out of more solid tissue than originally suspected. No biopsy of the mass was performed.

Conclusion

Conventional radiography remains the most commonly available imaging modality to the general practitioner. Not only it is relatively easy to perform, but it remains the least expensive alternative in practice. However, it is less sensitive than CT and MRI for the diagnosis of middle-ear disease and has little value in the diagnosis of otitis interna. Both CT and MRI are effective in outlining a disease process by eliminating superimposition of surrounding structures as they generate tomographic imaging of the middle ear. CT offers better anatomical detail of the middle ear than MRI because it excels in imaging bone. However, artifacts often obscure the pons, limiting its value for the diagnosis of vestibular disease, compared with MRI. Otitis interna cannot be diagnosed with CT. MRI does not use ionizing radiation and its tissue-contrast resolution is superior to that of CT. It also has the ability to image the animal in infinite planes; it can assess the pons more effectively than CT, and preliminary studies have shown good potential in the diagnosis of otitis interna. However, MRI is the most expensive and least available of the imaging modalities discussed in this chapter. MRI scanning takes longer and cannot image the normal bullae and petrosal portions of the temporal bone with the detail achieved with CT. The practitioner should view CT and MRI as complementary techniques rather than competitive imaging modalities. Finally, imaging of the ear is an evolving field. Ultrasound of fluid-filled bullae in an experimental setting has been reported.[20] However, this author speculates that MRI of the inner ear could become a more active area of research than ultrasonography.

References

1. Eom K, Lee H, Yoon J: Canalographic evaluation of the external ear canal in dogs, *Vet Radiol Ultrasound* 41(3):231-234, 2000.
2. Hofer P, MN, Bartholdi S, Kaserhotz B: A new radiographic view of the feline tympanic bullae, *Vet Radiol Ultrasound* 36(1):14-15, 1995.
3. Ziemer LS, Schwarz T, Sullivan M: Otolithiasis in three dogs, *Vet Radiol Ultrasound* 44(1):28-31, 2003.
4. Farrow CS: Known case conference, *Vet Radiol Ultrasound* 33:262-263, 1992.
5. Little CJ, Pearson GR, Lane JG: Neoplasia involving the middle ear cavity of dogs, *Vet Rec* 124(3):54-57, 1989.
6. Rogers KS: Tumors of the ear canal, *Vet Clin North Am Sm Anim Pract* 18(4):859-868, 1988.
7. Garosi LS, Dennis R, Schwarz T: Review of diagnostic imaging of ear diseases in the dog and cat, *Vet Radiol Ultrasound* 44(2):137-146, 2003.
8. Trower ND, et al: Evaluation of the canine tympanic membrane by positive contrast ear canalography, *Vet Rec* 142(4):78-81, 1998.
9. Russo M, et al: Computed tomographic anatomy of the canine inner and middle ear, *Vet Radiol Ultrasound* 43(1):22-26, 2002.
10. Love NE, et al: Radiographic and computed tomographic evaluation of otitis media in the dog, *Vet Radiol Ultrasound* 36(5):375-379, 1995.
11. Tidwell AS, Jones JC: Advanced imaging concepts: a pictorial glossary of CT and MRI technology, *Clin Tech Sm Anim Pract* 14(2):65-111, 1999.
12. Forrest LJ: The head: excluding the brain and orbit, *Clin Tech Sm Anim Pract* 14(3):170-176, 1999.

13. Seitz S, Losonsky J, Marretta S: Computed tomographic appearance of inflammatory polyps in three cats, *Vet Radiol Ultrasound* 37(2): 99-104, 1996.

14. Kaplan P, et al: Basic principles of musculoskeletal MRI. In *Musculoskeletal MRI,* Philadelphia, 2001, WB Saunders.

15. Chaljub G, et al: Projectile cylinder accidents resulting from the presence of ferromagnetic nitrous oxide or oxygen tanks in the MR suite, *AJR Am J Roentgenology* 177(1):27-30, 2001.

16. Garosi LS, et al: Results of magnetic resonance imaging in dogs with vestibular disorders: 85 cases (1996-1999), *J Am Vet Med Assoc* 218(3):385-391, 2001.

17. Allgoewer I, Lucas S, Schmitz SA: Magnetic resonance imaging of the normal and diseased feline middle ear, *Vet Radiol Ultrasound* 41(5):414-418, 2000.

18. Garosi LS, Lamb CR, Targett MP: MRI findings in a dog with otitis media and suspected otitis interna, *Vet Rec* 146(17):501-502, 2000.

19. Dvir E, Kirberger RM, Terblanche AG: Magnetic resonance imaging of otitis media in a dog, *Vet Radiol Ultrasound* 41(1):46-49, 2000.

20. Griffiths LG, et al: Ultrasonography versus radiography for detection of fluid in the canine tympanic bulla, *Vet Radiol Ultrasound* 44(2):210-213, 2003.

5

Primary Causes of Ear Disease

Louis N. Gotthelf, DVM

B y definition, otitis externa represents a spectrum of inflammatory changes that occur to the external acoustic canal in response to any insult to the ear canal epithelium. But what actually causes ear diseases? Can putting a bacterium or a yeast organism into a normal ear canal result in disease? Although there may be bacteria or yeasts found in the patient with otitis externa, these organisms are not the cause of the ear disease. The real reason for the ear disease is often overlooked. Primary causes of ear disease are those diseases of the skin that also have a direct effect on the skin lining the ear canal. Cutaneous diseases such as atopy, food hypersensitivity, parasites, foreign bodies, hypothyroidism, and seborrheic diseases frequently result in ear disease.

Trauma

Trauma to the ear canal from injury or inappropriate use of instruments in the ear can lead to primary inflammatory changes within the ear. Hair plucking with curved hemostats can result in traumatic inflammation of the ear canal and resultant infection. A more common reason for trauma to the ear canals is the use of cotton-tipped applicators to clean the ear. Cotton-tipped applicators (Q-tips) and applicators with synthetic materials are very irritating to the epithelium when pushed into an ear canal. Their abrasive effect essentially debrides the layer of surface keratinocytes, which is normally very thin. This results in ulceration of the ear canal and exposure of the dermal elements to the resident bacteria and yeasts in the ear, leading to infection. A Q-tip can also push accumulated material ahead of it as it goes deeper into the decreasing diameter of the ear canal. This may result in a hydraulic effect, with significant pressure and subsequent ruptured eardrum. Cotton-tipped applicators can be used to acquire a cytology sample and as an absorbent material. The cotton tip is laid onto liquid in the ear canal; the cotton absorbs the liquid and is then removed. Q-tips should never be used in a "mopping" motion, going in and out of the ear canal.

Atopic Dermatitis

The ear canal is an invagination of epidermis forming a hollow skin tube in the inside of the head that begins at the eardrum. Pathological mechanisms affecting the skin of the animal have the same effect in the epidermal tube lining the ear canal. Since many diseases found in the ear arise as a result of an underlying skin disease, the veterinarian evaluating the patient with otitis externa should also do a careful evaluation of the pet's skin to determine the underlying etiology of the ear disease, if possible. Often, proper diagnosis and appropriate treatment of the underlying skin disease diminish the severity of ear disease. The veterinarian should evaluate every otitis externa case for the primary underlying skin disease that has led to the otitis externa. Sometimes something as simple as *Otodectes* infestation acts as the inciting factor for the patient's ear disease. Sometimes a much more complicated, multiple-allergen atopic skin disease incites the otitis.

It has been estimated that almost 75% of all canine ear disease is related to atopic dermatitis. Atopy seems to be prevalent in many breeds, giving evidence that this disease may have a genetic origin. Most dogs show clinical signs after the first year of life. Atopic patients probably have a high immunoglobulin E (IgE) response from B-lymphocytes when exposed to individual allergens. IgE antibody binds to mast cells resulting in their degranulation and subsequent release of inflammatory mediators on subsequent exposure to that specific antigen. Often there will be a history of foot licking or chewing, face rubbing, and licking the groin area, in addition to scratching the ears. Many dogs with light-colored coats have the telltale red-orange saliva staining typically found with atopy. Cats may manifest their atopic dermatitis with miliary dermatitis, facial pruritus, or barbering of their hair on the belly and lower legs with their teeth in response to the pruritus. Often dental disease will accompany a pruritic skin disease as hairs get trapped between the teeth and in the gingival sulcus, resulting in gingivitis. Atopic dogs also frequently have secondary bacterial and yeast infections on their skin and in their ears.

Allergies can be seasonal or nonseasonal. In a seasonal allergy, the clinical signs are most intense during the period of high pollen counts and disappear with the reduction of the pollen. Atopic dogs and cats are not allergic to only one type of pollen, mold, or insect, so most allergic ears tend to be nonseasonal, with the severity extending for a long period from the spring to the fall, depending on which pollens, molds, or insects the patient is exposed to. In indoor-only dogs or cats with a nonseasonal history, or in a patient that flares up only during the winter, the atopic otitis may be due to indoor allergens such as house dust mites or molds. It is important to ask the owners about the times of the year in which the ear disease flares up. When clients move or relocate to a new geographical area, changes in pet environment may also cause flareups as the patient is exposed to new antigens.

Atopic dermatitis results from an inflammatory overreaction of the skin to antigenic stimulation. The antigens that remain on the surface of the skin maintain the reaction. In dogs, areas like the feet, face, pinnae, and ventrum have increased mast cell density than other parts of the skin. In cats, the mast cells are concentrated behind the ears and over the dorsum. The areas that are constantly contacting environmental allergens are more often involved in the inflammatory process. Unlike dogs, atopic cats tend to have allergies that also affect the respiratory system (bronchitis and asthma) and the eyes (conjunctivitis) as well as the skin.

Frequent bathing or rinsing of atopic patients with water helps to remove antigens physically from the surface of the skin and hair coat. Ear cleaners, flushes, and wet wipes help to remove antigens from the surface of the pinnae and ear canal. Many cats with ceruminous otitis are atopic, so ear cleaners help remove both the antigens and the cerumen from the ears.

Many patients get rapid relief from their ear disease when the atopic dermatitis is treated with corticosteroid therapy, systemically and/or topically. Most combination otic formulations contain corticosteroids to relieve the inflammation and pruritus in the ear. A new therapy for atopic dermatitis using oral cyclosporine-A–modified capsules (Atopica, Novartis) relieves the pruritic clinical signs without the side effects often seen with corticosteroids. Other dogs and cats get long-term benefit from successful immunotherapy to specific antigens identified through allergy testing. It is important to discuss atopic dermatitis as a cause of ear disease with clients so that they understand the value in pursuing a proper diagnosis. After the otic inflammation resulting from atopic dermatitis is controlled, the ear canal epithelium is not as likely to support bacterial or yeast growth, and the patient can remain comfortable.

Food Allergy

Another common primary cause of canine and feline ear disease is food allergy. Termed "cutaneous adverse food reactions," many components of this syndrome have a direct effect in the ear canal. Allergies in animals tend to become additive— that is, the severity of the clinical signs increases as the patient is exposed to more and more allergens, such as pollens, molds, insects, and foods. When the total antigen exposure is in excess to the tolerable antigen load, clinical signs develop. Some allergic animals can be controlled with a reduction in allergens. It is not uncommon to do a food trial with a hypoallergenic diet for 2 or 3 months with resultant reduction in otic signs. See Chapter 6 for a discussion of cutaneous adverse food reactions.

Ear Mites

Ear mites are the most common parasites found in the ear canals of dogs and cats. We are all too familiar with O*todectes* mites causing severe damage to the lining of the ear canal, with the resulting "coffee grounds" exudate composed of wax, blood, and epithelial cells. The ear mite has been identified in a number of animal species, both domestic and wild. A nonburrowing psoroptic mite, the ear mite feeds on epithelial cell lymph and blood. They have chewing mouthparts that can cause damage to the epithelium. In dogs and cats, ear mites can cause a severely pruritic parasitic otitis that is commonly associated with a bacterial infection and otitis media.

A unique result of *Otodectes* infestation in the cat is a systemic hypersensitivity reaction. Known as *otodectic mange,* this skin disease resembles miliary dermatitis, a papular, crusty eruption found around the neck and head, dorsolumbar area, and inguinal area. When an ear mite–infected cat sleeps with its ear in the flank, the ear mites can leave the ear canal and get on the skin. A similar transfer occurs when an infected cat scratches the ear and the mites get on the paw. Those mites in an ectopic location migrate along the skin and feed. This results in a hypersensitivity reaction to the mite antigens absorbed across the damaged epithelium. Experimentally, infected cats showed an immediate hypersensitivity reaction to an intradermal mite extract. Cats infected for 35 days showed an Arthus (Type III) reaction. Serum precipitating antibodies were noted 45 days after infection. When cats with miliary dermatitis do not respond to systemic steroids, such as methylprednisolone acetate (DepoMedrol, Pfizer), or to flea-control measures, otodectic mange should be considered and the cat should be treated for *Otodectes* using a systemic acaricide such as ivermectin, fipronil, or sealmectin.

A cat affected with ear mites shakes its head violently and scratches at the ears. Facial abrasions and hair loss may be evident between the lateral canthus of the eyelid and the ear. When examined, the ear canals display the typical reddish-brown to black, dried, crusty exudates. The brown color is presumed to be from dried wax mixed with blood products. On otoscopic examination, the mites can be seen as white insects crawling on the surface of the exudates.

If the otoscope is held very steady, the mite activity increases, because the light arouses the mites and makes them more active. When viewed with a video otoscope (Video Vetscope, MedRx, Inc., Largo, Florida), which has a high magnification and a bright light source, the mites can often be seen in colonies, with thousands of mites scurrying about (Figure 5-1).

In cases of ear mites in dogs, only a few mites may inhabit the ear canal. They often elude otoscopic or microscopic detection. It has been theorized that either severe inflammation in the ear drives the mites out of the ear or the exudates in the ear canal destroy them. In either case there is a local immune response to mite antigens in the dog's ears that makes the environment hostile to the mites. The severity of the symptoms associated with *Otodectes* may be due to the Arthus-like immediate hypersensitivity reaction provoked by the presence of very few mites.

One useful technique for diagnosing ear mite infection in patients in which *Otodectes* is suspected but no mites are seen otoscopically is a mineral-oil roll smear.

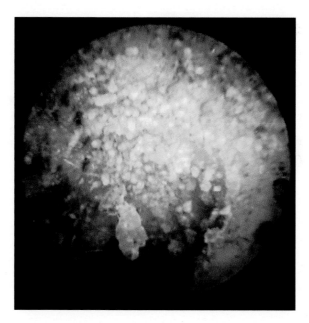

Figure 5-1

Otoscopic view of a cat's ear filled with hundreds of *Otodectes* mites. The dry, flaky ceruminous exudate is forming a crust in the ear canal.

A small cotton-tipped applicator is saturated with mineral oil and is used to swab out the exudates in the ear canal. The cotton tip is then placed into a drop of mineral oil on a microscope slide, and the tip is rolled back and forth to remove most of the harvested material from the cotton tip onto the slide. The slide is then coverslipped and examined under low-power (40× to 100×) magnification. Adult mites individually, or often in duos representing breeding pairs, can easily be seen crawling through the microscopic field. When few mites are present in the ear canal, the typical long oval brown eggs of *Otodectes* may be the only evidence of infection (Figure 5-2).

The ear mites live primarily in the ears, where they feed with their chewing mouthparts on epithelial cells and blood. Female *Otodectes* mites lay solitary eggs in the ear canal, and within 2 or 3 weeks of maturation adult mites begin feeding. Ear mites are very prolific, and in a short time after infection the mite infestation may be severe.

Although ear mites can live in the environment for a short time, direct transmission of *Otodectes* from animal to animal is accepted as the usual mode of transmission. Mites can jump onto any part of the body and then migrate into the ear canal. Many affected 6-week-old kittens have severe ear disease because they acquired *Otodectes* from their queens during the neonatal period. In situations of high animal density, such as shelters, pet shops, and breeding colonies, ear mites can affect the entire population. It is rare for a noninfected, solitary, indoor cat to acquire ear mites.

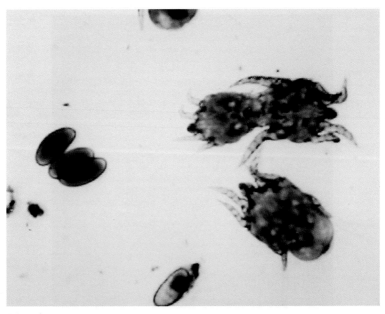

Figure 5-2

Otodectes mites in a mineral-oil swab of otic exudates. The presence of typical dark brown oval eggs of *Otodectes* may be the only indicator of infection in the absence of adult mites.

The aggressive feeding habits of *Otodectes* cause damage to the epithelium of the ear canal and the tympanic membrane. Ceruminous gland secretion is increased and contributes to the quantity of the exudates. Secondary bacterial infection may result from the loss of the protective epithelial barrier in the ear canal; a contributing factor is the high serum-protein substrates that are made available to the bacteria as a result. Damage to the germinal epithelium on the surface of the eardrum from ear mites prevents these cells from sliding across the eardrum as a cleansing mechanism. This results in the accumulation of waxy material on the eardrum, producing a wax plug. Ear mites at the eardrum can actually chew their way through the thin tympanic membrane and invade the middle ear, resulting in otitis media. Whether ear mites that reach the middle ear can be involved in the formation of nasopharyngeal polyps has yet to be determined.

Treatment of *Otodectes* has traditionally involved the use of ear drops containing a variety of insecticides in a number of different vehicles. Thorough cleaning of the ear canal, preferably with the patient sedated prior to the use of any topical medication, hastens the therapeutic effects of the topical medication. All ear mite medications contain insecticides, which are placed in the ear to kill the mites. Some preparations contain additional ingredients such as (1) ceruminolytics to help loosen the inspissated ceruminous material, (2) antibiotics to treat secondary bacterial infection, and (3) mineral oil, which is used as a vehicle to float the debris to the pinnal surface so it can be removed. Mineral oil may also have the beneficial effect of blocking the breathing tubes of the mites and suffocating them. Drops for ear mite infections need to be used for at least 14 days so that the mites hatching in the canal are killed before the life cycle starts over. Retreatment at monthly intervals has been recommended for free-roaming cats with chronic mite infestations.

Because the anthelmintic ivermectin has been demonstrated to be a good acaricide as well, it has been used for treatment of ear mites in dogs and cats. Ivermectin is only approved for use in dogs as a heartworm preventative. Injectable ivermectin (Ivomec 1% injection, Merial, Ltd.) is used at a dose of 250 µg/kg or 0.1 ml/10 lb of body weight. It is injected subcutaneously every 10 days to 2 weeks for two or three injections. Because it is well established that ear mites can live on the skin, these injections treat the entire body. All contact animals in the environment should be treated concurrently. Ivermectin can also be placed in each ear canal as a topical treatment for ear mites, but this preparation contains propylene glycol, which can be irritating to the ear canal.

Some severe neurological reactions and even deaths have been reported in cats treated with injections of ivermectin. Kittens under 12 weeks old treated with injectable doses that exceed 250 µg/kg may be more susceptible to the fatal reactions than adult cats. The reason for this may be linked to the age at which the blood-brain barrier develops in kittens. It is hypothesized that without an adequately mature blood-brain barrier, ivermectin can gain access to the brain in affected kittens and interact with gamma-aminobutyric acid (GABA) receptors in the brain, causing neurological signs to develop. Because of this, a topical aqueous ivermectin 0.01% solution (Acarexx, Idexx) has been developed for use in the ears of kittens 4 weeks of age and older. Another topical aqueous ear mite formulation safe for young kittens is a 0.1% milbemycin oxime solution (Milbemite, Novartis). These aqueous topical ear mite preparations are packaged in individual foil packs containing 0.5 ml of solution in two premeasured plastic applicator ampules.

Fipronil (Frontline TopSpot, Merial, Ltd.) and selamectin (Revolution, Pfizer) are monthly flea-control topical preparations that have demonstrated miticidal activity in both dogs and cats. In areas with high flea infestation rates, the use of either of these flea-control products may also aid in treatment of *Otodectes*. Free-roaming pets with these insecticides on their skin may acquire new *Otodectes* mites on their skin, but the mites will be killed by the residual insecticide prior to reproducing. This may act as a preventative against ear mites.

Treatment for otitis externa secondary to *Otodectes* infection must not be overlooked. Antibiotic and antibiotic-steroid ear drops are used until the epithelial surface heals and the infection subsides. If otitis media is present, the ear canal and the tympanic bulla should be flushed and suctioned carefully to remove any debris that may have gained access to the tympanic bulla.

Ticks

Ticks, with their deeply piercing, blood-sucking mouthparts, attach themselves in the ear canal and result in local inflammation and pain at the attachment site (Figure 5-3). Dogs with ticks on the body should be examined to see whether there are ticks in the ear canals.

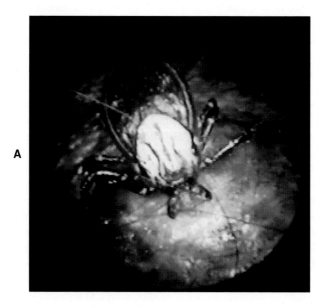

Figure 5-3

Ticks in the ear canal. **A,** *Rhipicephalus* tick attached to the epithelium.

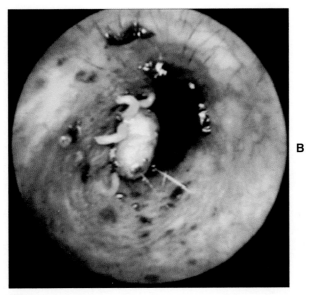

B

Figure 5-3—cont'd

B, *Otobius* tick in the ear canal. (Courtesy Dr. Richard Burrows, Kingman Animal Hospital, Kingman, Arizona.)

Demodectic Mange

Due to the high density of sebaceous glands in many breeds, *Demodex* mites can be found within the ear canal in ceruminous otitis cases, leading to both inflammation and secondary infection. The mites may be found using the mineral oil sampling technique described previously (Figure 5-4). Both *Demodex folliculorum* and *Demodex cati* have been reported as inhabitants of the ear canals. Amitraz in mineral oil has been advocated for topical treatment of *Demodex* mites in the ears.

Other Insects

Sarcoptes mites can be found anywhere along the ear canal from the pinna to the horizontal canal, resulting in severe pruritus.

Chiggers *(Trombicula)* are also found in the ears of dogs in some geographical areas.

Fleas are not generally thought of as a primary cause of ear disease, but the presence of fleas and the cutaneous sensation that they stimulate can cause a dog or cat to scratch the ears raw (Figure 5-5). Other types of insects can find the ear canal and can become lodged there, resulting in irritation or even a blockage of the ear canal.

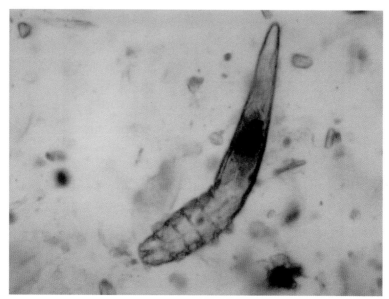

Figure 5-4

Demodex folliculorum in mineral oil.

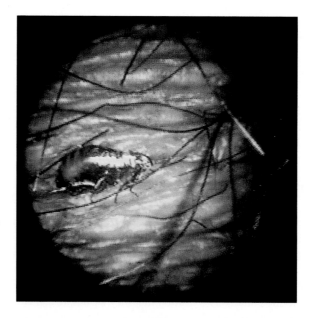

Figure 5-5

Dog and cat fleas can cause severely pruritic ears, although the fleas are rarely found in the ear canal.

Foreign Material

Patients presented with ear disease may have acquired foreign material in their ears that contributes to otitis. Foreign materials that get into the ear canal can cause local irritation and may be a primary cause of ear disease. Plant material that makes its way into the ear canal can migrate along the ear canal and even penetrate the eardrum, leading to otitis media. Small woody stems, plant awns, foxtails, and seed packets have been found in the ear canals and middle ears of dogs and cats (Figure 5-6). Plant material is often conical in shape, and the bases are smooth and round, so entrance into the ear canal is fairly easy. However, the other side of a plant awn or foxtail has a sharp, radiating crown of spikes; movement of the plant material out of the ear is prevented because the diameter of the clump of radiating spikes tends to increase with the outward directional movement. The plant awns migrate one way—deep into the ear canal—and gain access to the middle ear through a ruptured eardrum. Significant otitis media results. The ear canal may fill with a copious amount of mucus and pus, and the plant awns or foxtails are difficult to visualize through the material.

Good cleaning of the ear canals aids in uncovering and identifying the presence of plant material in the ear canal. A video otoscope helps facilitate the removal of plant awns and foxtails. Such an instrument allows clear visualization and good light for identification. The grasping type of endoscopic forceps can be inserted through the working channel of the instrument so that the plant awn or the foxtail

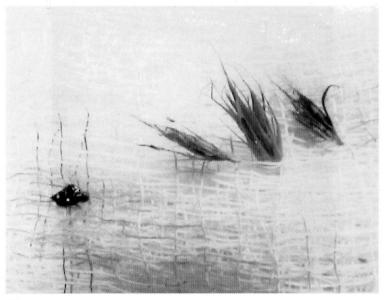

Figure 5-6

Plant awns (seed packets) retrieved from the middle ear of a Cocker Spaniel with otitis media.

can be removed. Gentle traction on the plant material collapses the radial spikes and allows its easy removal from the bulla or the ear canal.

Outdoor dogs that rub their ears into the ground may pick up sand and dirt that can fill the canal. Many medications applied into the horizontal canal can dry out, resulting in impaction. Thick ointment or cream otic formulations containing oils and particulate matter in drying agents (silicon dioxide) seem to result in more impactions when applied into the horizontal canal than do aqueous medications (Figure 5-7). These hardened concretions of medication remain in contact with the ear canal epithelium. When they are identified, these concretions can be gently flushed out of the ear canal using warmed water or warmed saline under pressure. They may also be curetted from the ear canal epithelium or removed with the use of a grasping-type endoscopic forceps to seize and remove the concretion.

Ectopic Hairs

Some dogs have very thick, ectopic bristly hairs emanating from a ring surrounding the eardrum. These bristles dig into the horizontal canal or move along the skin within the horizontal canal, resulting in cutaneous sensation and therefore itchiness to the ear. Plucking these hairs seems to relieve the itch and generally results in cure, as the hairs do not usually grow back. Often wax plugs develop surrounding these

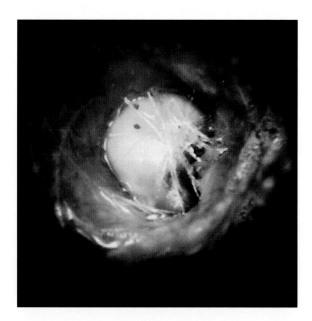

Figure 5-7

Dried medication causing a concretion to form in the horizontal canal. Oily and thick medications contribute to concretions more often than aqueous medications.

hairs resulting in large concretions, many of which harbor large numbers of *Malassezia* organisms.

Pets with itchy ears may not have ear disease seen on otoscopic examination at all but may be responding to a localized pruritus associated with an underlying pruritic disease. Mast cells degranulate in the external ear canal, as does the skin of the rest of the body, releasing vasoactive substances that exacerbate inflammation and pruritus. In addition, referred sensations from the throat may cause itchiness in the ear canals.

Otitis externa is not always complicated by an infectious organism. Many dogs and cats with itchy ears have only otic inflammation, which will respond to a topical corticosteroid alone, so in these cases the use of antibiotics and antifungals may not be appropriate. Bacterial and yeast infections within the ear canal occur secondarily to the primary skin disease and are considered to be perpetuating causes of ear disease (see Chapter 8). When infections are present, the internal environment of the ear canal becomes hospitable to these organisms. For example, the hyperemia associated with atopy increases the watery, lipid secretions from the ceruminous glands. The increased humidity allows attachment of yeasts to the macerated keratinocytes. They can actively reproduce and metabolize the fats within the ear, leading to an otitis externa complicated by yeasts.

Treatment of infections within the ear canals may give the patient temporary relief of its disease. However, without addressing the underlying mechanism responsible for the infection, the disease will return shortly after the antimicrobial treatment is stopped.

Other Causes

Other dermatological conditions can affect the skin lining the ear canal, making it susceptible to otitis externa. Examples of less common skin diseases that may also affect the ear canal include juvenile cellulitis; endocrine disorders, such as sex hormone imbalances; Cushing's disease; hypothyroidism; autoimmune diseases such as pemphigus and systemic lupus erythematosus; keratinization disorders, such as idiopathic seborrhea and sebaceous adenitis; and erythema multiforme, a systemic drug reaction.

Hypothyroidism

Hypothyroidism may be a common primary cause of otitis externa in breeds that are more prone to this disease.

Hypothyroidism is perhaps the most common endocrine imbalance found in dogs. It is responsible for many changes in the skin and ear canal that allow colonization by secondary invaders such as bacteria and yeasts. Lymphocytic thyroiditis is the most common type of thyroid deficiency in dogs. It has been proven to be a heritable disease in some dog breeds; many breeds are predisposed to hypothyroidism, suggesting a genetic predisposition. It seems to be a progressive disease that starts at a young age and progresses to destruction and fibrosis of the thyroid parenchyma. When thyroid hormone production is significantly impaired by fibrosis, the clinical signs of hypothyroidism begin to appear. As the disease progresses, destruction of the thyroid gland proceeds until the thyroid tissue is replaced by fibrosis.

Thyroglobulin autoantibody assays may be useful in determining which patients may be at risk for developing hypothyroidism due to lymphocytic thyroiditis. Even before the serum thyroxine levels fall, and prior to the onset of clinical disease, the destruction of the thyroid follicles results in increased levels of serum thyroglobulin autoantibodies.

Discussions concerning thyroid hormone assays and interpretation of thyroid test results can be found in numerous internal medicine and endocrinology references. The current standard of thyroxine measurement in the dog is the free or unbound thyroxine (T4) by equilibrium dialysis (fT4) or total thyroxine (tT4). An increased thyroid-stimulating hormone (TSH) level coupled with a low or borderline T4 level is often used to separate thyroidal from nonthyroidal illness.

Clinically, hypothyroidism is often misdiagnosed based solely on laboratory results because of the influence of nonthyroidal factors on the amount of thyroid hormone available to the test reagents. Many dogs with low serum thyroxine levels are not truly hypothyroid. Dogs that are being treated with corticosteroids or sulfa drugs may have a low total T4 level and yet may be euthyroid, as confirmed by a normal TSH level. When a dog is truly hypothyroid, the T4 level is low and the TSH value is elevated. Response to thyroid supplementation in true hypothyroid dogs is dramatic.

Certain breeds seem to be predisposed to hypothyroidism and also seem to pose the greatest challenge to the veterinarian dealing with their otitis externa. The Shar-Pei, Poodle, Cocker Spaniel, Golden Retriever, Chow Chow, and German Shepherd seem to be hypothyroid-prone breeds in which otitis externa is frequently a feature of their hypothyroid condition.

Hypothyroidism results in seborrheic dermatitis as well as seborrheic otitis. In the ear, the lower level of thyroid hormone alters the fatty acid composition of the lipids in the cerumen. When a dog is hypothyroid, the sebaceous glands may become overactivated, resulting in ceruminous otitis. On cytologic examination, there is a predominance of cornified epithelial cells, along with the presence of nonstaining sebaceous cellular debris. Yeasts and cocci bacteria are often found in the ears of hypothyroid dogs.

The bacterial degradation of the increased lipids found in seborrheic plaques results in more free fatty acids on the skin. *Malassezia* can utilize the free fatty acids as metabolic substrates. *Malassezia* can induce profound erythema and pruritus through the chemoattractant cytokines produced as well as their metabolic by-products, resulting in localized inflammation. Often the first presenting sign in a hypothyroid dog is the presence of a severely pruritic otitis externa, complicated with *Malassezia.*

Low circulating thyroid hormone levels are also associated with decreased activity of the B-lymphocytes responsible for humoral immunity. This diminishes the ability of the skin to respond to cutaneous bacteria. The effect of the bacterial colonization in concert with the altered lipid layer is that staphylococci normally held in check by the immune mechanisms have the ability to reproduce unchecked, causing staphylococcal pyoderma. Bacterial otitis externa with staphylococci is fairly common in hypothyroid dogs.

Proper diagnosis and treatment of hypothyroidism essentially removes this primary cause of otitis externa. Treatment for secondary bacterial and yeast infections reduces the perpetuating inflammatory reaction.

Thyroid testing should be done in dogs with otitis externa that have not responded to treatment for other primary causes of otitis, especially in the breeds prone to hypothyroidism. If this disease is diagnosed, future exacerbations of otitis externa can be prevented.

Without attention to the primary causes of ear disease, the veterinarian treating ear diseases in dogs and cats will find them very frustrating diseases to deal with. Successful management of ear cases depends on finding and correcting the primary causes of ear disease. When a case of otitis is presented for examination, the veterinarian should, rather than getting the otoscope, step away from the patient and look at the entire skin and take a good dermatological history from the owner before proceeding.

Suggested Readings

Boothe HW: Surgery of the tympanic bulla (otitis media and nasopharyngeal polyps), *Probl Vet Med* 3:254-269, 1991.

Fingland RB, Gratzek A, Vorhies MW, et al: Nasopharyngeal polyp in a dog, *J Am Anim Hosp Assoc* 29:311-314, 1993.

6

Adverse Food Reactions (AFR)

Paul Bloom, DVM, DACVD, DAB VP
(Canine and Feline Specialty)

Background

An adverse food reaction, specifically food allergy, is a phenomenon that has been studied in depth in humans. Unfortunately, very little scientific data have been collected for this disease in dogs and cats. Studies that have been performed in animals have not proven an immunologic mechanism. In addition, these studies were not consistent in their choice of an elimination diet (home prepared versus commercially prepared), the length of the trial, and whether rechallenging with the original diet was performed at the end, making interpretation of results and comparisons difficult.[1] Since it is possible that canine and feline food allergy is analogous to the human disease, it is important to review what is known about the pathophysiology in humans.

Immunopathogenesis in Humans

In humans, adverse food reactions may be either nonimmunologic or immune-mediated.[2,3] Nonimmunologically mediated reactions consist of toxic reactions and food intolerance. Toxic reactions typically are dose related and may affect many individuals without previous exposure or sensitization. An example of a toxic reaction is food poisoning. Food intolerance is mediated by a variety of nonimmunologic mechanisms, including metabolic, pharmacologic, and idiosyncratic mechanisms.[3] This reaction, like toxic reactions, does not require previous exposure and is typically dose related. In contrast to toxic reactions, food intolerance affects only a small population of individuals in a group. Examples of food intolerance include humans with lactase deficiency (metabolic mechanism), histidine conversion to histamine in poorly preserved fish, or reactions to foods that contain caffeine (pharmacologic mechanisms).[3]

There are four types of immunologically mediated adverse food reactions described in humans.[3,4] They are Type I hypersensitivity (including both immediate and late-phase reactions), Type III hypersensitivity (immune complex), Type IV hypersensitivity (delayed or cell-mediated immunity), and lastly a combination of both Type I and Type IV hypersensitivities (mixed reaction).[3-5]

Before hypersensitivity reactions are described, there are a few concepts that need to be understood. Lymphocytes are small round cells found in blood, lymph, lymphoid organs, and tissues. They are responsible for recognizing foreign antigens and mounting immune responses, both antibody mediated and cell mediated.[6] Lymphocytes are a heterogeneous group of cells that may be defined by their cell surface proteins. These proteins include cell surface receptors (e.g., CD4, CD8) and adhesion molecules (integrins, selectins or immunoglobulin superfamily). CDs (clusters of differentiation) are cell-surface molecules that have been detected with monoclonal antibodies. Adhesion molecules are cell-surface structures that mediate cell-to-cell or cell-to-matrix binding and interaction. These molecules help regulate cell-to-cell signaling and are also responsible for the movement of lymphocytes in tissues. Lymphocytes may also be differentiated by the types of cytokines they produce when activated (e.g., IL-2, IL-4). Cytokines are proteins or glycoproteins secreted from cells that function in cell-to-cell communication. They regulate the immune response by cells by controlling cellular interactions, cell growth, secretion, and function. Lymphocytes may also be segregated based on their organ of origin. Those that originate in the thymus are called *T-cells,* whereas those that originate in the bone marrow (bursa of Fabricius in birds) are known as *B-cells.*[6]

Major histocompatibility complex (MHC) molecules are specialized cell-surface glycoprotein receptors that are involved in antigen presentation to T-cells. MHC I receptors are present on most nucleated cells, while MHC II receptors are constitutively present only on professional antigen-presenting cells (macrophages, B-cells, dendritic cells). The presentation of antigen to T-cells must be in the context of antigen-MHC II in order to activate the T-cell.[6]

Type I hypersensitivity is biphasic, with an immediate reaction that is followed by a late-phase reaction. The immediate hypersensitivity Type I reaction is immunoglobulin E (IgE) mediated and requires prior exposure (sensitization phase). When a susceptible individual is exposed a second time to a complete antigen (elicitation phase), this antigen cross-links two IgE molecules that are bound to mast cells. This causes release of preformed molecules (histamine, serotonin, tryptase, chymases, carboxypeptidases, kallikreins, proteoglycans [chondroitin sulfate], eosinophilic chemotactic factor of anaphylaxis [ECF-A], neutrophilic chemotactic factor of anaphylaxis [NCF-A], and heparin) within seconds from the mast cell granules.[4] These preformed mediators, having vasoactive properties, are responsible for the wheal and flare associated with degranulation of mast cells. There are lipid metabolites (LTB4, LTC4, PAF, PGD_2), which are synthesized and secreted in minutes. Lastly, there are cytokines (IL2, IL6, IL13, TNFα), which are synthesized and secreted, but this occurs hours after the initial mast cell degranulation. These cytokines are responsible for the late-phase reactions. Symptoms associated with these inflammatory mediators include pruritus, urticaria, and anaphylaxis.[4,6,7]

Late-phase reaction is the second part of the biphasic Type I hypersensitivity reaction, and it is also dependent on mast cell degranulation. However, in contrast to the immediate reaction that occurs within minutes and resolves within an hour, this reaction occurs 2 to 8 hours after mast cell degranulation. The cytokines that are released from mast cells activate and attract neutrophils and eosinophils to the skin about 6 hours after exposure. Eight to 24 hours after cytokine release, the influx of inflammatory cells changes to primarily mononuclear cells. These are primarily CD4+ T-cells, specifically Th2 αβ cells and CD1+ dermal dendritic cells.[4,6,7]

Type III hypersensitivity (immune complex deposition, serum sickness) involves deposition of circulating antigen-antibody complexes. Soluble antigen needs to be in circulation for prolonged periods (typically more than 6 days) so that when the antibody is produced there is circulating antigen to bind. The immune complex typically involves immunoglobulin G (IgG) or immunoglobulin M (IgM), which are able to fix complement. The immune complexes are then deposited in tissues (blood vessels, kidneys, joints), and there is activation of complement, which attracts neutrophils. Neutrophils cause tissue damage by releasing proteases and reactive oxygen metabolites. Clinical signs may include arthralgias, fever, edema, and maculopapular or urticarial lesions.[4,6,7]

Type IV (delayed) hypersensitivity reaction is the only one of the hypersensitivities that does not involve antibody formation. Instead, it involves primarily macrophages and T-cells. An antigen (frequently an incomplete antigen known as a *hapten*) combines with a host molecule (frequently a protein) and forms a complete antigen. This antigen is phagocytized by antigen-presenting cells. The antigen-presenting cells process the antigen and then present the antigen on their surfaces via MHC II molecules. These antigen-bearing, antigen-presenting cells are poor stimulators of unprimed T-cells. These cells leave the gastrointestinal (GI) tract and migrate to the regional lymph node. During this journey they undergo profound phenotypic changes, thereby acquiring the ability to evoke a strong antigen-specific response in resting T-cells in the lymph node. Upon subsequent exposure (elicitation phase), the antigen-presenting cell will again phagocytize the antigen, process it, and present it on its cell surface complexed with a MHC II molecule. The antigen-presenting cell then presents this antigen–MHC II molecule to an antigen-specific, primed T-cell. This complex is very effective in activating primed T-cells. T-cells that have cutaneous lymphocyte antigen (CLA—a glycoprotein receptor on T-cells that is responsible for the migration of the T-cell through the skin) on their surfaces are then attracted to and migrate through the skin. These activated T-cells (CD4$^+$ Th1-cells) release cytokines that damage the tissues (IFNγ and TNFα) and also help activate cytotoxic T-cells (CD8$^+$) by up-regulating MHC I molecule expression on cells (IFNγ). Whether the first phase of a Type IV hypersensitization reaction (sensitization phase) occurs in the intestinal mucosa or to an absorbed antigen is unknown. Cutaneous signs include erythema, exudation, erosion, and ulceration.[4,6,7]

As in the skin, the GI tract has many defense mechanisms to prevent absorption of potential antigens.[3,4,7] These include the following:

- Intestinal mucosal barrier
- Seal formed by epithelial cells
- Digestion and breakdown of antigens by gastric acid and gastric, intestinal, and pancreatic enzymes
- Intestinal peristalsis
- Rapid cell turnover
- Surface (secretory) immunoglobulin A (IgA) binding of antigens

Many antigens that penetrate the GI tract elicit oral tolerance.[3,4] Tolerance is the immunologic unresponsiveness of an individual to an antigen.[6] Oral tolerance may involve active cellular suppression via T suppressor cells or suppressor cytokines (IL10, TGFβ). Tolerance may also occur via clonal anergy. Clonal anergy is the prolonged, antigen-specific suppression of a clone of T-cells. In order for an antigen-presenting cell to activate a T-cell, the T-cell must receive multiple signals. One signal is the binding of the antigen-presenting cell via its MHC II–antigen complex. Second signals are provided by the binding of CD80 or CD86 on the antigen-presenting cell to CD28 on the T-cell. If an antigen-presenting cell only binds its MHC II–antigen complex to the T-cell receptor without supplying a second signal, or if an antigen alone binds to the T-cell receptor without its MHC II molecule, anergy occurs. When low doses of antigen are present, active cellular suppression occurs. High doses of antigen exposure will provoke clonal anergy.[4,6]

Development of a food allergy occurs when there is a defect in the barrier function or digestive ability of the GI tract and subsequent absorption of foreign antigens. Complete digestion of food protein results in the production of free amino acids and small peptides, which are probably poor antigens. Thus an incompletely digested food protein has a greater potential to incite an allergic response. In the susceptible individual, one with a defective immune system, sensitization to these antigens then occurs. Most of these antigens that cause food allergy are water-soluble glycoproteins that are heat, acid, and protease stable. Multiple factors determine whether a substance is able to elicit an immune response. These include the following:

- *Molecular characteristics.* For a molecule to be immunologic, it must have a large molecular weight, usually greater than 5000 daltons. In humans, these antigens are usually between 10,000 to 60,000 daltons. A dalton is one-twelfth the mass of a carbon 12 atom, or ~1.66×10^{-24} of a gram.[3,4,8]
- *Immunogenetic ability.* The immune responses to a large variety of antigens are genetically controlled.

Food allergy in humans most commonly occurs in infancy and early childhood.[3] Factors in humans in this age group that may contribute to food allergy include the following:

- Lower gastric pH
- Lower proteolytic enzyme activity
- Immature intestinal barrier function
- Immaturity of the intestinal immune system (low levels of immunoglobulin A [IgA] production)

In humans, food allergy occurs in 33% to 38.7% of infants and young children with atopic dermatitis.[1,3] Food allergy, especially in children, is associated with a Type I (IgE-mediated) hypersensitivity reaction.[1,3,7,9] Not surprisingly, this reaction is characterized by an acute onset of symptoms (urticaria, angioedema, and anaphylaxis). There is also a subset of patients with a Type IV (cell-mediated) reaction that is characterized by subacute or chronic symptoms (eczema).[3]

Since the occurrence of food allergy—that is, an immunologically based reaction to food—has not been well documented in dogs and cats, *cutaneous adverse food reaction* is a more accurate term.[1] Even though there have been a few reports of naturally occurring IgE-mediated food allergy in dogs,[10,11] the immunologic pathogenesis of food allergy in dogs and cats has not been well established. Whether dogs and cats have the same immunologic basis for cutaneous adverse food reaction as occurs with food allergy in humans awaits determination.

Signalment and History

Whether the disease is called *cutaneous adverse food reaction* or a *food allergy* in dogs and cats, many things are known about this disease. The following discussion addresses the facts that are known concerning cutaneous adverse food reactions.

In dogs, there is no age, sex, or breed predilection.[4] The age of onset in dogs varies from as young as 4 months to as old as 12.5 years.[9] However, neonatal puppies exhibiting otitis externa due to a cutaneous adverse food reaction may be "cured" before seeing a specialist for their skin disease. The index of suspicion for cutaneous adverse food reactions exceeds environmental allergen–induced atopic dermatitis (atopy) when the onset of clinical signs occurs in geriatric dogs.

In cats, the Siamese may be predisposed, but any breed can be affected.[4,5] The age of onset ranges from 3 months to 11 years (mean 4 to 5 years).

Historical information that would be consistent with cutaneous adverse food reaction would include nonseasonal pruritus, recurrent or unresolved otitis externa, bacterial pyoderma, and *Malassezia* dermatitis. Responsiveness of pruritus to antiin-flammatory doses (¼ mg/pound q 12 hours orally) of prednisone or prednisolone varies from complete to poor. Therefore if a pruritic dog is poorly responsive to gluco-corticoids, diseases such as uncomplicated environmental allergen–induced atopic dermatitis (atopy) are very unlikely, while cutaneous adverse food reaction would still be likely. If a pruritic dog responds well to glucocorticoids, both environmental allergen–induced atopic dermatitis (atopy) and cutaneous adverse food reaction would be ruled out. The only consistent sign of cutaneous adverse food reaction is pruritus. The distribution of the pruritus is not much different than that of dogs with environmental allergen–induced atopic dermatitis (atopy) (face, feet, flexor surfaces of the limbs and folds) or with flea allergy dermatitis (rump and tail head). However some dogs have a propensity for otic and perineal pruritus. As with environmental allergen–induced atopic dermatitis (atopy), dogs with cutaneous adverse food reac-tion may only have otic disease. In one study, 20% of dogs with cutaneous adverse food reaction had only otitis externa as the presenting clinical sign.[12] Of these dogs, there were a number who had only unilateral disease.[13] Otitis externa as the only presenting sign is more common in dogs with cutaneous adverse food reaction than in environmental allergen–induced atopic dermatitis (atopy).[14] Dogs and cats with otitis externa may show very little, if any, clinical signs, in which case the diagnosis is established only by otoscopic examination. This occurs most commonly, in the author's experience, in dogs or cats having previous episodes of otitis externa. It appears that some animals become somewhat tolerant of otitis externa if they have experienced it previously. More commonly, dogs and cats show (any or all of) the following clinical signs:

- Odor or discharge from the ear(s)
- Scratching the ear(s)
- Shaking the head
- Otic pain or tenderness (this may be most apparent when the owner pets or manipulates the animal's head and ears).

In contrast to IgE-mediated food allergy in humans, systemic anaphylaxis from cutaneous food reaction has not been reported in cats or dogs.

Physical Findings

Physical examination findings in dogs may vary from normal (alesional) to the pres-ence of primary and secondary lesions, including papules, pustules, plaques, wheals, angioedema, erythema, ulcers, excoriations, urticaria (associated with eosinophilic vasculitis), lichenification, hyperpigmentation, posttraumatic alopecia, scale, crusts, and erosions. Otic findings may include discharge ranging from mild to copious; it may be black, tan, yellow, or cream colored. There may be hyperplasia of the ceruminous glands resulting in a "cobblestone" appearance of the vertical and/or horizontal ear canal. The external ear canals may also have erosions, ulcerations, hemorrhage or sanguineous discharge; fibrosis or calcification of the cartilage of the external ear canals; or proliferation of the epithelium of the vertical or horizontal canals, manifested as otic "masses." If there is involvement of the middle ear, the tympanum may be absent (ruptured), bulging, or necrotic in appearance. However, it has been reported that dogs may also have concurrent otitis media even in the presence of an intact and normal-appearing tympanic membrane.[3a] Pinnal marginal vasculopathy has also been associated with cutaneous adverse food reaction. As previously mentioned, the distribution of lesions may be focal or generalized, but the ears and rump are commonly affected. Due to the disruption of the normal barrier function of the epithelium that occurs with cutaneous adverse food reactions, secondary bacterial pyoderma, *Malassezia* dermatitis, bacterial or *Malassezia* otitis externa, and seborrheic skin disease are common.[4,7]

Cats, like dogs, vary in their physical examination findings. They too may be normal (alesional); more commonly, they have excoriations, papulocrusts, alopecia, crusts, erosions, ulcers, or exfoliative erythroderma. Miliary dermatitis, eosinophilic plaques, eosinophilic granulomas, and indolent ulcers have all been associated with cutaneous food reactions. Pruritus typically affects the face and neck (especially the pinnae and pre-aural region) but can affect any location.[4,5,7] Cats may have the same otic signs as dogs.

Adult humans may be affected by the oral allergy syndrome.[3] This occurs in patients with pollen allergies in which certain raw fruits and vegetables are cross-reactive with pollens. An immediate hypersensitivity response causes pruritus, tingling, and angioedema of the lips, tongue, palate, and throat. Occasionally there is otic pruritus.[3] Whether this may occur in dogs and cats is currently unknown.

The differential diagnosis of cutaneous adverse food reaction may include (depending on the presenting clinical signs) environmental allergen–induced atopic dermatitis (atopy), cutaneous drug reaction, flea-bite hypersensitivity, pediculosis, intestinal parasite hypersensitivity, scabies, and primary seborrhea.

Diagnosis

The "gold standard" for the diagnosis of food allergy in humans is a double-blind placebo-controlled food challenge.[3] When food allergy is caused by a Type I (IgE-mediated) immediate hypersensitivity, an in vitro serum testing for food-specific IgE antibodies is of diagnostic value. Intradermal testing with food extracts is not recommended in humans because of the poor specificity and the potential to induce systemic reactions. Skin-prick testing may also be positive in the cases of IgE-mediated food allergy. This is performed by applying drops of suspected antigen to the forearm of the patient and then scarifying the skin surface. A positive reaction is manifested as a wheal and flare. It has been reported that skin-prick testing has a positive predictive value (percentage of positive reactions that are true positives) of 50% and a negative predictive value (percentage of negative reactions that are true negatives) of 95%. Therefore a negative test greatly decreases the likelihood of food allergy, whereas a positive skin-prick test is more difficult to interpret. When food allergy is caused by a Type IV (delayed-onset) hypersensitivity reaction, patch testing with the suspected antigen is frequently positive while skin-prick testing is negative. Patch testing is performed by applying the suspected antigen to intact skin for 48 hours. The site is covered during this time. The site is evaluated 20 minutes and again 72 hours after removing the patch. A positive reaction will have erythema and induration at the site of the antigen.[3]

In contrast to the case with humans, serological testing or intradermal testing for cutaneous adverse food reaction is of no value in dogs and cats.[4,5] A previous study revealed that serum testing had a 40% positive predictive value (percentage of positive test results that were true positives) and a 60.9% negative predictive value (percentage of negative test results that were true negatives).[15] In a study performed with normal dogs, dogs with cutaneous food reactions, and those with skin diseases other than cutaneous food reactions, all the healthy dogs and 75% of the dogs with cutaneous food reactions had positive serum tests for food antigens. Unfortunately, the antigens identified by the serum test were not the antigens that were confirmed by a food trial.[16]

Such a finding may indicate that in dogs and cats cutaneous food reaction is not an IgE-mediated disease, or that the antigens tested are not the same as those that are causing the reaction. This may be due to changes in the antigens that occur during manufacturing and digestion. Also, test antigens for animal proteins, whether used for serologic or intradermal testing, are frequently derived from skeletal muscle, while chicken by-product meal is used in commercial dog and cat food. Chicken by-product meal from tissues from the neck, back, and viscera are antigenically different from skeletal muscle.[9]

Therefore, as in humans, the gold standard for diagnosing cutaneous adverse food reaction is an elimination-diet trial followed by a provocative challenge. Currently there are two schools of thought regarding how an elimination-diet trial may be performed. One group believes that a home-prepared diet consisting of a novel protein and novel carbohydrate is the only proper way to diagnosis cutaneous adverse food reactions. There is also a group that believes that a commercially prepared diet is appropriate to diagnosis cutaneous adverse food reactions. There are two types of commercially prepared "hypoallergenic" diets available on the market: novel protein source foods, and hydrolyzed proteins. The author believes that the commercially available diets may rule in adverse food reaction but cannot rule it out.

Novel protein diets contain such unique ingredients as venison, rabbit, duck, salmon, catfish, and kangaroo as protein sources, and either potato, rice, oat, or barley as carbohydrate sources. The basis of these diets is that individuals are allergic only to antigens to which they have been exposed previously. However, in one study of 40 dogs proven to have cutaneous adverse food reaction based on a home-prepared diet, recurrence of pruritus occurred in 52.5% fed a commercial chicken/rice dog food, 47% on a catfish/rice dog food, and 85% on venison/rice dog food, even though these ingredients were thought to be novel to them.[17] In another study, 50% of eight dogs with cutaneous adverse food reaction (also identified with home-prepared diets) were intolerant of a commercial catfish/rice diet.[18] In a double-blinded study of 20 cats with cutaneous adverse food reaction, the authors evaluated two commercial hypoallergenic diets.[19] The cats were diagnosed as having cutaneous adverse food reactions based on resolution of clinical signs when fed a home-prepared diet. The clinical signs then recurred after a challenge with their previous dietary components, and then resolved after the home-prepared diet was resumed. The cats were then challenged with two commercial hypoallergenic diets. Relapse of the clinical signs was seen in eight cats (40%) on a lamb and rice diet and in 13 cats (65%) on a chicken and rice diet ($P > 0.05$). Neither of the commercial diets was as effective in controlling the clinical signs as the home-prepared diet.

Hydrolyzed protein diets use common protein sources such as soy, chicken liver, or casein, which have been enzymatically hydrolyzed to such short peptide chains that, theoretically, the immune system should not be able to recognize them as the parent proteins. In food-allergic people, most major food allergens are water-soluble glycoproteins with molecular weights ranging from 10,000 to 70,000 daltons and are stable to treatment with heat, acids, and proteases. However, some proteins have been reported not to become antigenic until they are heated or digested.[3,4] In humans it has been reported that the immune system cannot recognize a molecule smaller than 12,000 daltons.[3] Although characterization of the physiochemical properties of most major food allergens in dogs and cats has not yet been performed, hydrolyzed products currently available in veterinary medicine have used a 5000- to 10,000-dalton particle size as their "ideal" cutoff. However, it is possible that the size of the antigens that may cause immunologic reactions in dogs may be smaller than in humans.[3] It has been reported that in a group of three casein-hypersensitive dogs, the antigen that was responsible for the reaction was between 1100 and 4500 daltons.[3] Products currently available use hydrolyzed chicken/chicken liver (Hill's Prescription Diet Z/D Low Allergen), hydrolyzed soy (Purina CNM LA Formula), and hydrolyzed casein and liver (DVM Exclude). The Hill's brand also has taken the potato and substituted it with potato starch to decrease the carbohydrate antigenicity (Hill's Prescription Diet Z/D Ultra Allergen Free). Along the same theory, Purina substituted corn with cornstarch (Purina CNM HA Formula). Of the products mentioned, only the Hill's Prescription Diet Z/D product is formulated for cats. In the cat product, the carbohydrate is rice. This is a concern since rice is a common ingredient in many maintenance cat foods.

The author is a firm believer that the only proper way to rule out a cutaneous adverse food reaction is by a home-prepared diet (Box 6-1). A certain percentage (not established, based on double-blinded, placebo-controlled trials) of dogs and cats respond to the novel protein or hydrolyzed diets. However, failure to respond to these diets does not rule out a cutaneous adverse food reaction. An explanation as to why the novel protein or hydrolyzed diets fail to identify dogs and cats with cutaneous adverse food reactions may include these factors:

- Sources of animal fats added to the diets may be from sources (e.g., beef or pork) other than those used for the hydrolyzed or novel protein.[3]
- The size of the antigen is still large enough to trigger an immunologic reaction (applies to hydrolyzed diets).

BOX 6-1   Home-Prepared Elimination Diet

We believe that your pet may have a food allergy—not an allergy to a particular brand of food, but to one of the individual ingredients. We therefore want to feed a diet that your pet *has not eaten* before. For this diet we will use ostrich, rabbit, goat, duck, or venison as the meat and potatoes, sweet potatoes (yams), or oats as the starch. It is very important that you adhere to the following guidelines:

1. The meat must be pure without any additives (e.g., spices, other meats [such as beef]). Be sure to mention to your butcher it *must* be *pure* meat. Make sure that if the butcher grinds the meat he uses a clean meat grinder.

2. The meat should be trimmed of any excess fat and then boiled or baked. If using duck, either skin it before cooking or poke large holes through the skin to allow the excessive fat to drain. If boiling meat, the water and fat should be drained. You can skim the fat off the water and let it harden into lard. This can then be used to help give your pet a pill. Nothing should be added to it (seasoning, etc.). Larger quantities may be prepared and then frozen for daily feeding.

3. Mix the meat and starch together and let them simmer, as you would stew. Large quantities may be prepared and then refrigerated for daily feeding.

4. Occasionally we will use pinto or kidney beans instead of or in addition to meat. To prepare them, soak beans in water overnight. Throw out this water and put in fresh water. Boil until cooked—typically approximately 1 hour.

5. Feed a one-quarter meat/three-quarters starch mixture daily. If using beans, mix 50/50 with the starch. You will need to feed 1 or 2 cups for a 10-pound dog per day. For cats we will *only* feed the meat, no starch!

6. It is very important that your animal not be allowed to put anything in his mouth except the home-cooked diet and water. This means no vitamins, chew toys, biscuits, rawhides, or table food—nothing! (If your pet is on any medication, however, please check with us *before* discontinuing.) If your pet is on a chewable form (i.e., beef-flavored biscuit) of heartworm medicine, please have your referring veterinarian change it to a nonchewable form.

7. Occasionally a change in diet may cause a digestive upset—either vomiting or diarrhea. Your pet may refuse to eat the above diet. If he/she does not eat for 2 days or a digestive upset occurs, please call us for instructions before giving up. Frequently they will only have a bowel movement every other day because the food is so well digested. Please call if your pet goes more than 2 or 3 days without a bowel movement.

8. In order to determine whether your pet has a food allergy, this diet must be *strictly* maintained for 4 to 12 weeks. You may not see complete relief from itching, scratching, or licking, but you should see some improvement. It is very important that you keep a daily "itch" calendar. Please contact us before you change your pet's diet, regardless of whether improvement is noted.

9. Your pet will *not* be on the elimination diet for the rest of his life. Once we have established that your pet has a food allergy, we will outline procedures to determine which foods cause an allergic response. When we know which pure foods cause a problem and which do not, we can choose a commercial preparation that your pet will tolerate.

10. Please schedule a reexamination/evaluation for 30 days from now. Bring your "itch" calendar with you.

Other explanations may be extrapolated from lessons learned about humans with food allergies. These explanations include the following:
- Contamination from other food prepared at the manufacturing plant by jointly used equipment or even aerosolization of antigens[20-23]
- Contact with humans (or even cats or dogs) that have recently eaten the offending food[24]

Whatever method is used for the elimination-diet trial, it should be fed for a minimum of 8 weeks in dogs and 12 weeks in cats. One possible explanation for the need for such a prolonged trial is the presence of histamine-releasing factors. Histamine-releasing factors are a heterogeneous group of cytokines generated by chronic antigenic exposure that may cause histamine release in the absence of an antigen. This release may continue for weeks after the antigen is removed.[4]

Of 265 dogs reported collectively by 12 different studies, beef, dairy products, and wheat accounted for two thirds of reactions. Reactions to corn, pork, rice, and fish were rarely reported in dogs. Of 56 cats reported collectively by 10 studies, beef, dairy products, and fish accounted for 80% of reactions.[8]

Treatment

Elimination of the sensitizing antigen(s) may not be the only treatment necessary for dogs and cats with cutaneous adverse food reaction. During the early stages of the food trial, many dogs and cats require a short course of glucocorticoids to break the itch-scratch-itch cycle. Also it is essential that secondary bacterial pyoderma, *Malassezia* dermatitis, or otitis externa/media be resolved during the initial portion of the food trial. The patient should be able to maintain the test diet alone, without any ancillary therapy, for 3 or 4 weeks before ending the trial. If the clinical signs (e.g., pruritus, otitis externa) have resolved during the trial, a challenge with the former diet should be performed (Box 6-2). Pruritus or otitis externa should recur within 14 days of exposure to the original diet. The diet is then changed back to the test diet, at which point all clinical signs should resolve. At that time, the dog or cat is placed on a commercially prepared restricted diet for 14 days. If clinical signs do not recur during this time, this diet is used as the base diet. Individual ingredients (beef, chicken, egg, pork, cottage cheese, dairy, wheat, soy, corn, fish) are fed for up to 14 days. If a recurrence of clinical signs occurs when the new ingredient is added, the ingredient is removed from the base diet and the patient is fed only the base diet until the clinical signs resolve. At that time, a new ingredient is added to the base diet. If after 14 days the patient's clinical signs do not recur, this ingredient is placed on the "safe to feed" list (see Box 6-2). After all ingredients have been tested, the owner is able to feed whatever commercial diet is preferred as long as it avoids ingredients that cause a reaction in the dog or cat. However, it has been reported that up to 20% of dogs cannot be managed on any commercial food.[25,26]

BOX 6-2   Guidelines for Determination of Specific Food Allergies

Your animal has shown improvement on the home-prepared elimination diet. We must now continue with the next phase of the program.

1. Start your pet back on *all* the *same* things he/she ate prior to the special home-made diet. We are doing this to establish that there is a definite food allergy and that the improvement was not due to other factors. If after feeding the original diet for 14 days the itching has not increased, please call us for the next step. However, if the itching increases, *immediately stop* the pet food and reinstitute the home-made elimination diet. Continue this homemade diet trial until the itching has again reduced, then proceed to the next step. If after 14 days the itching does not decrease, please call us.

2. Now we want to try [_____] commercial "hypoallergenic" pet food for 14 days. If your pet does not experience an increase of itching, go to step 3.

3. Now that we have established for *certain* that your pet has a food allergy, we must determine what individual ingredients are causing the problem. Make a list with two columns—one column "safe" food and the other column "unsafe" food. Each week add a new ingredient to the above commercial pet food as directed below. If no increase in itching is noted after 1 week, list this food in the column labeled "safe." You may immediately start on the next food mixture on the list, following the same procedure. If your pet's itching increases, list the new food in the "unsafe" column. Stop that food and resume feeding [_____] commercial pet food (only) until the animal is as itch-free as prior to adding the offending food. Once the itching has subsided, resume feeding as directed below. When you have completed the list, schedule a follow-up examination and evaluation (please bring your list of "safe" and "unsafe" foods), *and one of the following* (depending on the week): _____

Weeks 1 & 2	Ground beef
Weeks 3 & 4	Chicken
Weeks 4 & 5	Pork
Weeks 5 & 6	Cottage cheese
Weeks 6 & 7	Boiled eggs (one egg per 25 pounds)
Weeks 7 & 8	Ground whole wheat flour
Weeks 9 & 10	Corn oil (half-tablespoon per 25 pounds)
Weeks 11 & 12	Soybean

When you return for your reevaluation, please do not forget to bring your list of safe and unsafe foods.

References

1. Hiller A, Griffin CE: The ACVD task force on canine atopic dermatitis (X): is there a relationship between canine atopic dermatitis and cutaneous adverse food reactions? In Olivry T, ed: *Veterinary immunology and immunopathology. Special issue. The American College of Veterinary Dermatology Task Force on Canine Atopic Dermatitis,* Oxford, UK, 2001, Elsevier.
2. Ring J, Vieluf D: Adverse reactions to food, *Curr Probl Dermatol* 20:187, 1991.

3. Nowak AW: *Pathophysiology of food allergy,* 18th Proc Ann Meeting AAVD/ACVD, Monterey, CA, 2003, Hill's Pet Nutrition, Inc.
3a. Cole LK, Kwochka KW, Lowalskin JJ, et al: Microflora and antimicrobial susceptibility patterns of isolated pathogens from the horizontal ear canal and middle ear in dogs with otitis media, *J Am Vet Med Assoc* 212:534-538, 1998.
4. Scott DW, Miller WH, Griffin CE, eds: *Mueller and Kirk's Small animal dermatology,* ed 6, Philadelphia, 2001, WB Saunders.
5. Guaguere E, Prelaud P: Food intolerance. In Guaguere E, Prelaud P, eds: *A practical guide to feline dermatology,* Paris, 1999, Merial.
6. Tizard IR: *Veterinary immunology: an introduction,* ed 6, Philadelphia, 2000, WB Saunders.
7. Reedy LM, Miller WH, Willemse T: *Allergic skin diseases of dogs and cats,* ed 2, Philadelphia, 1997, WB Saunders.
8. Roudebush P: Ingredients associated with adverse food reactions in dogs and cats, *Adv Small Anim Med Surg* 15(9):1-3, 2002.
9. Rosser EJ, White SD: Diet and the skin in companion animals. In Kwochka KW, Willemse T, von Tscharner C, eds: *Advances in veterinary dermatology,* vol 3, Oxford, UK, 1998, Butterworth-Heinemann.
10. Ishida R, Masuda K, Sakaguchi M, et al: In vivo and in vitro evidence of Type I hypersensitivity to food allergens in atopic dogs, *Vet Dermatol* 11:32, 2000.
11. Jackson HA, Cates C, Hammerberg B: Total and allergen specific serum and fecal IgE responses to dietary changes in dogs with suspected food hypersensitivity, *Vet Dermatol* 11:33, 2000.
12. Griffin CE: Otitis externa and otitis media. In Griffin CE, Kwochka KW, MacDonald JM, eds: *Current veterinary dermatology: the science and art of therapy,* St Louis, 1993, Mosby.
13. Muse R, Griffin C, Rosenkrantz WS: *The prevalence of otic manifestations and otitis externa in allergic dogs,* 12th Proc Ann Meeting AAVD/ACVD, Las Vegas, 1996.
14. Bigler B, Merchant SR: Otitis externa. In von Tscharner C, Halliwell REW, eds: *Advances in veterinary dermatology,* vol 1, London, 1990, Bailliere Tindall.
15. Jeffers JG, Shanley KJ, Meyer EK: Diagnostic testing of dogs for food hypersensitivity, *J Am Vet Med Assoc* 198(2):245-250, 1991.
16. White SD, Mason IS: Dietary allergy. In von Tscharner C, Halliwell REW eds: *Advances in veterinary dermatology,* vol 1, London, 1990, Bailliere Tindall.
17. Leistra MH, Markwell PJ, Willemse T: Evaluation of selected-protein-source diets for management of dogs with adverse reactions to foods, *J Am Vet Med Assoc* 219(10):1411-1414, 2001.
18. Tapp T, Griffin C, Rosenkrantz W, et al: Comparison of a commercial limited-antigen diet versus home-prepared diets in the diagnosis of canine adverse food reaction, *Vet Therap* 3(3):244-251, 2002.
19. Leistra MH, Willemse T: Double-blind evaluation of two commercial hypoallergenic diets in cats with adverse food reactions, *J Feline Med Surg* 4(4):185-188, 2002.
20. Gonzalez-Galan I, Garcia-Menaya JM, Jimenez-Ferrera G, et al: Anaphylactic shock to oysters and white fish with generalized urticaria to prawns and white fish, *Allergol-Immunopathol* 30(5):300-303, 2002.
21. Furlong TJ, DeSimone J, Sicherer SH: Peanut and tree nut allergic reactions in restaurants and other food establishments, *J Allergy Clin Immunol* 108(5):867-870, 2001.
22. Jeebhay MF, Robins TG, Lehrer SB, et al: Occupational seafood allergy: a review, *Occup Environ Med* 58(9):553-562, 2001.
23. Taylor AV, Swanson MC, Jones RT, et al: Detection and quantitation of raw fish aeroallergens from an open-air fish market, *J Allergy Clin Immunol* 105(1):166-169, 2000.
24. Steensma DP: The kiss of death: a severe allergic reaction to a shellfish induced by a good-night kiss, *Mayo Clin Proc* 78(2):221-222, 2003.
25. Rosser EJ: Diagnosis of food allergy in dogs, *J Am Vet Med Assoc* 203(2):259-262, 1993.
26. White SD: Food hypersensitivity in 30 dogs, *J Am Vet Med Assoc* 188(7):695-698, 1986.

7

Factors that Predispose the Ear to Otitis Externa

Louis N. Gotthelf, DVM

Careful examination of a clean, dry ear canal in a dog or cat with otitis externa may reveal many conditions that affect the ear canal. Because the ear canal lining is actually modified skin, the same basic types of lesions found on the skin of the trunk may be found in the ear canal. Certain conditions, called *predisposing factors,* are responsible for altering the anatomy and physiology of the ear canal and increasing the likelihood of otitis externa. These factors increase the susceptibility of the ear canal to support bacteria and yeast growth.

For example, excessive skin folds at the base of the tail may predispose the English Bulldog to a tail fold pyoderma. In the ear of this breed, excessive skin folds also predispose to otitis. The presence of a predisposing factor in a patient makes the ears more susceptible to otitis externa even when the patient is not exhibiting symptoms of otitis externa. By analogy, not all English Bulldogs with excessive tail folds suffer from tail fold pyoderma. Because such dogs have the predisposing factor (the excessive folds), tail fold pyoderma is more likely to occur in this breed than in the Beagle, which has no tail folds.

The floppy ear carriage common to many dog breeds may predispose them to otitis because of inadequate ventilation of the ear canal, which ultimately leads to higher humidity there. The dark, warm, moist area increases the chance that bacteria and yeasts will have a more favorable environment for growth and reproduction. It is not surprising that the incidence and severity of otitis externa are greater in dog breeds with floppy ears. However, there are many floppy-eared breeds that do not have increased incidence of ear disease. The decrease in cosmetic ear trimming in recent years has not resulted in increased otitis in the Miniature Schnauzer or the Doberman Pinscher. Some of the predisposed floppy-eared breeds such as the Cocker Spaniel, the Labrador Retriever, and the Springer Spaniel have increased densities of glandular tissue, also contributing to the increased humidity. Many of the floppy-eared breeds have the predisposing factor of excessive hair growth in their ears. Excessive hair can matt or knot and seal the ear canal. Hairs can also accumulate wax, creating a plug. Cats and many dog breeds have erect ears that are well ventilated, and these pets have a lower incidence of otitis externa.

In developing a therapeutic plan for otitis externa, the veterinarian must give attention to the treatment of predisposing factors that effectively reduce the likelihood that the patient's ear disease will become chronic or recurrent. Some treatments to remove predisposing factors are very simple, such as plucking the excessive hairs found in a Poodle's ears to reduce the humidity within the ear canal. Some breeders and veterinarians advocate taping or fixation of the ears of a Cocker Spaniel over the top of its head to allow ear canal ventilation. Lateral canal ear resection in a nondiseased ear opens it up and provides ventilation as well as prevents accumulation of exudates that may form. Treatment of other predisposing factors is not such a simple matter. Diffuse cerumen gland adenocarcinoma, for example, requires total ear canal ablation to resolve.

Among the conditions found in the ear canals of dogs and cats that are considered to be predisposing factors favoring the development of otitis externa are the following:

- Stenosis
- Excessive hair

- Excessive cerumen production
- Any trauma to the ear canal
- Obstruction by tumor, polyp, or excessive granulation tissue

These anatomic and physiologic alterations create favorable climates for the proliferation of infectious organisms. High temperature and humidity in the ear canal, greater amounts of substrates for growth of bacteria and yeasts, and damaged epithelium result in the failure of the ear's normal immune mechanisms. Commensal bacteria and yeasts may be induced to reproduce in the favorable climate created. Otitis externa is the eventual result.

How does the presence of a predisposing factor in a patient's ear canal affect the course of otitis externa? Some pathophysiologic mechanisms have been explained, but other mechanisms remain a challenge. An understanding of the mechanisms involved in how these predisposing factors affect the normal physiology of the ear canal helps clinicians formulate more complete therapeutic plans for the treatment of otitis externa.

The normally smooth epithelial surface of the ear canal has a mechanism for clearing surface debris out of the ear canal; the process has been termed *epithelial migration*. Surface keratinocytes slowly slide along the epidermal layer of the ear canal, carrying cerumen and microorganisms out of the ear canal. When the anatomy of the epithelium of the ear canal is altered by the presence of abnormal tissue, the movement of kerotinocytes is also altered. The smooth surface of the normal ear canal becomes roughened or obstructed, and the debris accumulates at the point where the epithelial movement stops (Figure 7-1). Inflammation and colonization of microorganisms occur at these points.

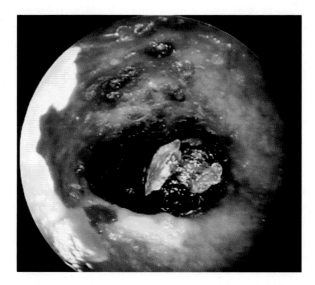

Figure 7-1

Dry wax accumulating in the ear canal. When the skin cells lining the ear canal do not migrate toward the facial opening of the ear canal, wax and other debris accumulate.

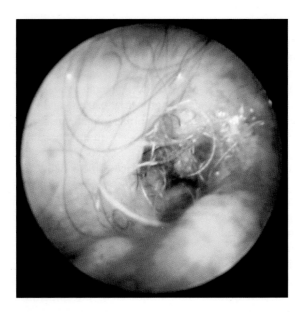

Figure 7-2

Stenotic ear canal as the result of trauma. Swelling from inflammation or increased tissue mass from fibrosis in the ear canal closes off the lumen.

Stenotic Ear Canals

A common finding in dogs with otitis externa is a narrowed ear canal. Within the tube of skin that makes up the external ear canal, any swelling translates to decreased lumen diameter. When the lumen of the ear canal becomes narrowed or occluded, stenosis results (Figure 7-2). The stenosis magnifies the severity of the ear disease, making examination and treatment of the otitis externa more difficult.

A brief review of the anatomy of the external ear canal is helpful in delineating the mechanisms involved in creating the stenotic ear canal. The ear canal of the dog is lined by keratinizing stratified squamous epithelium.

Vertical Ear Canal

The skin of the vertical canal is approximately 1 mm thick and contains a well-developed dermis and subcutaneous layer. Numerous long, coarse hairs are present along the vertical canal. Surrounding the hair follicles are numerous sebaceous and ceruminous glands (modified apocrine glands). No eccrine sweat glands are located in the external ear canal. Hairs are most numerous toward the opening of the ear canal; they decrease along the ear canal toward the eardrum. Conversely, the ceruminous glands increase in density in the vertical canal distally.

The external acoustic meatus and the skin on the pinna contain numerous adnexal structures and have a significant subcutaneous layer, which can respond to disease. Frequently, the stenotic portion of the ear is limited only to the external

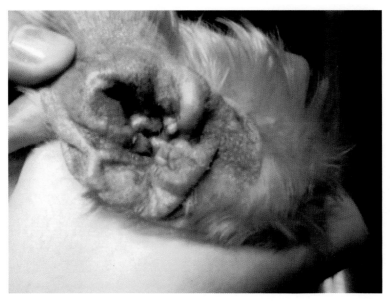

Figure 7-3

Hyperplastic epithelium on the concave pinna closes off the opening to the vertical ear canal.

acoustic meatus (Figure 7-3). In that situation, the otoscope tip may be passed through the stenosis, revealing a normal vertical canal beyond it.

The ear canal of the Shar-Pei has an abundant mucinous dermis under the epithelial layer that increases the thickness and folding of the dermal-epidermal layer. Owing to the anatomically normal thick lining, the lumen diameter in this breed is decreased. The Shar-Pei's ear canal is thus predisposed to higher humidity and greater glandular secretions, promoting bacterial and yeast colonization.

Anatomically, the vertical canal is more prone to becoming stenotic because of the vascularity and glandular structures found there. The inflammation and edema lead to narrowing of the ear canal. The stenosis prevents drainage of exudates out of the ear canal and complicates therapy by preventing topical medications from achieving therapeutic levels beyond the stenotic portion. Increases in fluid and air pressure beyond the stenosis can cause excessive pressure on the eardrum, predisposing it to rupture.

Inflammation and edema increase the thickness of the subcutaneous layer of the ear canal, leading to stenosis. Chronic otitis externa leads to progressive pathologic changes of the lining epithelium such as hyperkeratosis and hyperplasia (Figure 7-4). The marked thickening of the epithelial layer may significantly reduce ear canal diameter. Increases in the number and size of sebaceous glands (Figure 7-5) and dilated apocrine glands also reduce lumen diameter (Figure 7-6). In addition, pathologic changes that lead to calcification (Figure 7-7) and thickening of the auricular cartilage (especially in American Cocker Spaniels) or to fibrosis and formation of excessive granulation tissue resulting from chronic infection also lead to narrowing of the ear canal lumen (Figure 7-8). Tumors such as ceruminous adenocarcinoma may also occlude the ear canal lumen (Figure 7-9).

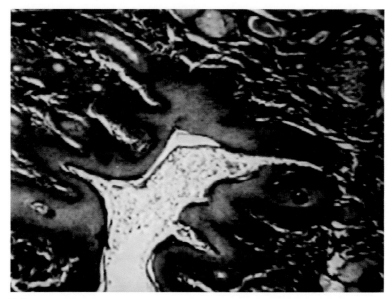

Figure 7-4

Histopathologic section of an ear canal with extensive fibrosis below a hyperplastic epithelium. Numerous epithelial folds are present and there is an exudate in the stenotic ear canal.

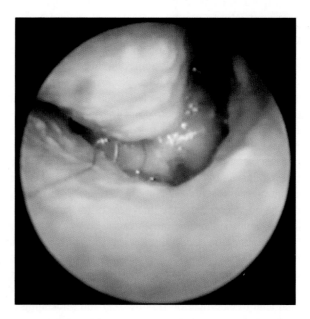

Figure 7-5

Sebaceous hyperplasia usually results in a smooth, stenotic canal. In this Shetland Sheepdog's ear, the epithelium is also hyperplastic.

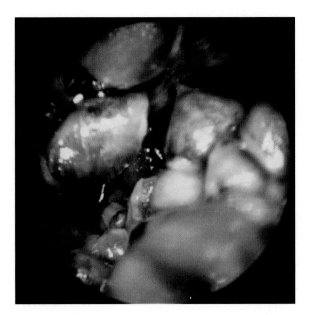

Figure 7-6

Ceruminous gland hyperplasia causes a stenosis in the vertical ear canal of this Cocker Spaniel.

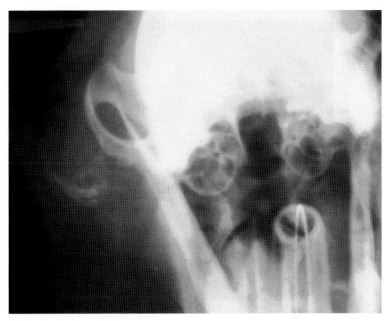

Figure 7-7

Radiograph of a stenotic, calcified ear canal in an American Cocker Spaniel. This radiographic sign of pathology indicates a nonreversible, end-stage ear that will require surgical removal.

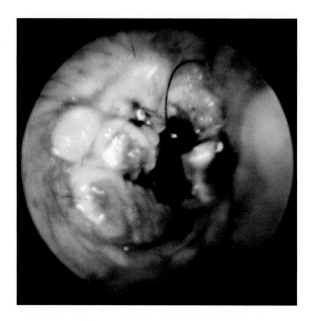

Figure 7-8

Fibrosis and granulation tissue can result from chronic otitis externa.

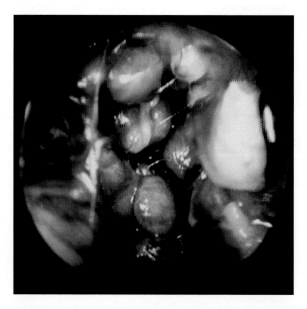

Figure 7-9

Cerumen gland adenocarcinomas in an American Cocker Spaniel. This ear was also secondarily infected with *Staphylococcus intermedius,* which remained until surgery was performed. Laser ablation of these tumors opened up the ear canal.

Horizontal Ear Canal

Fortunately, the skin of the horizontal canal is often spared the devastating effects of inflammation associated with otitis externa. The thin epidermis lining the horizontal canal firmly attaches to the underlying auricular cartilage in the lateral aspect of the horizontal canal (cartilaginous portion) and is approximately 0.2 mm thick. The ventral portion of the horizontal canal has an extension of the pertrous temporal bone underlying the thin epidermis (bony portion). The thin epithelium of the bony horizontal canal is continuous with the epithelium on the lateral aspect of the tympanic membrane, which is one or two cells thick. Epidermal rete ridges, skin adnexal structures, and a subcutaneous layer are absent in the skin of the horizontal canal. Because the skin is adherent to the underlying cartilage and to the periosteum of the bony portion of the horizontal canal, pathologic changes of the horizontal canal are usually limited to hyperplasia. The exception to this anatomic feature is the American Cocker Spaniel. This breed supports much more glandular tissue in the horizontal canal than other breeds. This has been verified by an analysis of histopathologic specimens from the horizontal canal of several breeds.

Overtreatment

Long-standing overtreatment of ears with ear cleaners may macerate the epithelium, causing swelling and greater folding of the epithelial surface. Ear cleaners usually contain a combination of several ingredients, including alcohols, acids, detergents, propylene glycol, and water. Prolonged contact of these substances with the ear canal causes the cells to swell as the ear canal skin loses its waterproof properties. Drugs such as neomycin and silver sulfadiazine are known to trigger a contact dermatitis within the ear canal, leading to erythema and swelling in the ear canal. If any of these causes is suspected, suspending all topical treatment for 1 or 2 weeks may decrease the tissue reaction and relieve the swelling.

Stenosis

Stenosis presents a special problem in examination of the ear canal. Instruments cannot be inserted through the narrowed canal, and the integrity of the eardrum cannot be determined otoscopically. Occasionally, a short course of potent corticosteroids, applied topically, injected directly into the stenotic tissue, or administered parenterally, decreases the inflammatory infiltrates and reduces edema (Figure 7-10). In addition, corticosteroids decrease the amounts of glandular secretions, making them less viscous so that they are easier to flush out of the ear canal; they also reduce the secretion and dilation of ceruminous glands. If corticosteroids successfully increase the lumen diameter, adequate visualization of the ear canal and tympanic membrane becomes possible.

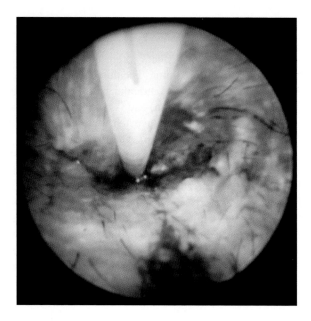

Figure 7-10

Potent corticosteroids can be infused through a small catheter through a stenotic portion of the ear canal to reduce inflammation.

When medical therapy for stenosis is ineffective because of severe pathologic changes to the ear canal, surgical ablation of the vertical canal, horizontal canal, or both is required. Surgical treatment of stenotic ears relieves the pain associated with chronic otitis and allows the remaining ear canal to be ventilated.

Hair in Ear Canals

In some of the haired breeds, such as the Poodle and many of the terriers, long hairs normally grow from the skin of the ear canal. The number of hair follicles in predisposed breeds gradually decreases along the length of the external ear canal. The highest density of hair follicles occurs at the entrance to the ear canals at the pinna and along the proximal portion of the vertical canal. Occasionally hairs may be found along the deeper parts of the canal.

Excessive hair or knots of ear hair may occlude the ear canals and interfere with adequate drying of the canal. The excessive moisture created by hair plugs predisposes these breeds to otitis externa. Certain bacteria such as *Pseudomonas* and *Proteus* thrive in a humid ear canal. When long hairs become matted and tangled in the ear canal, cerumen, exudates, and other secretions mold to the hair mass and form an occlusion.

Routine plucking of hairs by groomers may not be necessary in a dog whose ears are normal, and it can sometimes be detrimental. Plucking the hairs with curved hemostats can create an inflammatory reaction that can predispose the ear to infection. In a dog that has recurrent ear infections and excessive hair growth in the ear canal, however, the hair should be routinely removed to prevent a mass of tangled hairs from blocking the ear canal lumen. Plucking the excessive hairs from the ears in patients predisposed to otitis externa is recommended for the prevention and management of otitis externa.

Excessive Cerumen Production

The external ear canal is lined with both sebaceous and apocrine glands. The sebaceous glands are relatively superficial, surround hair follicles, and have ducts that open into the hair follicle below the surface of the epithelium. The apocrine (tubular) glands are located in the deeper dermis, are unassociated with hair follicles, and are often referred to as the *ceruminous glands* (Figure 7-11).

Cerumen is primarily a lipid-containing material produced by the secretory products of both of these types of glands. The sebaceous gland is a holocrine gland. Its secretion is composed of disintegrating desquamated glandular epithelial cells. The apocrine glandular secretion is a waxy acellular liquid. Cerumen, then, is composed of a mixture of sebaceous epithelial cells suspended in apocrine lipid secretion.

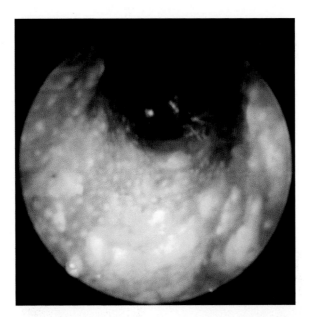

Figure 7-11

Ceruminous gland hyperplasia in its early stage. Polka dots indicate the glands with their ducts above the level of the ear canal epithelium. Clumps of the apocrine lipid secretion accumulate in this ear.

Increased ceruminous gland secretion in response to inflammation results in a more watery, humid cerumen. Imbalances in the ratio and concentration of the secretions of these two types of glands may play a role in allowing otitis externa to provide substrates necessary for infectious organisms to grow. That is why the use of ceruminolytic ear cleaners alone can result in effective treatment for otitis externa.

As the number of hairs decreases along the length of the vertical ear canal, the number of sebaceous glands also decreases. The ceruminous glands are numerous along both the haired and nonhaired portions of the vertical ear canal.

Some authorities suggest that there are actually two types of cerumen, liquid and dry. In humans, it is thought that residents of arctic climates favor the dry cerumen, whereas those who reside in temperate or equatorial climates tend to have more liquid cerumen. The author has observed both dry and wet cerumen in dogs and cats (Figures 7-12 and 7-13). Whether this is a genetic predisposition, as is suggested in the case of humans, or a feature of certain ear diseases, has not been determined.

The hydrophobic properties of normal cerumen make it an important barrier to the entry of excessive moisture to the epithelial cells of the external ear canal. Certain components of normal cerumen such as lysozyme and interleukins are thought to provide an antibacterial and antiviral characteristic to cerumen. Routine ear cleaning in normal dogs and cats, which removes these important immunologic factors, is not necessary and may even predispose to otitis externa.

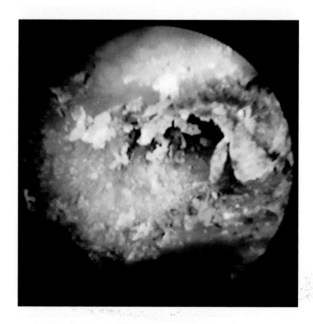

Figure 7-12

As the thick liquid lipid secretion from the apocrine glands dries out, it darkens. This is a dry cerumen.

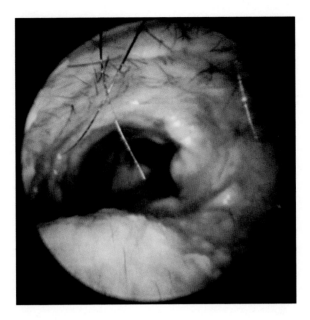

Figure 7-13

Wet cerumen tends to stay moist in the ear canal.

Under normal circumstances, cerumen that is produced along the vertical canal is transported laterally along the canal wall toward the pinna in conjunction with normal epithelial migration and is subsequently extruded. If cotton-tipped applicators are used to clean an ear canal full of cerumen and other debris, the material can be pushed toward the horizontal canal and eardrum, resulting in cerumen impaction. This condition is best treated with ceruminolytic agents or curettage of the inspissated cerumen.

A condition known as *failure of epithelial migration* results when the normal cerumen clearance mechanism is disrupted. Normally, keratinocytes originating from the central portion of the eardrum slide along the basal epithelium in the superficial layers along the entire ear canal and carry cerumen from the eardrum to the pinna. Damage to the eardrum prevents the migration of these cells, allowing layering rather than promoting clearing of cerumen. The resulting accumulation can become quite large (Figure 7-14). Such ceruminoliths may be removed from the surface of the eardrum with a grasping forceps. Occasionally, soft cerumen makes grasping the entire cerumen plug impossible. These plugs are best prepared for removal by using warm flushing solution to soften the wax. Curettes and large-bore catheters connected to suction aid in their removal.

Certain breeds predisposed to otitis externa, such as the Cocker Spaniel, Springer Spaniel, and Labrador Retriever, have a higher number of apocrine glands in the dermis of their ear canals than other breeds. A greater area of apocrine glands may be a predisposing factor in otitis externa. The density of glandular tissue is significantly

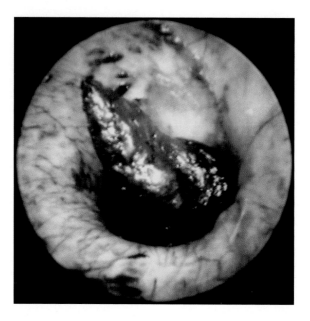

Figure 7-14

Cerumen plug extends from the eardrum into the vertical ear canal in this Miniature Schnauzer with vestibular disease. The plug put pressure on the eardrum resulting in circling. Removal of the wax plug resolved the vestibular signs immediately.

higher in the vertical (distal) ear canal, with a scarcity of glandular tissue and hair follicles in the horizontal (proximal) ear canal. In the presence of otitis externa, however, the proximal ear canal may also become infiltrated by distended apocrine glands. Cystic ceruminous glands called *apocrine cysts* are sometimes found in the ear canal (Figure 7-15).

Apocrine tubular glands are the major secretory glands in otitis externa. These glands increase substantially in size in response to the severity of otitis (Figure 7-16). The sebaceous glands apparently do not proliferate in otitis externa and do not increase in size. In fact, in chronic otitis the sebaceous glands are less active and are displaced by distended apocrine tubular glands. The apocrine tubular glands secrete their lipids and often dilate, but the total amount of cerumen produced may not increase because of the reduction in sebaceous secretions.

The secretion of the apocrine tubular glands may provide a nutrient-rich medium for microorganisms. It has been speculated that the presence of excessive apocrine tubular gland secretion coupled with the decreased sebaceous secretion in predisposed breeds facilitates growth of microorganisms. Many endocrinologic skin conditions affecting the ear stimulate the secretion of the apocrine tubular glands. Many of these same diseases are also immunosuppressive and may encourage the growth of microorganisms.

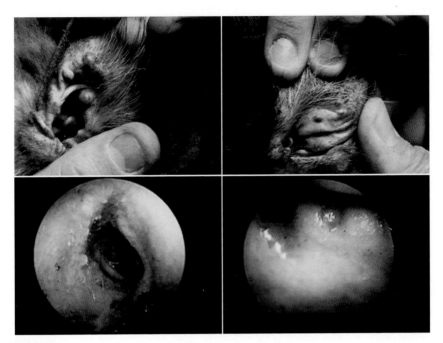

Figure 7-15

Ceruminous cysts in a Persian cat. Often seen as dark blue to black cystic structures on the pinna and in the ear canal, cystic apocrine glands may have a genetic predisposition in this breed.

Because cerumen is a hydrophobic lipid material, excessive cerumen production associated with otitis externa provides an occlusive coating of the infected epithelial tissues. Bacteria, yeasts, proteolytic enzymes, and other vasoactive substances in exudates remain sealed under the thick lipid coating. Treatment of bacterial or yeast otitis externa must include the use of ceruminolytic flushes to remove this lipid covering, to allow the topical antimicrobial agent to contact the organisms inhabiting the infected epithelium. Ear flushes also serve to remove (1) the pro-inflammatory fatty acids produced as a result of bacterial degradation of ceruminous lipids and (2) the proteolytic enzymes released by inflammatory cells.

After the ceruminous glands enlarge, they rarely return to pre-otitis size, and the ears produce excessive cerumen. Routine ear care must include frequent home ear flushes. Flushing the ears of affected patients to remove excessive cerumen becomes a preventive treatment. If the excessive cerumen is not removed, ceruminous otitis results. This condition is characterized by excessive buildup of ear wax, with bacterial degradation of the lipids. The resultant free fatty acids become triggers for inflammation, leading to erythema and pruritus. They are also the substrates that favor *Malassezia* growth.

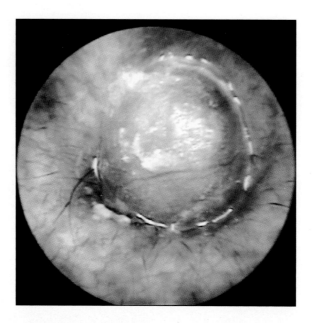

Figure 7-16

Apocrine cyst completely occluding the vertical ear canal. When this cyst was decompressed using a laser, there was significant debris accumulation between the cyst and the eardrum that had to be removed.

Trauma

Trauma from any external cause can affect the ears. Whether due to fight wounds, trauma to the pinna from being hit by a car, or surgical trauma, a tissue reaction triggered by a traumatic injury may lead to problems in the ear canals.

Wounds

Underlying the ear canal epithelium is a subcutaneous layer of dermis and a cylindrical to conical layer of elastic cartilage surrounded by muscles, blood vessels, and nerves. Trauma to any one of these tissues causes intense inflammation and bleeding, and may lead to acute stenosis of the ear canal from the edema that follows inflammation. In most cases the stenosis resolves when the tissue in the damaged portion of the ear canal heals. In other cases, especially in traumatic injury to the cartilage, the healing may be very slow and return of normal anatomic architecture incomplete. The stenotic canal that remains is the result of contracture of fibrous connective tissue or deformation of cartilage during healing. An example of the deformity of cartilage can be seen in an untreated aural hematoma in which the shape of the pinnal cartilage has been permanently changed. When the cartilaginous cylindrical shape has been compromised, the lumen of the ear canal may be obliterated. Fistulous tracts may appear around the site of facial trauma that may communicate with the ear canal (Figures 7-17 and 7-18).

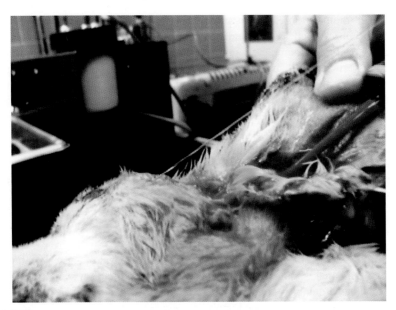

Figure 7-17

Traumatic facial wound of a Beagle resulted in a communication from the facial wound to the ear canal. A red rubber catheter has been placed in the ear canal and dilute povidone-iodine is being flushed into the ear canal. As the ear canal is being flushed, the flush solution exits from the facial wound in a forceful stream parallel to the red rubber catheter.

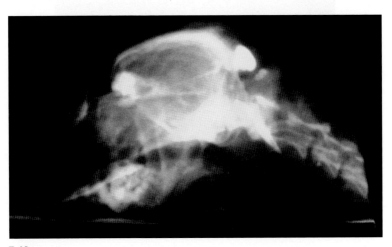

Figure 7-18

Radiograph showing infusion of iodinated contrast medium into the facial wound shown in Figure 7-17. Contrast material can be seen filling the facial wound site, the ear canal, the tympanic bulla, and the subcutaneous region in the occipital area.

Surgical trauma from ear canal surgery can also lead to postoperative complications. Procedures such as total ear canal ablation often result in fistulous tracts emanating from the incompletely removed lining of the middle ear with unresolved infection. Vertical ear canal ablation or the Zepp lateral ear resection surgery requires cutting through cartilage. Suturing through cartilage incites an inflammatory reaction. Hyaluronic acid, which is released into the surrounding tissue from the cut cartilaginous matrix, stimulates intense inflammation and swelling; therefore, suturing skin to skin over the cartilage is advised.

Trauma induced by blunt force injury to the head and neck can result in a ruptured eardrum (Figure 7-19). Fresh bleeding from the ear may be seen on examination. The ear canals in such cases must be examined for the presence of an eardrum and accumulation of blood behind the eardrum.

Trauma from Cotton-Tipped Applicators

Cotton-tipped applicators (Q-tips) are often used for removal of ear wax in humans. The dog's ear canal is long, bent, and tapered, so the tip of an ear swab inserted into the vertical canal quickly approaches the diameter of the ear canal as it is advanced.

Trauma from the cotton-tipped applicator occurs as the ear canal is plugged by the cotton tip. The ear canal is "scraped" by the abrasive cellulose or synthetic fiber.

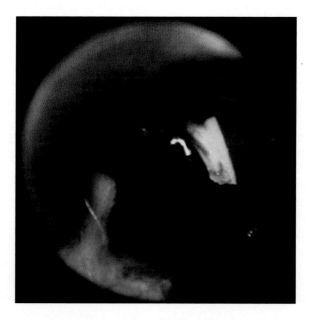

Figure 7-19

The patient, a mixed terrier, was hit by a car and had blood coming out of the ear. Examination showed that the patient had a ruptured eardrum. The manubrium of the malleus is prominently displayed.

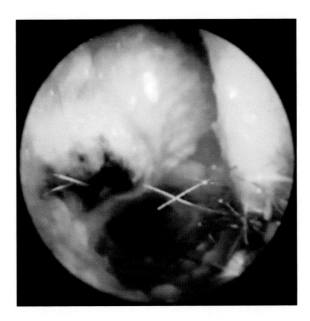

Figure 7-20

A cotton-tipped applicator used in this ear resulted in denuding the epithelial surface with the abrasive material. Acid-type ear cleaners will cause severe pain when they contact the ulcer.

In an infected ear, the epithelium is edematous and very often friable, so that only mild pressure from a cotton-tipped applicator can result in ulceration (Figure 7-20). When the ear canal becomes ulcerated, microorganisms can flourish as growth-enhancing nutrients, such as blood components and serum proteins, are released into the ear canal.

Cotton-tipped applicators also tend to push any material that may be ahead of the cotton tip farther down the ear canal, packing cerumen into the horizontal canal. If enough pressure is applied, this material may be pushed right through the eardrum. Cotton-tipped applicators themselves may perforate the eardrum if they are pushed too quickly into an ear, creating a traumatic myringotomy (Figure 7-21).

Cotton-tipped applicators are available in a variety of tip sizes. Veterinarians should use only the small applicators in the ears of small animals. Obtaining roll-smear cytologic samples (see Chapter 2) for determining the organisms present in otic exudates can be accomplished by inserting the small cotton-tipped applicator into the horizontal ear canal through an otoscope cone and pulling the swab slowly along the ear canal toward the pinna.

Use of cotton-tipped applicators should be restricted to removal of liquids. The absorptive capacity of the cotton tip allows liquid to be absorbed. Simply inserting the tip very carefully into an ear filled with liquid (e.g., flush solutions, pus, mucus) while restricting movement of the applicator enables liquids to be absorbed into the tip. Repeated insertions of applicators are required until a tip is dry when removed.

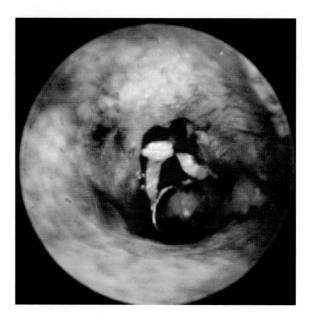

Figure 7-21

This cat's ear was filled with wax and debris associated with ear mites. The material was flushed out, but when a cotton-tipped applicator was put into the ear, it popped the eardrum.

Trauma from Instrumentation

Many instruments are used in the ear canal by veterinarians, groomers, and pet owners. Curettes are used to remove wax and tenacious material from the epidermal layer. Various rigid catheters are put into the ear canals for flushing and suctioning debris; sharp edges on cut urethral or feeding tubes will cut the epithelium of the ear canal. Curved hemostats are used for pulling hair from the ear canals; hemostats tend to crush tissue and, when improperly used, may cause damage to the ear canal. Water pumps, such as the Water Pik, provide a forceful stream of ear cleaning solution; increased water pressure in the ear canal can rupture an already macerated, friable eardrum.

Because most procedures done in the ear canal are performed without good visibility, trauma invariably occurs. Instruments and catheters are fairly small, and some bleeding and discomfort may be evident after the procedure. Various medications and ear cleaners may burn the ear tissue when applied. Most traumatic injuries from instruments heal rapidly. The exception is perforation of the eardrum (Figure 7-22).

When traumatic perforation of the eardrum occurs, it is intensely painful. The patient exhibits clinical signs and pain that were not previously present. The amount of exudates in the ear canal may rapidly increase, and the otitis externa being treated appears worse. Traumatic myringotomy heals in approximately 2 to 3 weeks, if iatrogenic otitis media has not been created. In the presence of an otitis externa, however, pushing exudates into the middle ear predisposes to otitis media.

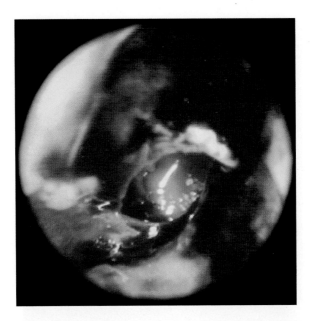

Figure 7-22

Ulceration and iatrogenic perforation of the eardrum in a Poodle's ear. This large hole in the eardrum may never completely heal. Medications that may be potentially ototoxic should not be used in this ear.

Neoplasia of the Ear Canals

When a dog or cat with chronic otitis externa that does not respond to routine therapy is presented to the veterinarian, the clinician should be alert to the possibility of a tumor or growth in the ear canal. Medical treatment for otitis externa may offer palliative relief, but the chronic recurrent nature of the disease is indicative of an underlying condition.

When cytologic examination of otic exudates reveals large sheets of epithelial cells, neoplasia must be considered as a diagnosis. Chronic purulent otitis complicated by bacterial or yeast infection may also be obvious. Tumors occlude the ear canal and prevent drainage of exudates and therefore are often complicated by infection.

Symptomatology

Tumors arising in the external ear are often diagnosed only when they become large enough to be obvious. A tumor in the more distal portions of the ear canal may be obscured by wax (Figure 7-23), or the examiner may not look past the bend in the ear canal to see a tumor in the horizontal canal. Many tumors are extremely small, and in an ear canal with a very small diameter, they predispose to infection. The tumors

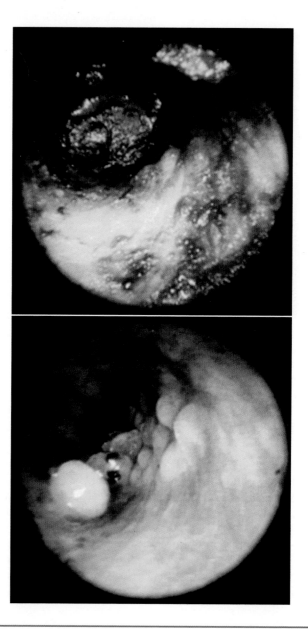

Figure 7-23

Many cerumen gland tumors are functional, producing wax in great quantities *(top)*. The wax obscures the tumors until the ear is cleaned with a ceruminolytic *(bottom)*.

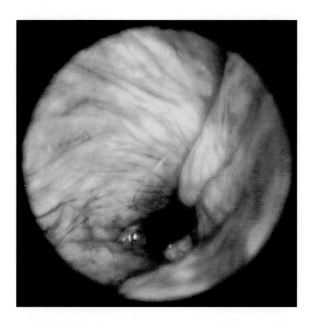

Figure 7-24

Ulcerated cerumen gland adenomas. This Golden Retriever had recurrent aural hematomas. The dog had been operated on three times previously for aural hematoma. When this dog was presented to the author for the fourth aural hematoma, a careful examination of the otherwise normal ear canal revealed these small ulcerated tumors. Removal of these tumors at the time of aural hematoma surgery cured this dog of its head shaking.

often have an ulcerated tip (Figure 7-24). Occlusion of the ear canal by a tumor can cause pain and discomfort. If the patient shakes the head excessively, aural hematoma may result. It is difficult to examine the horizontal canal for tumors without an instrument such as a video otoscope (Video Vetscope, MedRx, Inc., Largo, Florida), but if a tumor is found in the horizontal canal, it may explain the extreme discomfort the patient evidently experiences (Figure 7-25).

A tumor of the middle ear may present as vestibular disease with head tilt or nystagmus. If visualization is possible, as with a video otoscope, the tumor mass can be seen and samples taken for further diagnostic testing. Open-mouth rostrooccipital radiographs or lateral views of the tympanic bullae (Figure 7-26) showing opacity of the osseous tympanic bulla may indicate a tumor or polyp of the middle ear. Osteolysis or fluid densities may also be seen. Computed tomography scans are also used to identify lesions within the middle ear.

Routine cleaning of the ear canal and careful examination of the skin surface of the ear canal may reveal small tumors. Good visualization and magnification are mandatory in identifying these very tiny early growths. Larger tumors may be confused with stenoses because they are large and occlude the lumen of the ear canal. Flat tumors may look like edematous ear canals, and sessile tumors have

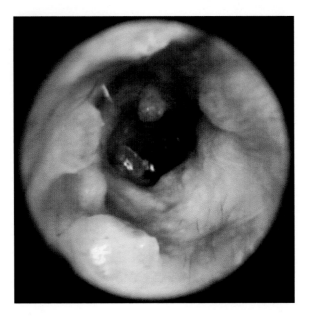

Figure 7-25

In addition to the tumors in the vertical ear canal of this Labrador Retriever, small cerumen gland tumors can be seen in the horizontal ear canal near the intact eardrum. These small tumors are hard to see with conventional otoscopy.

a cobblestone appearance (Figures 7-27 and 7-28). Some tumors are seen only when the otoscope is placed beyond a stenotic portion of the vertical ear canal.

Secondary infection is common in ears that harbor tumors. An obstructive tumor mass allows accumulation of cerumen and debris beyond it. Because the smooth, uniform epithelial surface has been permanently changed, accumulations of wax and serum are found in the deep recesses created by the uneven surface. These crevices promote bacteria and yeast growth. Continued antibiotic or anti-yeast treatment is warranted in the presence of tumors because of the secondary infections and inflammation commonly associated with aural neoplasms. If the eardrum is intact, flushing the ear canal with detergent ear cleaners is beneficial for removing the cerumen and debris. If the eardrum cannot be visualized, however, caution in selecting a non-ototoxic ear cleaner is warranted.

Gross Examination

On gross examination, tumors of the ear canal can have a variety of topographic features. They may be raised (Figure 7-29), pedunculated, broad based, lobulated, irregular (Figure 7-30), or ulcerated, or they may have a combination of these features.

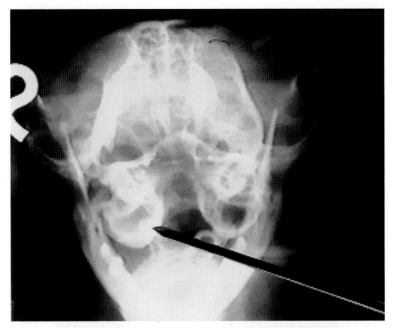

Figure 7-26

Open-mouth rostrooccipital radiograph of a cat with a unilateral nasopharyngeal polyp and otitis media. Notice the thickened tympanic bulla and the opacified bulla lumen *(pointer)*. (Courtesy Dr. Gary Lantz, Purdue University.)

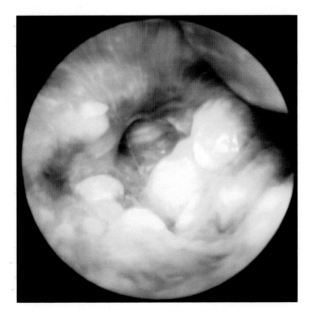

Figure 7-27

Flat, broad-based cerumen gland adenomas can be confused with edema or tissue maceration.

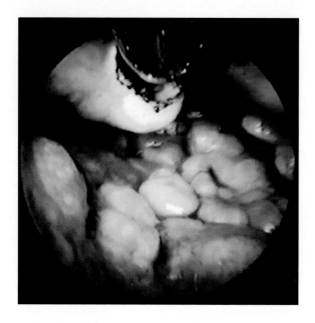

Figure 7-28

Protruding cerumen gland adenoma and cobblestone adenomas in the same ear canal as in Figure 7-27.

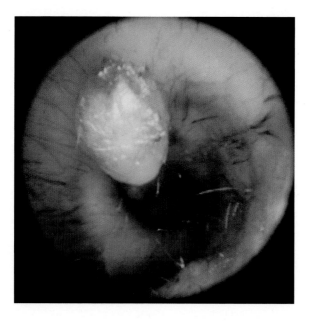

Figure 7-29

Solitary cerumen gland adenoma in an otherwise normal ear canal.

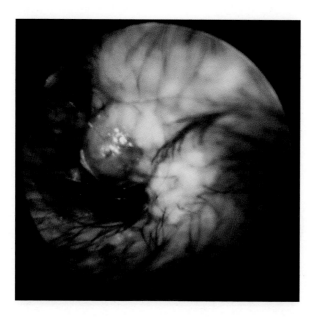

Figure 7-30

Irregular, broad-based cerumen gland adenoma. Smaller tumors surround the larger tumor mass.

For small tumors, tissue for histopathologic evaluation may be obtained by curetting the tumor with a sharp-edged curette (Figure 7-31). An endoscopic biopsy tool may be used to grasp and remove a section of tumor (Figure 7-32). In the case of a large solitary tumor or a diffuse spreading tumor mass, a portion of the ear canal is removed surgically, and the entire section of ear canal is submitted to the pathologist. Tissue architecture is preserved in this manner, and the pathologist can better characterize the lesion as benign or malignant. Fortunately, the circumferential cartilage of the external ear canal provides a limiting barrier to the spread of most malignant tumors. If the ear tumor and the cartilage can be submitted to the pathologist, the invasiveness of the tumor can also be determined.

Exfoliative cytologic evaluation is often adequate for differentiating inflammatory from hyperplastic and neoplastic lesions. A curette is used to obtain scrapings from a suspected tumor. If the cells indicate an inflammatory lesion (neutrophils, macrophages, lymphocytes, plasma cells, and eosinophils), appropriate antiinflammatory treatment may be instituted. If, however, clumps and clusters of large round cells are found, an epithelial neoplasm is a diagnostic possibility and the slide should be submitted to the pathologist for evaluation. Single spindle-shaped cells may indicate fibrosis or a nonepithelial type of neoplasm.

It has been theorized that chronic inflammation, more common in the dog than in the cat, may initiate progression of otic lesions from hyperplasia to dysplasia to neoplasia. It has also been speculated that bacterial degradation of the apocrine

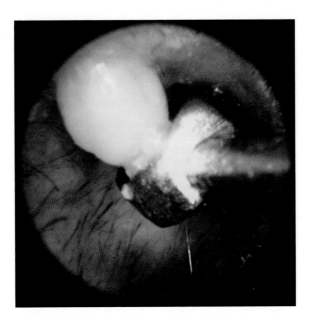

Figure 7-31

Removal of the tumor mass shown in Figure 7-29. A 6-mm dermal curette with a sharp edge has been placed over the mass. Angling the curette to cut the base of the tumor allows its removal.

secretions from the cerumen glands that become inspissated in the ear canal during episodes of otitis externa may result in increased carcinogenesis. Whether the presence of a tumor leads to the chronic inflammation or chronic inflammation leads to dysplastic changes and eventually to neoplastic changes is not known.

Ear canal tumors can develop in any of the skin structures lining the ear canal, including the squamous epithelium, ceruminous or sebaceous glands, and the mesenchymal structures (Figure 7-33). Tumors arising from the external ear canal and pinna are much more common than tumors arising from the middle or inner ear.

Much controversy exists concerning the incidence of the various tumors reported in dogs and cats. Because of the difficulty in obtaining samples from the ear canal, most samples submitted to diagnostic laboratories are submitted from university or referral surgeons and not from general practitioners. The number of tumors of the ear submitted for evaluation is therefore low.

Tumors of the ear canal are relatively uncommon in dogs and cats. In one report, of all tumors found in cats, only 1% to 2% were derived from aural tissue. In a second report, of all the canine aural tissue sent to different laboratories for histopathologic evaluation, 2% to 6% contained tumors. Generally, tumors of the ear canal in dogs tend to be benign, and tumors of the ear canal in the cat tend to be more malignant. Fortunately, malignant neoplasms of the ear canal rarely metastasize. Failure to remove a wide en bloc section of the ear canal, however, often results in

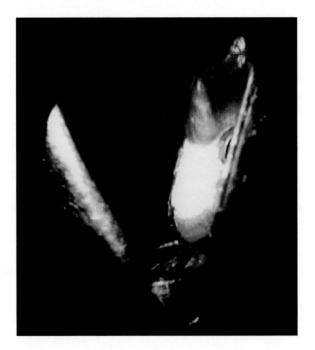

Figure 7-32

A 1.8-mm endoscopic biopsy tool was placed through the 2-mm working channel of the Video Vetscope to take a "bite" of the tumor for histopathologic evaluation.

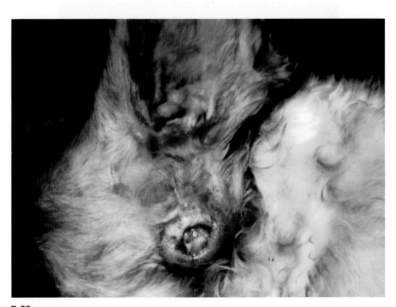

Figure 7-33

Tumor mass protruding from the horizontal canal of this Cocker Spaniel that had a previous vertical ear canal ablation. The mass was described by the pathologist as a liposarcoma.

local recurrence of tumor. Total ear canal ablation may be the best surgical solution to ear neoplasia.

Most reports indicate that benign cerumen gland adenoma is the most common tumor of the dog's ear and that malignant ceruminous gland adenocarcinoma is the most common neoplasm of the cat's ear. However, histopathologic differentiation of the two types of ceruminous neoplasms is not always clear. Other benign tumors found in the ear canal of dogs are polyps, papilloma, sebaceous gland adenoma, histiocytoma, plasmacytoma, benign melanoma, and fibroma. Malignant canine neoplasms of the ear that have been reported are ceruminous gland adenocarcinomas, carcinoma of undetermined origin, squamous cell carcinoma, round cell tumor, sarcoma, malignant melanoma, and hemangiosarcoma.

Benign tumors of the cat's ear include polyps, cerumen gland adenoma, and papillomas. Malignant tumors of the cat's ear are ceruminous gland adenocarcinoma, squamous cell carcinoma, carcinoma of undetermined origin, and sebaceous gland adenocarcinoma.

Tumors found in the middle ear are rare and include fibrosarcoma (Figure 7-34) and lymphoma.

Treatment of neoplasia found in the ear canals of dogs and cats requires surgical intervention so that the tumor mass can be completely excised. Newer modalities such as electrosurgery and laser surgery through a video otoscope (Video Vetscope, MedRx, Inc., Largo, Florida) make removal of ear canal tumors easier.

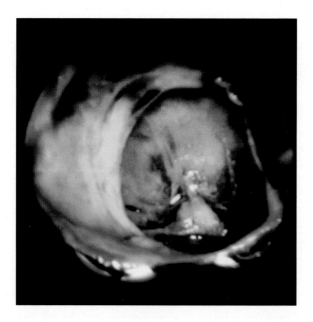

Figure 7-34

Middle ear fibrosarcoma. A fleshy mass was seen in the middle ear. Myringotomy revealed a large infiltrating mass filling the tympanic bulla. Histopathologic analysis of a biopsy specimen revealed fibrosarcoma.

Histopathologic evaluation of removed tissues helps in providing a prognosis of the disease. For malignancies, follow-up radiation therapy has been shown to be effective in preventing recurrence of many ear canal tumors, especially cerumen gland adenocarcinoma of cats.

Suggested Readings

Gotthelf LN: Secondary otitis media: an often overlooked condition, *Canine Pract* 20:14-20, 1995.

Logas D, Rosychuck RAW, Merchant SR: Diseases of the ear canal, *Vet Clin North Am Small Anim Pract* 24(5):905-980, 1994.

London CA, Dubilzeig RR, Vail DM, et al: Evaluation of dogs and cats with tumors of the ear canal: 145 cases (1978-1992), *J Am Vet Med Assoc* 208:1413-1418, 1996.

Moisan PG, Watson GL: Ceruminous gland tumors in dogs and cats: a review of 124 cases, *J Am Anim Hosp Assoc* 32:449-453, 1996.

Rogers KS: Tumors of the ear canal, *Vet Clin North Am Small Anim Pract* 18:859-868, 1988.

Theon AP, Barthez PY, Madewell BR, et al: Radiation therapy of ceruminous gland carcinomas in dogs and cats, *J Am Vet Med Assoc* 205:566-569, 1994.

van der Gaag I: The pathology of the external ear canal in dogs and cats, *Vet Q* 8:307-317, 1986.

8

Perpetuating Factors and Treatment of Otitis Externa

Louis N. Gotthelf, DVM

Otitis externa is a common malady, occurring in 15% to 20% of dogs and 5% to 7% of cats seen in veterinary practice. Otitis externa is also one of the most frustrating diseases for veterinarians and owners to treat effectively. Treatment regimens vary widely, and a myriad of products containing a variety of ingredients are available for the treatment of ear disease.

Effective treatment of otitis externa often varies from one patient to another; treatments successful in one patient may not help in the next. Each patient and each ear must be considered individually, and treatment regimens must be tailored to the specific case.

In addition, dermatologic conditions often affect the ear canal, making it susceptible to otitis externa. The ear canal is an invagination of epidermis forming a hollow skin tube inside the head; it begins at the eardrum. Pathologic mechanisms affecting the skin of the animal also affect the epithelial tube lining the ear canal. For example, a dog with atopy may also show inflammation of the ear canal, resulting in redness, swelling, heat, and pain (Figures 8-1 and 8-2). In a cylindrical tube such as

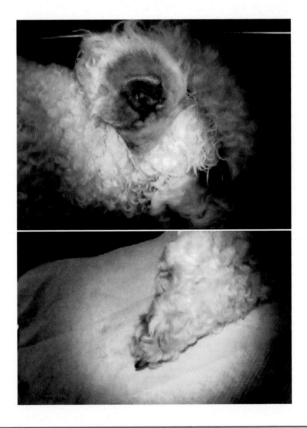

Figure 8-1

Top, Red, hot, itchy ear in a Miniature Poodle with otitis externa. *Bottom,* Salivary staining on the foot of the same dog indicates atopic dermatitis as the cause of the otitis. Often there is concomitant *Malassezia* dermatitis between the toes of these dogs.

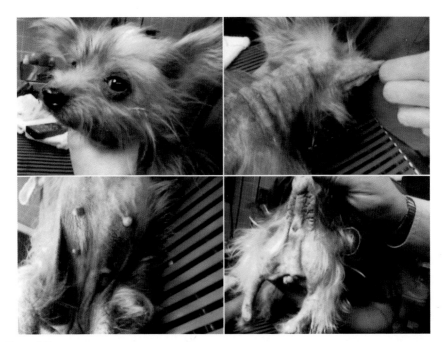

Figure 8-2

Underlying skin disease predisposes the ear to secondary bacterial or yeast infection. The patient, a 5-year-old Yorkshire Terrier with severe allergic skin disease complicated with *Malassezia* dermatitis, also had severe *Malassezia* otitis externa.

the ear canal, inflammation decreases the lumen diameter, tending to reduce both the ventilation and drying of the ear canal. Without ventilation, the humidity level of the ear canal rises, a factor favorable for bacterial growth.

Papules, pustules, crusts, ulcers, and alopecia that may occur on the skin of the trunk may also occur on the skin of the ear canal. Because the ear canal is L-shaped, exudates from these lesions tend to accumulate in the horizontal portion of the ear canal (Figure 8-3). In the treatment of skin disease, shampoo therapy, using a variety of compounds formulated for specific purposes, acts to remove irritating substances and improve healing. In the ear canal, ear flushing solutions containing a variety of ingredients are also used for adjunctive therapy of disease of the ear canal.

New approaches to the medical management of otitis externa in dogs and cats have now been introduced. They include (1) cytologic evaluation of exudates to identify disease processes and determine the type of disease organisms that may be present; (2) flushing products to remove exudates and to disinfect the canal epithelium; and (3) elucidations of pathophysiologic mechanisms showing that otitis externa is a secondary manifestation of underlying skin disease. New combinations of topical medications have been formulated to be effective against bacteria, fungi, and inflammation. The fluoroquinolone antibiotics, injectable ivermectin, and topical fipronil

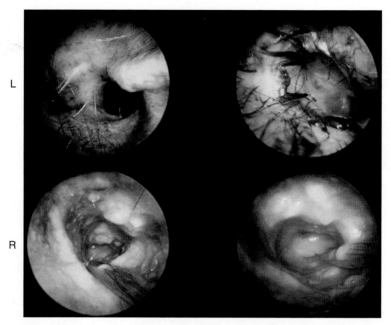

Figure 8-3

Left and right ear canals from a dog with atopic dermatitis. *Top,* The left ear canal *(left)* and eardrum *(right)* are normal. *Bottom,* The right ear canal *(left)* is severely inflamed and ulcerated and there is a thick exudate composed cytologically of rods and neutrophils. Culture revealed *Pseudomonas.* When the ear canal was flushed, there was no eardrum in that ear. Infection had moved through the eardrum into the tympanic bulla, resulting in secondary otitis media. Hyposensitization of this dog allowed complete resolution of this dog's otitis after 1 year.

for ear mite infestations have reduced the use of potentially ototoxic antibiotics, oils, and insecticides in the ear canal.

Cytologic Evaluation

The first stop in approaching ear disease is to examine a cytologic preparation of the otic exudates. Examination of a prepared ear smear gives the clinician a starting point for treatment based on the presence of yeasts, cocci, or rod bacteria.

Obtaining samples and preparing a slide to examine constitute a simple procedure that should be a part of the minimum approach to every case of otitis presented to the veterinarian. A sample is obtained with the use of a small cotton-tipped applicator. The swab is inserted through a disinfected otoscope cone positioned near the horizontal canal. The swab is extended beyond the plastic cone, and pressure is applied to the ear canal epithelium as the swab is drawn back through the cone. Every attempt is made to sample from the horizontal canal epithelium only because the vertical canal is often contaminated with a number of commensal organisms unrelated to the ear disease.

The material collected on the swab is rolled onto a clean microscope slide, with the exudates from the left ear on the left part of the slide and the sample from the right ear on the right side. The slide is appropriately labeled with the patient's name, the date of the collection, and which sample is from which ear. It is then heat fixed and stained with a modified Wright's blood stain. A drop of slide-mounting medium is placed over the dried, stained material. Then a coverslip is placed on top of the drop, and the glue is allowed to set. The use of slide-mounting medium makes a permanent record of the cytologic characteristics, which can be stored for comparison at subsequent examinations. Alternatively, immersion oil can be smeared along the stained slide and examined.

Examination of the slide under low-power magnification allows an overall view of the cellular debris. High-power examination can help identify and quantify organisms. Cytologic evaluation is very helpful in detecting bacteria and yeasts responsible for secondary infection. Normal commensal bacteria may be found, but in otitis, abnormal increases in numbers of organisms to the point of almost a pure culture, the presence of neutrophils, or both indicate secondary bacterial infection. Often only one ear is affected clinically, but the same organism may be found in the unaffected ear. Sometimes each ear of the same animal has a different organism and needs a different treatment. The severity of the otitis may also be different in the two ears.

When infectious organisms are seen under high-power (400×) magnification, cocci are usually *Staphylococcus,* and rods are usually *Pseudomonas* or *Proteus.* Budding yeasts of *Malassezia* may be seen individually in the background on a roll smear, but large numbers of yeasts colonizing on exfoliated epithelium indicate secondary yeast infection. *Staphylococcus* and *Malassezia* are often found together in the same ear, and there is evidence to suggest that *Malassezia* growth is stimulated by *Staphylococcus.*

Bacterial culture and sensitivity testing of exudates may be useful in cases of resistant otitis externa. Many organisms have developed resistance to the routinely used antibiotics, and they should be identified. A limitation of bacterial sensitivity testing is that the organism's sensitivity or resistance is reported by the laboratory on the basis of the minimum inhibitory concentration (MIC) of the antibiotic in the blood required to kill the bacteria. Topical antibiotics can achieve significantly higher concentrations in the ear canal than systemic antibiotics can in the blood. The high topical antibiotic concentration may actually be effective at killing a bacterium that was reported as resistant. Samples for culture should be taken from the horizontal canal if possible, so that contaminant bacteria are not mistaken for the offending organism. Routine culture of exudates in all cases of otitis is often unrewarding and extremely misleading because four or five bacterial isolates are often reported.

Roll-smear cytologic evaluation becomes useful in determining the etiology of cases of otitis externa without secondary infection. Sheets of epithelial cells may indicate neoplasia as the cause of otitis externa, and the presence of numerous intact nonstaining epithelial cells may indicate a seborreic condition. Parasites such as *Otodectes* and *Demodex,* which may be present in the ceruminous exudates, may be found on cytologic preparations, but these parasites are better viewed on a direct mineral oil preparation; this type of preparation is made by rolling the ear swab sample in a drop of mineral oil on a slide. Negative findings on cytology may indicate the need for antiinflammatories only, without the antibiotic or antifungal therapy.

Flushing of the Ear Canal

After the class of disease and the type of infection are determined, the next step is to sedate or anesthetize the animal so that a thorough flushing and suctioning of the ear canal can be done. It is imperative that exudates and dried medications that have accumulated in the ear canal be removed so that the canal epithelium itself can be evaluated. Good visualization of the ear canal after flushing helps to ensure that the vertical and horizontal canals are clean and free of debris (Figure 8-4). The efficacy of otic medications is enhanced when they are applied directly onto the cleaned epithelial surface.

Care must be taken in the selection of a flushing agent because so many ear cleaners contain materials that are potentially ototoxic when the eardrum is not intact (see Chapter 17). Prior to using an ear cleaner, the veterinarian should read the label to see whether it can be used when the eardrum is damaged. Many manufacturers are now placing a warning about this issue on their labels.

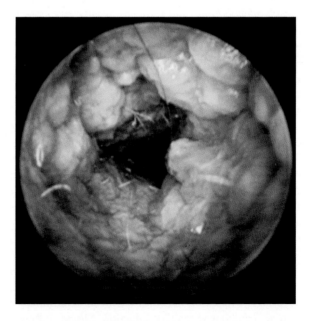

Figure 8-4

Chronic otitis externa is characterized by permanent pathologic changes to the glands and the epithelium. Epithelial proliferation, cerumen gland hyperplasia, and fibrosis result in an uneven surface contour. This photo was taken after the ear canal was cleaned and dried.

Mechanical Ear Cleaning

When the ear canal is full of liquid exudates such as pus, warmed saline or warmed, very dilute povidone-iodine solutions (not iodine scrub, which contains detergents) are safe flushing materials to use. Many types of high-pressure irrigation systems are available that can be used to loosen the exudates, but the pressures in such instruments can be very high, necessitating extra caution to avoid rupturing the eardrum. Many of these new irrigation instruments have controls to adjust the flush pressure. Ear curettes, designed to remove debris firmly attached to the epithelium, are useful for scraping the ear canal to dislodge large pieces of wax and epithelial shreds. Curettes are also useful for harvesting cells for cytologic evaluation when a tumor mass is suspected.

After the external ear canal is flushed, it is cleaned with a catheter attached to suction. With good visualization, small pieces of wax, epithelial flakes, and foreign material can be removed. Flushing and suctioning may need to be repeated several times to ensure that the ear canal is thoroughly cleaned.

Cotton-tipped applicators should never be used to clean ears! When a cotton-tipped applicator is pushed into an ear canal full of exudates, the exudate is pushed farther toward the eardrum, making cleaning more difficult and possibly rupturing a weakened eardrum. Cotton swabs are also very irritating to a friable epithelium, and their use may result in painful abrasion or ulceration of the canal epithelium.

Chemical Cleaning

After it is established that there is an eardrum present, ceruminous exudates can be emulsified by using ceruminolytics. Most of these agents are detergents, which require an aqueous medium to function. Many combination ear cleaners contain dioctyl sodium sulfosuccinate (DSS) as a wax remover. Detergents can be very irritating to ulcerated ears, and they should not be used in ulcerated ear canals. In addition, most detergent ear cleaners are ototoxic.

Only after the ear canal has been cleaned and dried can a determination of the integrity of the eardrum be made. Unfortunately, severely stenotic ear canals often prevent adequate visualization of the eardrum through the otoscope.

Examining the Ear Canal

For examination of the cleaned, dry ear canal, it is helpful to determine whether the otitis externa is acute or chronic. Chronic otitis externa is characterized by epithelial hyperkeratosis, glandular hyperplasia, fibrosis, stricture, and inflammatory cell infiltration of the dermis of the external auditory canal. The changes in surface contour of the ear canal caused by chronic otitis lead to the formation of folds; routine flushing helps uncover offending organisms hidden deep in these folds so that topical antibiotics can gain access to the deeper epithelium.

Pathologic changes associated with otitis externa may extend the entire length of the ear canal and may affect the tympanic membrane. One report involving histopathologic evaluation of postmortem specimens from dogs with chronic otitis demonstrated that hair and keratin originating from the external ear were often found in the middle ear. The tympanic membrane in these specimens could not be identified histologically in a significant number of cases, and when it could be identified, it was often thickened.

When the eardrum is ruptured, exudates drain from the external ear canal into the tympanic bulla. The mucous membrane lining the bulla, the mucoperiosteum, becomes inflamed and can produce copious exudates, complicating the continued treatment of otitis externa. Liquid medications placed into the external ear canal cannot reach the bulla if the canal is already filled with mucus and pus.

Perpetuating Factors

The perpetuating factors that prevent the ear canal from effectively healing include infections with bacteria and yeasts, improper treatment of the ear, overtreatment of the ear with ear cleaners and medications, and otitis media.

Because of the changes in the ear canal that occur as a result of disease, bacteria and yeasts colonize and reproduce. Otitis externa is complicated by the growth of these infectious organisms, which is secondary to a primary disease process. Although antimicrobial therapy may temporarily relieve the symptoms of otitis externa, they may recur unless the underlying disease is identified and treated as well. Concomitant growth and colonization by these organisms are considered to be perpetuating factors in ear disease.

Improper treatment of infectious organisms is a problem and may be the most important reason for treatment failures. Applying ointment medications directly into an ear full of wax results in the ointment being layered on the wax and not penetrating through to the skin of the ear canal, where the infection is present. Treatment of a yeast infection with an antibiotic alone results in failure. Treatment of pseudomonal ear infections with drugs such as cephalexin, clindamycin, and neomycin also results in failure. Treatment with effective systemic antibiotics and antifungals that cannot get into the ear canal to affect the organisms will result in failure.

Colonizing organisms associated with otitis externa include bacteria and yeasts. Members of the genera *Malassezia, Staphylococcus,* and *Pseudomonas* are the organisms most commonly isolated from the ears of dogs. *Corynebacterium, Enterococcus,* and *Proteus* are also frequently isolated. The prevalence of one organism over another is determined by a variety of factors. For example, excessive cerumen production from cerumen gland hyperplasia permits *Malassezia* growth. Water in the ears often leads to *Pseudomonas* infections, whereas the decreased immune function seen with hypothyroidism allows colonization by *Staphylococcus*.

Epidemiologic reports from investigators around the world indicate a wide variety of prevalent organisms found in the ears of dogs with otitis externa. *Malassezia pachydermatis* is commonly found in the author's Alabama practice, but a report from Spain indicates that *Candida albicans* is the most prevalent otic fungal organism isolated there. Interpretation of the literature concerning the most prevalent organisms isolated from ear disease may therefore need to be regionalized. In addition, prevalent organisms may be determined by breed susceptibility to certain primary disease states that result in otitis. For example, acute otitis externa or otitis media in German Shepherds frequently is perpetuated by a secondary *Pseudomonas* infection.

Isolates from the external ear canal do not always correlate with the isolates from the middle ear. *Pseudomonas* may be found more often in the middle ear than the external ear, whereas *Malassezia* is rarely found in the middle ear when the eardrum in intact. Some organisms rarely isolated from the external ear canal of dogs, such as B-hemolytic streptococci, may be found as the prevalent organism in otitis media.

Frequently, otitis externa resists topical treatment because infection extends through the tympanic membrane into the tympanic bulla, causing otitis media. This secondary otitis media occurs in approximately 16% of cases of acute otitis externa and in as many as 50% of cases of chronic otitis externa. Primary otitis media (extension of infection from the nasopharynx through the auditory tube to the tympanic bulla) is rare in the dog but is often seen in cats with nasopharyngeal polyps.

Studies in dogs have suggested that otitis media may be more common than previously recognized. In many dogs with otitis externa with intact eardrums, significant bacterial populations may also be isolated from the middle ear. These dogs may have had eardrum rupture that healed, trapping bacteria in the tympanic bulla.

Treatment

Corticosteroids have a definite place in the treatment of otitis externa. Systemic corticosteroids reduce both the intense pruritus associated with acute otitis externa and the inflammation in the epithelium of the ear canal. High-dose systemic corticosteroids (prednisone, 1 mg/lb daily for 2 weeks, then reduce) are used for several days to reduce the edema and stenosis that prevent adequate examination of the ear canal. If the ear canal is patent, a potent topical corticosteroid such as dexamethasone, triamcinolone, betamethasone, or fluocinolone may be used to relieve the intense pain and itching. Otic corticosteroids can be absorbed systemically from the ears, especially if they are severely inflamed or ulcerated, and they can depress the pituitary-adrenal axis, resulting in iatrogenic hyperadrenocorticism. As the otitis resolves, a less potent corticosteroid such as 1% hydrocortisone may be used in the ear to prevent inflammation in atopic dogs that may have recurrent otitis.

Antibiotics that kill *Staphylococcus, Pseudomonas,* and other gram-negative bacteria are used in many otic preparations. They may be formulated with other topical pharmaceuticals such as antifungals, corticosteroids, insecticides, and topical anesthetics. Antibiotics such as gentamicin, neomycin, and polymyxin B are potentially ototoxic, so if the patient has no eardrum, these antibiotics should be avoided. In addition, neomycin has been implicated as a sensitizer in contact dermatitis in the ear. If the ear becomes worse with neomycin treatment, the antibiotic should be stopped immediately. Although an aminoglycoside antibiotic, ophthalmic tobramycin solution can be safely instilled into the external ear canal to treat resistant bacterial infections.

Fluoroquinolones are used in otic formulations, but their use should be reserved for *Pseudomonas* infections that do not respond to other antibiotics. Because of the resistance problem emerging due to the improper use of fluoroquinolones, they should not be the first choice for bacterial otitis externa. Enrofloxacin/silver sulfadiazine (Baytril Otic, Bayer) is an effective formulation for otitis externa. The ototoxicity of silver is unknown at this time, but it has been known to cause inflammation and flaking of the skin of the ear canal and pinna. Although not labeled for otic use, injectable fluoroquinolones are used by the author in a variety of forms. The drug may be instilled directly into the ear as a bulla infusion to obtain very high tissue levels quickly. An enrofloxacin topical otic solution can be made by mixing 2 ml of injectable enrofloxacin with 13 ml of artificial tears. Also, 2 ml of injectable enrofloxacin (Baytril Inection, Bayer) mixed in an 8-ml bottle of dimethyl sulfoxide (DMSO) with fluocinolone (Synotic) provides a potent antibiotic, antiinflammatory combination. This solution is unstable and should not be used for more than 5 days. Ciprofloxacin 0.3% eye drops can also be used in the ear. A new topical otic fluoroquinolone, ofloxacin, has been shown to be safe and effective in children with suppurative otitis media. In Europe, a marbofloxacin/clotrimazole/dexamethasone combination veterinary product is available to treat otitis externa (Aurizon, Vetoquinol).

Ticarcillin has been used in severe cases of *Pseudomonas* otitis externa, both as a topical infusion into the tympanic bulla and as an intravenous antibiotic. This antibiotic is very expensive, and the intravenous route of administration requires the patient to be in the hospital for treatment. A treatment regimen is described using 1 to 2 mg/kg prednisolone orally once daily and a cleansing and drying ear cleaner, followed by topical administration of injectable ticarcillin solution four times daily. The patient with a ruptured eardrum receives 15 to 25 mg/kg ticarcillin three times daily intravenously until the membrane heals. Topical ticarcillin and the ear cleaner are continued twice daily for 14 days after clinical resolution. The duration of treatment ranges from 14 to 36 days. Reactions to intravenous ticarcillin have been seen in dogs.

Silver sulfadiazine cream has been used to treat resistant *Pseudomonas* infections. A small amount of the cream is dispersed in a volume of normal saline to make a 1% solution and is used as an ear drop twice daily. This compound has the potential to cause inflammation in the ear canal and may be ototoxic.

Another useful compound for resistant ear infections is ethylenediamine tetraacetic acid–tris (tris-EDTA) in alkaline solution. The solution can be mixed up in the veterinary hospital and dispensed fresh (Box 8-1). This mixture is also available commercially for the treatment of otitis externa (TrizEDTA, DermaPet, Inc., T8 Solution, DVM). Tris-EDTA is particularly useful for otitis externa caused by gramnegative bacteria. It affects the cell membranes of bacteria by chelating minerals such as calcium and magnesium, essentially "stripping off" the outer membrane layer, rendering the membranes more porous so that the antibiotic can diffuse into the bacteria and kill them. Even if culture and sensitivity results indicate that a gram-negative bacterium is resistant to a certain antibiotic in vitro, pretreatment with tris-EDTA may render the organism sensitive to the antibiotic in vivo. Tris-EDTA is used as a pretreatment in the external ear 5 minutes before the

---

BOX 8-1   Tris-EDTA Ear Solution for Gram-Negative Ear Infections

---

HOW TO MAKE

1. Mix:
   EDTA (disodium salt) 1.2 g
   Tris (tromethamine) (Trizma, Sigma Chemical) 6.05 g
   Distilled water 1 L
   Glacial acetic acid 1 ml
2. Adjust pH to 8.0 with additional glacial acetic acid.
3. Autoclave and store sterile.
4. Dispense in 4-ounce bottles. Keep refrigerated.

HOW TO USE (TWICE DAILY)

1. Fill ear canal with tris-EDTA solution.
2. Wait 5 minutes, then wipe out any excess with a cotton ball.
3. Immediately instill antibiotic solution into the ear canal.

---

instillation of topical antibiotics, most of which require an alkaline medium for maximum efficacy.

Alterations in cerumen lipid composition caused by underlying skin diseases such as atopy or hypthyroidism may play a role in the pathogenesis of *Malassezia* otitis externa. Low levels of free fatty acids in surface lipids coupled with increased levels of surface triglycerides favor *Malassezia* infections. *Malassezia* growth is inhibited in an acid medium, so manufacturers of otic products directed against *Malassezia* usually formulate them with organic acids that provide an intra-otic pH in the range of 4.5 to 5.0. Lactic, acetic, salicylic, malic, citric, boric, and benzoic acids are all used to acidify the ear canal. For otitis externa complicated by *Malassezia*, the author prefers the use of a combination of acetic acid and boric acid solution (Malacetic Otic, DermaPet). The cleansing and desquamating effects of the acetic acid solution essentially remove fatty acid substrates necessary for the metabolism and reproduction of *Malassezia*. This organism produces a chemotactic factor for neutrophils that is a hydrophilic protein. The presence of this factor may help explain why only a few *Malassezia* organisms can cause such profound erythema and pruritus. The cleansing effect of the acetic acid–boric acid solution removes this chemoat-tractant and may account for the reduction in inflammation. Boric acid, which is hygroscopic (drying out the humid ear canal), removes moisture necessary for this hydrophilic chemoattractant. Boric acid also dehydrates the surface of the epithelial cells lining the ear canal so the *Malassezia* yeasts cannot reattach to them. Wiping the ear cleaner on the lower part of the concave pinna also aids in decreasing the numbers of yeasts in the ear canal.

It has been demonstrated that more than 50% of atopic dogs with pruritic skin disease may have increased cutaneous *Malassezia* populations. Humans with atopic dermatitis also demonstrate *Malassezia* infections. With *Malassezia* otitis externa, treatment failures are frequent even though there appears to be temporary resolution of symptoms. Presumably, these "relapses" are often related to the initial diminution of inflammation due to the corticosteroid used in the ear medications or administered parenterally in atopic patients. The reduction in inflammation reduces clinical symptoms, but when the topical medication is discontinued and the infectious organism is still present, symptoms of erythema and pruritus reappear.

Follow-Up

Because veterinarians rely on pet owners to follow their prescribed therapeutic protocols, time spent explaining proper ear care to clients helps them treat their animals' ears as prescribed. Clients should understand the need for frequent rechecks to monitor the progress of the pet with otitis externa. Too often patients are sent home with ear drops and then are not seen again until the otitis externa flares up. Scheduling a recheck visit allows the veterinarian to change therapy if there is no response.

The external canal can be cleaned by the owner at home to facilitate removal of excessive exudate accumulation associated with otitis externa or otitis media. The author prefers an acetic acid–boric acid solution for *Malassezia* infection and tris-EDTA for bacterial otitis for home use, because they are antiseptic and non-ototoxic. The procedure is as follows:

- The ear canal is filled with the cleaning solution until it overflows.
- The canal is externally massaged for 5 minutes.
- The loosened debris is wiped off the external opening of the ear canal and pinna with a dry cotton ball.
- Limit the daily use of ear cleaners to 14 days. After the ear is clean, a maintenance ear cleaning once or twice weekly will prevent maceration of the ear canal epithelium.

This procedure is repeated daily at home until the recheck visit. An anti-yeast or antibacterial medication can be applied after the ear cleaning.

A 2-week recheck is required to determine the success of the therapy. If there is progress, then the regimen is continued until the cytology is negative and the patient is free of symptoms. If there are bacteria, yeasts, or white blood cells on subsequent recheck, the therapy needs to be changed accordingly.

Overtreatment of otitis externa with ear cleaners and liquid medications may indeed clear up the infection, but because the surface epithelium is macerated from all of the liquid, the ear canal remains swollen. If the cytology is negative and the inflammation has subsided, intensive ear cleaning should be stopped completely, or a maintenance schedule should be provided to the owner. Overcleaning of the normal ear canal removes much of the cerumen, which is beneficial to the ear canal, providing a moisture barrier for the ear.

A good prognostic sign that uncomplicated otitis externa is resolving is to see regrowth of hair in the vertical canal. Most of the exudates formed in the acute phase of otitis externa have a depilatory effect on the hair, so the hair falls out. When the inflammation subsides and the exudates are not dissolving hairs, hair regrowth can occur.

Frequently, after the otitis externa has resolved, the client is willing to allow the veterinarian to look for the underlying cause of the ear disease with a hypoallergenic food trial, allergy testing, or endocrine assays. Failure to identify and treat any underlying disease results in chronic otitis externa.

Suggested Readings

Foster AP, DeBoer DJ: The role of *Pseudomonas* in canine ear disease, *Compend Cont Ed* 20:909-918, 1998.

Gotthelf LN, Young SE: New treatment of *Malassezia* otitis externa in dogs, *Vet Forum* 14:46-53, 1997.

Harvey RG: *Aspects of the interaction between skin and staphylococci,* Bayer Selected Proceedings of the North American Veterinary Conference, January 1998.

Kiss G, Radvanyi S, Szigeti G: New combination for the therapy of canine otitis externa: microbiology of otitis externa and efficacy in vivo and in vitro, *J Small Anim Pract* 38:51-60, 1997.

Merchant SR, Bellah JJ: Otitis symposium, *Vet Med* 92:517-550, 1997.

Nuttall TJ: Use of ticarcillin in the management of canine otitis externa complicated by *Pseudomonas aeruginosa, J Small Anim Pract 39*:165-168, 1998.

Powell MB, Weisbroth SH, Roth L, et al: Reaginic hypersensitivity in *Otodectes cyanotis* infestation of cats and mode of mite feeding, *Am J Vet Res* 41:877-882, 1980.

Trevor PB, Martin RA: Tympanic bulla osteotomy for treatment of middle-ear disease in cats: 19 cases (1984-1991), *J Am Vet Med Assoc* 202:123-128, 1993.

9

Microbiology of the Ear of the Dog and Cat

Sandra R. Merchant, DVM

Otitis Externa

Otitis externa is a very common problem in the dog. It is seen less often in the cat. The prevalence of disease in the dog has been reported to be between 10% and 20% of total patient admissions, with the prevalence in the cat being 2% to 10%. Many factors may predispose an animal to ear disease, including allergy, disorders of keratinization, parasites, foreign bodies, autoimmune diseases, treatment errors, nutritional factors, hormonal factors, and any process that interferes with epithelial migration and desquamation, including benign and malignant tumors. All of these factors serve to alter the microenvironment of the ear canal.

Successful treatment relies on proper diagnosis and correction of any primary, predisposing, or perpetuating factors. It is important to evaluate and correct, if possible, any alterations in the microclimate of the external ear canal. The normalization of the microclimate aids in keeping an ear disease free, after all other factors have been identified and addressed.

Structure of the External Ear Canal

The epidermis of the ear canal is similar in structure to that of the interfollicular epidermis of the skin. However, from a gross anatomic standpoint, this epidermis is rolled into a tube, forcing the glandular secretions of the sebaceous and apocrine glands into a canal instead of to the skin, where the secretions can be more easily removed by the normal keratinization and desquamation process of the epidermis. Further modifications of the anatomy such as pendulous ears or excessive ear canal hair result in significantly more otitis externa than that seen with other ear types. Dogs with erect ears, regardless of the amount of ear canal hair, have less risk of developing otitis externa than mongrel dogs. In humans and in the guinea pig, and presumably in the dog and cat, the superficial epidermis and keratinized stratum corneum migrate laterally from the tympanum. This process keeps the proximal ear canal and tympanum free from cerumen and debris.

Microclimate of the External Ear Canal

The principal factor affecting the microflora within the external ear canal is the microenvironment. In several studies the temperature within the external ear canals of dogs measured between 38.2° to 38.4°C (100.7° to 101.1°F). There was no significant difference between breeds of dog or whether the pinnae were pendulous. The temperature within the external ear canal rises if otitis externa is present, to a mean of 38.9°C (102°F). Even when environmental temperature increased, there was only a small rise in the temperature of the external ear canal, illustrating how the environment within the ear canal is buffered to a degree from the external environment.

The relative humidity of the external ear canal in one study of 19 dogs was 80.4%. This was stable through the day, rising only 2.3%, compared with the 24% rise in the humidity of the external environment. However, this increase in average humidity from a relatively high baseline may predispose the canal epithelium to becoming over-hydrated and macerated, creating a more ideal environment for bacterial proliferation.

The pH of the external ear canal in normal dogs is 4.6 to 7.2, with a mean of 6.1 in males and 6.2 in females. The pH is seen to change in otitis externa, with a mean of 5.9 (range 5.9 to 7.2) in acute cases and 6.8 (range 6.0 to 7.4) in chronic cases. The data from this study were analyzed by another author, who showed that in cases of otitis externa associated with *Pseudomonas* spp. the pH was significantly higher (mean of 6.85) than in cases of otitis externa in which no *Pseudomonas* was isolated (mean of 5.7). Thus pH either seems to play an important role in the predominant type of bacteria colonizing the ear canal, or the bacteria and its products alter the pH of the environment.

Cerumen coats the lining of the external ear canal. It is composed of lipid secretions from the sebaceous gland and apocrine (ceruminous) glands mixed with sloughed epithelial cells. The lipid content of cerumen from a normal ear canal of a dog can vary widely (18.2% to 92.6%), as does the type of lipid within the cerumen. The types of cerumen lipids found in normal dog ears were cholesterol, 100%; cholesterol esters, 93.8%; free fatty acids, 93.8%; fatty aldehydes, 93.8%; waxes, 93.8%; triglycerides, 68.8%; lecithin, 56.3%; and sphingomyelin, 18.8%. The methodology used in the study was not able to detect small amounts of lipids; therefore this list of lipids accounts for only the major lipids found in the canine ear canal.[1]

The total amount of lipid in the cerumen also varies considerably in dogs with otitis externa (4.3% to 69.6% of cerumen) and is significantly lower than that from healthy ears. This may be due to pathologic changes in the glands responsible for the formation of cerumen. The apocrine glands are thought to maintain the consistency of the cerumen, although they probably contribute little in the way of lipids. Lipids excreted by sebaceous glands probably constitute a large proportion of cerumen lipids. In chronic otitis externa the apocrine glands become hyperplastic and cystic, whereas the sebaceous gland can vary from hypertrophic to atrophic. This may cause pathologic changes of the cerumen in otitic ears, producing a generally lower lipid yield. The high lipid content of normal cerumen helps maintain normal keratinization of the epidermis and aids in the capture and excretion of debris that is produced within. The high lipid content also results in a relatively lower humidity within the lumen of the ear canal. With a decrease in secretion by the sebaceous glands or a dilutional effect by increased production by the apocrine glands, humidity within the ear canal rises, and maceration, followed by otic inflammation and infection, results.

Microbiology of the External Ear Canal

Common diagnostic tests used to evaluate an animal with ear disease include otoscopy, cytology, and bacterial culture and sensitivity. Since the normal ear canal is not a sterile environment, cytologic results, as well as results from culture and sensitivity testing, must be viewed in conjunction with information obtained from a thorough otoscopic examination. On otoscopic examination of the normal ear canal, a small amount of yellowish-brown wax may be seen. There should be no erosion, ulceration, or inflammation of the epidermal lining. The ear canal should be able to accommodate an average-size otoscopic cone without undue pressure on the sides of the canal. The tympanic membrane should be easily visualized in a willing patient.

A cytologic examination of exudate from the ear of a patient with otitis externa should be performed during each examination. Samples can be taken with a dry, cotton-tipped swab placed as far into the canal as is comfortable and safe—usually to the junction of the vertical and horizontal canals. Obtained exudate is placed on a slide and mixed with mineral oil to examine for ear mites. A second sample should be rolled on a slide and stained with either a Wright-Giemsa stain, modified Wright-Giemsa stain, or Gram's stain. If the exudate is greasy or waxy, heat fixation before staining may be helpful. The stained slides should be examined with the low- (100×) and high- (1000×) power objectives of the microscope. A low-power scan permits rapid evaluation of the smear and identification of the best area(s) of the slide for high-power examination. Otic parasites will be seen at low power (Figure 9-1). High-power oil immersion (1000×) evaluation permits quantitation of yeast and examination for bacteria.

Smears should be evaluated for (1) the number and morphology of bacteria, (2) the number of yeasts, (3) the presence of fungal elements, (4) the presence of parasites, (5) the number and types of leukocytes and whether they contain phago-cytized microorganisms, (6) the presence of excessive cerumen, (7) the presence of excessive keratinaceous debris, and (8) the presence of neoplastic cells.

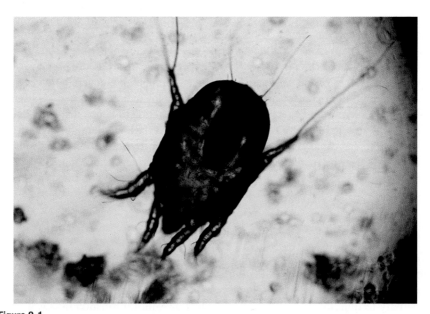

Figure 9-1

Gravid female *Otodectes cynotis* from a dog ear smear (magnification 100×).

The physical characteristics of the material collected from the external ear canal may provide clues as to the underlying cause. The normal ear canal should have small quantities of yellowish to light brown nonodiferous ceruminous discharge. Dark yellow to light brown discharge is seen in ears infected with gram-positive cocci. Pale yellow, thick, sweet, or sewer-smelling purulent exudates are noted in ears infected with gram-negative rods. Copious, dark brown, waxy, or "yeasty" smelling exudates are seen with the yeast *Malassezia canis*. Dark brown or black, crumbly exudate resembling coffee grounds suggests the presence of the parasitic mite *Otodectes cynotis*. A white exudate with no odor, resembling melted candle wax, is often seen after resolution of infection in cases of chronic otitis externa. There is no evidence cytologically of any microorganisms in this exudate, just continued excessive oily or waxy cerumen of hyperplastic ears. Combinations of the various etiologic agents lead to alterations of the characteristics listed previously.

On microscopic evaluation, gram-positive cocci, most often staphylococci, occur singly, in pairs, or in short chains. Streptococci will also be gram positive, but the cocci are usually smaller. Streptococci do not commonly form chains when observed in smears from ear infections. Medium sized gram-negative rods are most likely to be *Pseudomonas, Proteus,* or *Escherichia coli.* Small beaded or club-shaped gram-positive rods are likely to be *Corynebacterium.* The presence of large gram-positive rods in gram-stained smears suggest the presence of *Bacillus* or its anaerobic counterpart *Clostridium. Malassezia canis* occurs as an oval-shaped yeast in which the buds are broad based. As a result of budding the *M. canis* often appear peanut-shaped. In the Gram's stain, *M. canis* is gram variable.

The normal cytology of the external ear canal is characterized by the presence of squamous epithelial cells and low numbers of commensal but potentially pathogenic microorganisms, including *M. canis* and *Staphylococcus intermedius.* There is some debate as to whether *M. canis* is a primary pathogen; however, it is found three times more frequently in ears with otitis externa than in normal ears. *M. canis* is the most common organism demonstrated in ear specimens. It has been isolated in up to 49% of normal dogs and 23% of normal cats. In dogs, *M. canis* has been isolated in up to 80% of otitis externa cases and is probably the most common complicating factor of allergic otitis. In one study it was proven that *M. canis* in the presence of extraneous influences of atraumatic manipulation or moisture enhanced the conditions necessary for proliferation of the organisms and gross and microscopic evidence of otitis externa, establishing this organism as an opportunistic pathogen.[2] On cytologic examination, there are usually few to no leukocytes unless bacteria are also present with the broad-based budding yeasts.

The significance of numbers of *M. canis* or bacterial organisms found on cytologic evaluation varies among authors. Few pure quantitative studies concerning populations of bacteria and yeast residing in the external ear canal are published in the veterinary literature.

A semiquantitative cytologic evaluation of the exudate from normal ears and from ears with otitis externa in the dog and cat has been performed.[3] In this study it was shown that numbers of cornified squamous cells are not consistently correlated with clinical findings, as animals with high counts may not show any clinical sign of otitis externa. In the above mentioned study, the results indicated that two or fewer *M. canis* yeast cells per high-power dry field (400×) should be considered normal in the dog or cat. Mean counts of greater than or equal to five yeast cells per high-power dry field in the dog and greater than or equal to 12 yeast cells per high-power dry field in the cat should be considered abnormally increased. It was theorized that *Malassezia* otitis may be a more common clinical entity in the cat than previously reported in the literature and that clinical signs are associated with higher mean yeast counts than in the dog.[3]

In reference to bacteria, mean counts per high-power dry field (400×) less than or equal to five bacteria per field in the dog and less than or equal to four bacteria per field in the cat should be considered normal, whereas mean counts greater than or equal to 25 bacteria per field in the dog and greater than or equal to 15 bacteria per field in the cat were abnormally increased.[3] Degenerating neutrophils are seen most often with significant bacterial disease and may indicate the need for systemic antibiotic therapy.

Relying on bacterial culture alone without considering the results of cytologic evaluation to determine the significance of bacteria or yeast in an inflamed ear may lead to inappropriate use of antimicrobials, because normal and acutely infected ears may harbor the same organisms. It is the opinion of many authors that cytologic evaluation of otic exudate provides greater diagnostic information about the significance of bacteria and yeast in ear disease than do culture results, especially since it is unlikely that pathogenic organisms will be cultured if they are not seen on cytologic examination. However, cultures should be considered in recurrent or refractory cases, especially those involving gram-negative bacteria and when otitis media is suspected.

The most common gram-positive organism isolated from cases of canine otitis externa is *Staphylococcus intermedius* (Figure 9-2). Other gram-positive bacteria isolated include *Streptococcus* spp., *Micrococcus* spp., *Staphylococcus aureus, Staphylococcus epidermidis, Corynebacterium* spp., and *Bacillus* spp. Gram-negative organisms isolated from cases of canine otitis externa include *Pseudomonas* spp., *Proteus* spp., *Klebsiella* spp., *E. coli,* and *Pasteurella* spp. These gram-negative organisms, particularly *Pseudomonas,* are seen more commonly in chronic cases of otitis externa (Figure 9-3).

Pseudomonas aeruginosa is perhaps the most difficult to manage of the bacteria that infect the ear canal. *Pseudomonas* is intrinsically insensitive to many antimicrobial drugs because of the low rate of passage of antibiotics across its outer membrane. There is evidence accumulating that *P. aeruginosa* isolates from dogs with otitis externa are becoming resistant to a number of antibacterial agents, including the fluoroquinolones. *Pseudomonas* thrives in an environment created by chronic inflammatory changes of the ear canal.

The most common yeast agent cultured from canine ears is *M. canis* (Figure 9-4). Other yeast organisms isolated from cases of canine otitis externa include *Candida, Cryptococcus, Rhodotorula, Trichosporon,* and *Saccaromyces. Malassezia sympodialis* has been isolated from the external ear canals of both normal cats and those with mild otic pruritus.

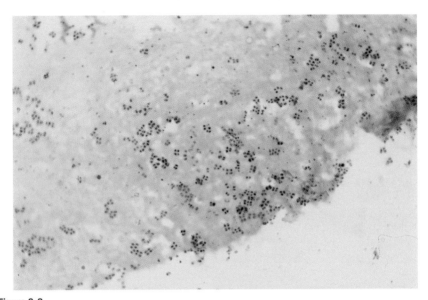

Figure 9-2

Modified Wright-Giemsa stain of staphylococci from a dog ear smear (magnification 1000×).

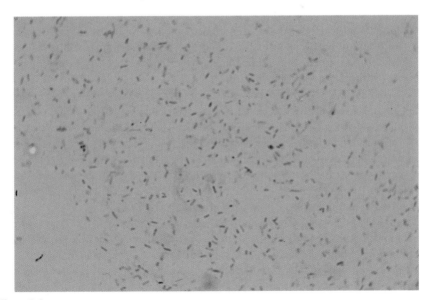

Figure 9-3

Gram's stain of *Pseudomonas* from a dog ear smear (magnification 1000×).

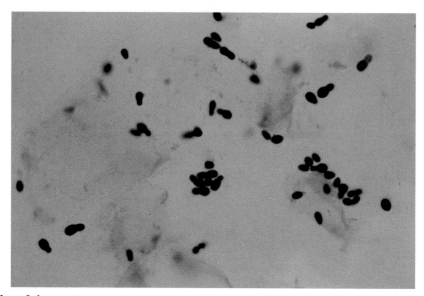

Figure 9-4

Modified Wright-Giemsa stain of *Malassezia* from a dog ear smear (magnification 1000×).

Many qualitative studies have been published concerning the microflora of the dog's ear canal in health and disease. Tables 9-1 and 9-2 summarize the studies in the literature performed to evaluate qualitatively the microbial flora in dogs with normal ears and dogs with otitis externa.

Few studies have been performed to evaluate the microflora of the cat's ear canal in health and disease. The most common bacteria recovered from otitis externa in cats' ears are coagulase-positive staphylococci. Gram-negative bacteria such as *Pseudomonas* and *Proteus* spp. are only rarely recovered from cats with otitis externa.

Unfortunately, neither cytology nor culture are perfect diagnostic tests. In a recent study, cytology agreed with culture results only 68% of the time, but even more disturbing is that samples taken simultaneously from the same area of the ear canal gave different culture results 20% of the time.[4]

From a clinical standpoint, determining the significance of a yeast or bacterial population in animals with otitis externa is difficult because of the multifactorial origin of otitis externa. Many dogs and cats with otitis externa do not have increased numbers of microbes in the external ear canal. In addition, it has been theorized that microbes in the ear canal cannot proliferate unless inflammation or maceration occurs within the ear canal. Because of this, August considered microorganisms as perpetuating causes rather than primary or predisposing causes of otitis externa.[3] In the semiquantitative cytologic evaluation study cited previously, the conclusion was that the pathogenic role of these organisms always depends on considerations other than only their numbers.[3]

Pathophysiology of Otitis Externa

Otitis externa has many etiologies. However, after the acute inflammatory stage has been initiated, there is a common pathway for the development of chronic otitis externa, regardless of the inciting cause. In the acute stage the ear canal becomes erythematous and swollen. Epidermal changes impede epidermal migration and decrease the self-cleansing function. The epidermis continues to thicken, and the sebaceous glands initially appear to become hyperplastic. These changes result in an increase in sebaceous secretion and desquamated cells, causing excessive wax production. As the otitis becomes more chronic, the apocrine glands begin to dilate and secrete. The addition of this low-lipid material decreases the concentration of the lipids secreted by the sebaceous glands. The lipid concentration of the cerumen decreases and the humidity in the ear increases.

Ultimately, the ear canal microclimate can be permanently altered. Stenosis of the canal and increased cerumen production can continually favor microbial overgrowth. Connective tissue proliferates in the dermis and subcutis, leading to fibrosis and additional thickening of the integument. The auditory cartilages may undergo calcification and possibly ossification, which further decrease the expansibility of the ear. All of these changes continue to cause further occlusion of the ear canal, which further impedes the normal cleansing function. It is likely that these altered ear canals will suffer from intermittently to constantly increased numbers of microbes, with attendant inflammatory changes, thus continuing the vicious cycle of chronic otitis.

Otitis Media

Otitis media is a recognized cause of recurrent otitis externa. The presence of bacteria in the middle ear acts as a source of reinfection of the outer ear canal. The presence on examination of an intact tympanum does not rule out the possibility of previous rupture and repair of the tympanic membrane in the presence of otitis media. Conversely, the most common cause of otitis media is infection extending through a compromised tympanic membrane from an infected external ear canal. Hematogenous spread of bloodborne pathogens to the middle ear and extension of infection from the nasopharynx through the auditory tube to the tympanic bulla are rare. Obstruction of the eustachian tubes in cats and dogs has been shown experimentally to result in a middle ear effusion. Cats can develop otitis media via extension through the auditory tubes as a sequela to an upper respiratory infection, but this also occurs infrequently. Foreign bodies, trauma, and tumors may also induce otitis media.

Middle ear defense mechanics include a mucociliary system and a cellular defense system. The epithelium in the middle ear can function actively in clearing foreign material. In addition, these cells also secrete lysozymes to aid in defense mechanisms. Fibroblasts, when activated, secrete increased amounts of collagen and ground substance, which participate in protection and repair. A surfactant that lowers surface tension has been found in the auditory tubes of dogs. This substance may be

Text continued on p. 200.

TABLE 9-1 Summary of Microbial Flora (% Incidence) Isolated from the External Ear Canal of Dogs with no Evidence of Ear Disease

STUDY #	NUMBER OF EARS	NO GROWTH	COAGULASE-POSITIVE STAPHYLO-COCCUS	COAGULASE-NEGATIVE STAPHYLO-COCCUS	CORYNE-BACTERIA SPP. OR BACILLUS	STREPTO-COCCUS SPP.	PROTEUS SPP.	PSEUDO-MONAS SPP.	COLI-FORMS	MALAS-SEZIA
1	156	40	42.9	Combined	0	0	0	0	<0.5	ND
2	70	ND	54.3	Combined	15.7	32.9	0	0	5.7	ND
3	124	1.6	47.6	74.2	25.8	15.3	1.6	2.4	42.7	35.9
4	279	ND	9.6	13.6	1.8	3.6	0	0	0.4	15.8
5	600	22.7	28.7	73.7	11.0	14.3	0	0	1.6	20.7
6	60	ND	1.6	3.2	5	0	0	0	0	28.3
7	42	26.2	19.0	ND	ND	ND	ND	ND	ND	14.3
8	51	41	9.8	Combined	9.8	2	0	0	0	31.4
9	70	ND	54	Combined	31	33	0	0	6	36
10	101	45.5	9.9	0	20.7	1.9	0	0	0	16.8
11	60	61.7	2	3.3	5	0	0	0	0	28.3
12	58	ND	15	Combined	ND	2	0	4	1	6
13	60	53	19	Combined	0	0	0	0	2	7

ND, Either not done, not recorded, or not specifically recorded (e.g., no genus species given in certain studies; recorded only as gram-negative or gram-positive coccobacilli).

1. Gustafson B: Otitis externa hos hund, *Nordic Veterinaermedicin* 6:434-442, 1954.
2. Fraser G: Factors predisposing to canine external otitis, *Vet Rec* 73:55-58, 1961.
3. Grono LR, Frost AJ: Otitis externa in the dog, *Aust Vet J* 45:420-422, 1969.
4. Sharma VD, Rhodes HE: The occurrence and microbiology of otitis externa in the dog, *J Sm Anim Pract* 16:241-247, 1975.
5. McCarthy G, Kelly WR: Microbial species associated with the canine ear and their antibacterial sensitivity pattern, *Irish Vet J* 36:53-56, 1982.
6. Marshall MJ, Harris AM, Horne JE: The bacteriological and clinical assessment of a new preparation for the treatment of otitis externa in dogs and cats, *J Sm Anim Pract* 15:401-410, 1974.
7. Chengappa MM, Maddux R, Greer S: A microbiological survey of clinically normal and otitic ear canal, *Pet Pract* 78:343-344, 1983.
8. Dickson DB, Love DN: Bacteriology of the horizontal ear canal of dogs, *J Sm Anim Pract* 24:413-421, 1983.
9. Fraser G, Gregor WW, MacKenzie CP, et al: Canine ear disease, *J Sm Anim Pract* 10:725-754, 1970.
10. Gedek B, Brutzel K, Gerlach R, et al: The role of *Pityrosporum pachydermatis* in otitis externa of dogs: evaluation of a treatment with miconazole, *Vet Rec* 104:138-140, 1979.
11. Marshall MJ, Harris AM, Horne JE: The bacteriological and clinical assessment of a new preparation for the treatment of otitis externa in dogs and cat, *J Sm Anim Pract* 15:401-410, 1974.
12. Sampson GR, Bowen RE, Murphy CN, et al: Clinical evaluation of a topical ointment, *VMSAC* 68:978-982, 1973.
13. Matsuda H, Tojo M, Fukui K, et al: The aerobic bacterial flora of the middle and external ears in normal dogs, *J Sm Anim Pract* 25:269-274, 1984.

TABLE 9-2 Summary of Microbial Flora (% Incidence) Isolated from the External Ear Canal of Dogs with Otitis Externa

STUDY #	NUMBER OF EARS	NO GROWTH	COAGULASE-POSITIVE STAPHYLOCOCCUS	COAGULASE-NEGATIVE STAPHYLOCOCCUS	CORYNE-BACTERIA SPP.	STREPTO-COCCUS SPP.	PROTEUS SPP.	PSEUDO-MONAS SPP.	COLI-FORMS	MALAS-SEZIA
1	—	—	79.3	Combined	ND	56.0	3.4	3.4	3.4	ND
2	62	ND	80.6	ND	19.4	6.5	12.9	12.9	7.7	ND
3	716	9.9	30.9	8.0	3.1	12.6	20.8	34.6	7.3	35.9
4	115	18.3	32	ND	1.0	1.0	9.0	9.0	4.0	54.2
5	69	ND	22.6	1.9	1.8	4.2	3.9	18.1	5.6	34.8
6	116	ND	37.9	20.7	6.0	8.6	3.4	16.4	2.5	82.8
7	160	26.2	19.0	ND	ND	ND	ND	ND	ND	14.3
8	60	ND	51.8	Combined	ND	29.6	14.8	3.7	25.9	63
9	371	ND	66.6	Combined	ND	25.8	14.8	11.3	15.6	51.5
10	87	ND	32	ND	1	1	9.0	9.0	ND	56
11	669	22.3	16.3	Combined	ND	ND	ND	ND	ND	19.3
12	389	ND	32.1	0.5	0.5	9.0	13.4	20.1	ND	2.1
13	59	ND	47.5	3.4	1.7	25.4	13.6	5.1	ND	ND
14	293	ND	33.8	Combined	ND	6.5	3.1	3.8	ND	35.8
15	36	ND	41.6	Combined	ND	25	19.4	25	13.8	50
16	49	2	53	ND	ND	6	ND	ND	ND	86
17	47	ND	34	27.7	ND	8.5	19.2	14.9	ND	ND
18	500	ND	61	Combined	ND	22	16	13	13	44
19	158	0	17.7	3.1	0	6.8	0.6	12.6	1.2	56.9
20	68	ND	35	Combined	ND	6	5	5	2	23

ND, Either not done, not recorded, or not specifically recorded (e.g., no genus species given in certain studies; recorded only as gram-negative or gram-positive coccobacilli).

1. Gustafson B: Otitis externa hos hund, *Nordic Veterinaermedicin* 6:434-442, 1954.
2. Fraser G: Factors predisposing to canine external otitis, *Vet Rec* 73:55-58, 1961.
3. Grono LR, Frost AJ: Otitis externa in the dog, *Aust Vet J* 45:420-422, 1969.
4. Sharma VD, Rhodes HE: The occurrence and microbiology of otitis externa in the dog, *J Sm Anim Pract* 16:241-247, 1975.
5. McCarthy G, Kelly WR: Microbial species associated with the canine ear and their antibacterial sensitivity patterns, *Irish Vet J* 36:53-56, 1982.
6. Marshall MJ, Harris AM, Horne JE: The bacteriological and clinical assessment of a new preparation for the treatment of otitis externa in dogs and cats, *J Sm Anim Pract* 15:401-410, 1974.
7. Chengappa MM, Maddux R, Greer S: A microbiological survey of clinically normal and otitic ear canals, *Pet Pract* 78:343-344, 1983.
8. McKellar QA, Rycroft A, Anderson L, et al: Otitis externa in a foxhound pack associated with *Candida albicans*, *Vet Rec* 127:15-16, 1990.
9. Fraser G, Withers AR, Spreull JSA: Otitis externa in the dog, *J Sm Anim Pract* 2:32-47, 1961.
10. Baxter M, Lawler DC: The incidence and microbiology of otitis externa of dogs and cats in New Zealand, *New Zealand Vet J* 20:29-32, 1972.
11. Krogh HV, Linnel A, Knudsen PB: Otitis externa in the dog: a clinical and microbiological study, *Nordic Veterinaermedicin* 27:285-295, 1975.
12. Blue JL, Wooley RE: Antibacterial sensitivity patterns of bacteria isolated from dogs with otitis externa, *J Am Vet Med Assoc* 171:362-363, 1977.
13. Nesbitt GH, Schmitz JA: Chronic bacterial dermatitis and otitis: a review of 195 cases, *J Am Anim Hosp Assoc* 13:442-450, 1977.
14. Rycroft AK, Saban HS: A clinical study of otitis externa in the dog, *Can Vet J* 18:64-70, 1977.
15. Hallu RE, Gentilini E, Rebuelto M, et al: The combination of norfloxacin and ketoconazole in the treatment of canine otitis, *Canine Pract* 21:26-28, 1996.
16. Blanco JL, Guedeja-Marron J, Hontecillas R, et al: Microbiological diagnosis of chronic otitis externa in the dog, *J Vet Med B* 43:475-482, 1996.
17. Webster FL, Whyard BH, Brandt RW, et al: Treatment of otitis externa in the dog with Gentocin Otic, *Can Vet J* 15:176-177, 1974.
18. Fraser G, Gregor WW, MacKenzie CP, et al: Canine ear disease, *J Sm Anim Pract* 10:725-754, 1970.
19. Gedek B, Brutzel K, Gerlach R, et al: The role of *Pityrosporum pachydermatis* in otitis externa of dogs: evaluation of a treatment with miconazole, *Vet Rec* 104:138-140, 1979.
20. Sampson GR, Bowen RE, Murphy CN, et al: Clinical evaluation of a topical ointment, *VMSAC* 68:978-982, 1973.

important in decreasing cohesive forces between the coapting walls of the auditory tube. In otitis media, the auditory tubes may be more resistant to opening during the act of swallowing, which results in a lack of aeration of the middle ear.

When otitis media is present, the lamina propria of the middle ear cavity often thickens and forms loose vascular and edematous granulation tissue, sometimes maturing into dense connective tissue. Occasionally spicules of bone can be found within the connective tissue. New bone or bone remodeling can be seen on the intraluminal and extraluminal aspect of the tympanic bulla.

Microbiology of the Middle Ear

Cytology and culture should be performed from exudate retrieved from the middle ear. The exudate can be retrieved via myringotomy or the more invasive bulla osteotomy. The most common pathogens cultured from the middle ear include *Staphylococcus intermedius* and *Pseudomonas aeruginosa. Streptococcus* spp., *Escherichia coli, Proteus mirabilis, Enterobacter* spp., *Pasteurella* spp., *Corynebacterium* spp., *Enterococcus* spp., *Klebsiella* spp., *Citrobacter* spp., *Lactobacillus* spp., *Clostridium* spp., and anaerobes have also been cultured from the middle ear. Yeast *(Malassezia, Candida)* and *Aspergillus* spp. have also been cultured from the diseased middle ear. *Otodectes cynotis* will occasionally cause middle ear disease.

In a study comparing the microbial flora of the horizontal ear canal and middle ear of dogs with otitis media, a difference in types of isolates and/or susceptibility patterns between the horizontal ear canal and middle ear was found 89.5% of the time.[5] Therefore, it is important that specimens for bacterial culture be taken from the horizontal ear canal and the middle ear in dogs with chronic otitis externa in which otitis media is suspected.

Conclusion

Otitis externa is a very common problem in the dog. It occurs less often in the cat. Otitis media is most often a sequela to chronic otitis externa. Many factors have been identified as predisposing an animal to ear disease. All of these factors alter the microenvironment of the ear canal. Successful outcome of treatment relies on proper diagnosis, correction of any primary predisposing or perpetuating factors, and restoration of the microclimate of the ear canal to normal.

References

1. Huang HP, Fixter LM, Little CJL: Lipid content of cerumen from normal dogs and otitic canine ears, *Vet Rec* 134:380-381, 1994.
2. Mansfield PD, Boosinger TR, Attleberger MH: Infectivity of *Malassezia pachydermatis* in the external ear canal of dogs, *J Am Anim Hosp Assoc* 26:97-100, 1999.
3. Ginel PJ, Lucena R, Rodriguez JC, et al: A semiquantitative cytological evaluation of normal and pathological samples from the external ear canal of dogs and cats, *Vet Derm* 13:151-156, 2002.

4. Graham-Mize CA, Rosser EJ: *Comparison of microbial isolates and susceptibility patterns from the external ear canal in canines with otitis externa,* 18th Proceedings of AAVD/ACVD Meeting, Monterey, CA, April 2003.
5. Cole LK, Kwochka KW, Kowalski JJ, et al: Microbial flora and antimicrobial susceptibility patterns of isolated pathogens from the horizontal ear canal and middle ear in dogs with otitis media, *J Am Vet Med Assoc* 212:534-538, 1998.

Suggested Readings

August JR: Otitis externa, *Vet Clin North Am Small Anim Pract* 18:731-742, 1988.
Colombini S, Merchant SR, Hosgood G: Microbial flora and antimicrobial susceptibility patterns from dogs with otitis media, *Vet Derm* 11:235-239, 2000.
Logas DB: Disease of the ear canal, *Vet Clin North Am Small Anim Pract* 24:905-919, 1994.

10

Ceruminous Diseases of the Ear

Norma White-Weithers, MS, DVM

Histopathology of the External Ear Canal

The epithelium of the external auditory meatus is composed of components similar to those of normal skin. The stratum corneum is the outermost layer; keratinocytes make up this layer of squamous anuclear cells. There are no rete ridges in the epithelium of the ear canal. The sebaceous glands are the outermost glands; they become progressively more numerous deeper into the meatus. Underlying the sebaceous glands are simple, coiled, tubular, apocrine glands called *ceruminous glands,* with ducts that open directly into hair follicles or onto the surface of the ear canal (Figure 10-1). During inflammatory reactions, sebaceous glands become hyperactive and hyperplastic; the ceruminous glands become dilated, thickened, and filled with secretions (Figure 10-2). Under normal physiologic conditions, ceruminous secretions (cerumen) combine with sebum produced by the sebaceous glands and epidermal debris to form earwax, the normal secretion of the ear.

Etiology of Ceruminous Otitis

When ceruminous glands and sebaceous glands of the ear canal become chronically irritated, the results are cystic dilation of ceruminous glands, hyperplasia, and increased activity of the overlying sebaceous glands. The excessive amount of cerumen produced by ceruminous glands forms a favorable medium for the growth of secondary bacteria and yeast. These organisms are normal flora of the ear and include *Pseudomonas* spp., *Proteus* spp., and *Malassezia pachydermatis* (see Chapter 9).

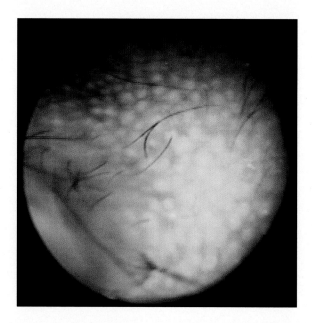

Figure 10-1

Multiple openings of the cerumen glands along the ear canal.

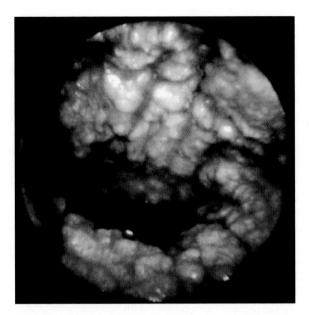

Figure 10-2

Many diseases cause increased blood supply to the ears, increasing the metabolism within the ceruminous glands. Bacteria and yeasts secondarily grow on the roughened ear canal surface, using the glandular secretions as their nourishment.

With improper drainage and lack of air circulation (due to pendulous ears in some breeds), excessive growth of these organisms may occur within the ear canal.

In most cases of ceruminous otitis, the epidermal hyperplasia and inflammatory reaction occlude the external ear canal, making visual examination difficult. In both the dog and cat, hyperplasia of the ear canal can simulate neoplastic conditions that may lead to misdiagnoses and improper treatment. When hyperplasia does not respond to treatment and hardening of the ear canal ensues, surgical intervention is often the treatment of choice. Surgical opening of the ear canal allows proper drainage. The identification and treatment of underlying infections are important for surgical success.

Ceruminous otitis is inflammation of the glandular structures of the ear canal, with subsequent excessive epidermal proliferation and otitis externa that requires medical or surgical management. The causes of ceruminous otitis are many, and each condition is accompanied by other dermatologic or systemic manifestations.

Disorders of Keratinization

Primary Idiopathic Seborrhea

Ceruminous otitis can be due to an inherited or acquired keratinization defect. Inherited disorders include idiopathic primary seborrhea, commonly seen in West Highland White Terriers, American Cocker Spaniels, English Springer Spaniels,

Basset Hounds, Irish Setters, Dachshunds, Chinese Shar-Peis, and German Shepherds. Primary idiopathic seborrhea, epidermal dysplasia of West Highland White Terriers, and lichenoid-psoriasiform dermatosis of English Springer Spaniels are examples of primary keratinization defects with ceruminous otitis externa. Secondary or acquired keratinization defects include vitamin A–responsive dermatosis, zinc-responsive dermatosis, and fatty acid deficiency.

The epidermis of the canine ear canal undergoes proliferation, differentiation, and desquamation with renewal of the viable epidermis in approximately 22 days. In American Cocker Spaniels that have idiopathic primary seborrhea, the proliferative, differentiative, and desquamative stages take an average of 8 days. This rapid turnover of epidermal cells increases the renewal stage that produces seborrhea (manifested as seborrheic dermatitis, ceruminous otitis, or both). This defect in differentiation includes hyperkeratosis or hypokeratosis and dyskeratosis.

Clinical Signs. The clinical signs of primary and secondary ceruminous otitis are the same and can only be diagnosed on the basis of response to therapy. In-depth clinical and diagnostic evaluations are mandatory for animals that present with chronic ceruminous otitis. These animals usually present with other primary or secondary dermatologic manifestations.

Clinical signs can be mild or chronic, with secondary bacterial or *Malassezia* infections complicating the primary problem. Ears with ceruminous otitis are malodorous, and there is often secondary epidermal hyperplasia of the ear canal and pinna that may occlude the auditory meatus. Other presenting signs are usually generalized, focal to multifocal, seborrheic dermatitis with secondary bacterial and/or *Malassezia* infections.

In the author's experience, animals with moist vertical canals due to pendulous ears and poor ventilation are presented more often with chronic ceruminous otitis that requires general anesthesia for proper ear examination. Examination under general anesthesia allows the clinician to visualize thoroughly, clean, and obtain biopsy specimens from the ear.

A biopsy is often necessary to differentiate chronic epidermal hyperplasia with chronic ceruminous otitis from ceruminous gland tumors. Secondary bacterial and *Malassezia* infections respond when the underlying cause is properly treated. If there is no response, evaluation should consist of bacterial and fungal culture and sensitivity testing.

Diagnosis. Histologic evaluation of noninfected seborrheic areas usually supports a diagnosis of primary seborrhea. After identification of secondary invaders and appropriate medical management, diagnosis is most frequently confirmed by response to treatment.

Treatment. Because ceruminous otitis is only the manifestation of a more serious problem, finding the underlying cause should be the clinician's primary goal. Treatment of primary seborrhea should attempt to control the disease rather than produce a complete cure. Treatment of the ears should focus on (1) control of secondary infections and of production of scales and crust, and (2) reduction of inflammation. Frequent ear cleaning with appropriate topical medication can control the odor associated with this condition. Steroids, cytotoxic drugs, and retinoic acid have variable effects. Results with the use of synthetic retinoid (etretinate) in Cocker Spaniels and other breeds to treat idiopathic seborrhea are disappointing. In the Cocker Spaniel, for example, there is a reduction of scales, crust, and alopecia, but the ceruminous otitis is not responsive to this therapy. It is less effective in other breeds affected with this condition.

Endocrine Dermatosis

The most common endocrine diseases associated with ceruminous otitis are hypothyroidism and hyperadrenocorticism.

Hypothyroidism. Breed predilections for hypothyroidism include Golden Retrievers, Alaskan Malamutes, Chow Chows, Boxers, English Bulldogs, Chinese Shar-Peis, Great Danes, Afghan Hounds, Doberman Pinschers, Newfoundlands, Dachshunds, and Cocker Spaniels. Hypothyroidism in cats is extremely rare.

Etiology. The causes of hypothyroidism are classified as primary, secondary, tertiary, and congenital. Examples of causes of primary hypothyroidism include lymphocytic thyroiditis, thyroid atrophy, thyroid gland hyperplasia, neoplasia, and thyroid cell destruction due to radioactive iodine treatment or antithyroid drug therapy. Secondary hypothyroidism in the dog is the result of pituitary destruction and malformation or suppression of thyrotropic cell function. There are no known causes of canine tertiary hypothyroidism. Defects in iodine organification and thyroid gland dysgenesis are the two most common causes of congenital hypothyroidism in the dog.

Clinical Signs. Thyroid hormone is an important regulator in the body's metabolic function. A deficiency causes a decrease in the normal cellular metabolic functions of the body. The clinical signs of hypothyroidism in the dog are extremely variable, being those of metabolic, dermatologic, reproductive, neuromuscular, ocular, gastrointestinal, cardiovascular, hematologic, and behavioral disorders.

Serum and cutaneous fatty acid concentrations are affected by thyroid hormones. Thyroid hormones stimulate the synthesis, mobilization, and degradation of lipids, with the most dramatic effect being a decrease in degradation. This may present as an increase in serum low-density lipoprotein (LDL).

Thyroid hormone increases the sebum production necessary for the normal lipogenesis and synthesis of sterol by keratinocytes and increases cutaneous linoleic acid, with a decrease in gamma linolenic and arachidonic acid concentrations. The decrease in arachidonic acid concentration alters epidermal proliferation. This alteration is responsible for the seborrhea, seborrheic dermatitis, and ceruminous otitis so often present in hypothyroid dogs. This may be the only presenting sign in a hypothyroid dog. The dryness or greasiness associated with the alteration of cutaneous fatty acid levels can manifest as a dry or a greasy form of seborrhea.

Secondary bacterial and *Malassezia* infections are complicating factors in ceruminous otitis and can be a dermatologic nightmare if not treated properly. Other dermatologic abnormalities in dogs with hypothyroidism are myxedema, thin skin, hyperkeratosis, seborrheic ear pinnae, pyoderma, symmetrical or patchy endocrine alopecia, and various degrees of hyperpigmentation. Otic pruritus is often present with secondary bacterial or *Malassezia* infection.

Diagnosis and Treatment. The resolution of the ceruminous otitis largely depends on the proper diagnosis and control of hypothyroidism. History and physical examination findings are important in the diagnosis of hypothyroidism. A complete blood count, serum biochemistry profile, urinalysis, and thyroid stimulation test are some of the few laboratory tests used to diagnose hypothyroidism.

Because the availability of thyroid-stimulation hormone is limited due to factors of price and supply, in most cases the interpretations of total tetraiodothyronine (T4), free T4, and thyroid-stimulating hormone (TSH) in combination with clinical manifestations are the only diagnostic tools at the clinician's disposal. For this reason, it is important to note that misdiagnosis of this disease can be easily made if the appropriate tests are not performed. Drugs such as glucocorticoids, anticonvulsants, trimetoprim/sulfamethoxazole, phenylbutazone, quinidine, salicylates, and radiocontrast agents can adversely affect thyroid levels in the body. It is recommended that these medications be withdrawn, if possible for up to 2 weeks, before a thyroid test is performed. These drugs can reduce the conversion of T4 to triiodothyronine (T3), inhibit thyroxine synthesis in the gland, inhibit TSH secretion from the pituitary gland, and interfere with the binding of serum thyroxine to binding proteins. Thyroid testing should not be performed immediately after anesthesia. Due to its adverse effect on serum thyroid levels, a waiting period of up to 1 or 2 weeks is recommended before performing a thyroid profile on these animals. A free T4 using the equilibrium dialysis (ED) method is recommended in veterinary medicine. This test measures the quantity of T4 in the dialysate and does not use the thyronine-binding globulin as a high-affinity binding protein, as in the radioimmunoassay (RIA) test. The level of this binding protein is low in the dog, compared with humans. The free T4 by the ED method as compared with the RIA method is a more specific and sensitive test in the dog.

Epidermal hyperplasia and pain often occur in the treatment of ceruminous otitis. Topical steroid preparations are useful in controlling pain and inflammation and reducing epidermal hyperplasia. Because steroids affect baseline thyroid levels, thyroid profiles should be performed before or 1 or 2 weeks after discontinuing any topical otic medications with steroids.

Hyperadrenocorticism. Bilateral adrenocortical hyperplasia due to pituitary adenoma is the most common cause of hyperadrenocorticism in the dog. The excessive production of cortisol by the adrenal gland results in systemic as well as dermatologic abnormalities. The prolonged exogenous use of oral, intramuscular, or intravenous (and possibly otic and ophthalmic) corticosteroids may also cause iatrogenic hyperadrenocorticism. Other causes are adrenal adenomas and carcinomas.

The cutaneous manifestations of excessive serum cortisol are as follows:
- Alopecia
- Failure or slowness of hair growth after clipping
- Thin skin
- Pyoderma
- Seborrhea
- Comedone formation
- Bruising
- Striae formation

Seborrhea dermatitis may manifest as ceruminous otitis with secondary bacterial or *Malassezia* infections.

Glucocorticoids inhibit epidermal proliferation and sebum production through antimitotic, protein-catabolic, and antienzymatic effects. The decrease in hair growth is manifested clinically through bilateral symmetrical or "moth-eaten" alopecia. The antimetabolic and antiproliferative effects on fibroblasts are evident as poor wound healing. There is also an increase in susceptibility to infections. Because animals with hyperadrenocorticism show signs of secondary hypothyroidism, clinical signs of seborrhea and skin infection may be exaggerated due to the dermatologic effects of low thyroid levels.

The combination of seborrhea and bacterial or *Malassezia* infections can be manifest as ceruminous otitis, which is not as common in the cat as in the dog.

Diagnosis and Treatment. Diagnosis of hyperadrenocorticism is based on history, complete blood count, serum biochemistry, urinalysis, adrenocorticotropic hormone (ACTH) stimulation test, low- or high-dose dexamethasone suppression tests, and ultrasonographic and radiographic findings. Because steroids affect thyroid levels, a thyroid stimulation test, if available, or a thyroid profile (T4, free T4 [ED], and TSH) is part of the diagnostic plan. However, a thyroid profile should be performed after hyperadrenocorticism has been diagnosed and controlled to minimize the adverse effects of steroids outlined previously. Treatment of otitis externa secondary to hyperadrenocorticism depends on proper diagnosis and treatment of the hyperadrenocorticism. Any secondary bacterial or *Malassezia* infection should also be treated.

Several factors are important in the treatment of hyperadrenocorticism. Most animals with this disease are presented with other problems such as a secondary bacterial, parasitic *(Demodex),* or fungal skin infection, as well as otitis. When these are encountered, individual treatment modalities are recommended for each specific problem. Therefore, in treating an animal with hyperadrenocorticism, secondary problems can complicate the picture, making therapy prolonged and complicated at times.

Other Endocrine Dermatoses. Other causes of endocrine dermatosis include Sertoli cell tumors, seminoma, interstitial cell tumor, estrogen-responsive dermatoses, and hyperandrogenism in intact male dogs.

Nutritional Deficiency

Nutritional keratinization disorders that can cause ceruminous otitis are fatty acid deficiency, vitamin A–responsive dermatosis, and zinc-responsive dermatosis.

Fatty Acid Deficiency

Fatty acid binds water into the stratum corneum of normal skin, helping to maintain the permeability properties of the skin barrier. Fatty acids also function as antioxidants.

Prolonged storage of dry dog and cat food causes degradation of fatty acids, fatty acid deficiency, and reduced levels of antioxidants. Animals fed home-cooked diets or reduced-fat diets may develop fatty acid deficiency. Gastrointestinal diseases that cause poor absorption will result in fatty acid deficiency in spite of an adequate diet. In dogs, the essential fatty acids linolenic and arachidonic acid, can be synthesized from linoleic acid. Cats lack the enzyme omega-6-desaturase, so they cannot convert linoleic acid to arachidonic acid. Therefore, cats require linolenic and arachidonic acid in their diets. Fatty acid deficiency in cats does not become clinically apparent until many months of feeding a fatty acid–deficient diet.

Deficiency of fatty acids, especially arachidonic acid, in the diet may result in abnormalities in keratinization with microscopic epidermal changes (hypergranulosis, epidermal hyperplasia with orthokeratotic or parakeratotic hyperkeratosis).

Clinically, animals with acute fatty acid deficiency produce a dry, dull hair coat with generalized fine scaling of the skin. This also affects the ear, with involvement of the pinna and horizontal ear canal. In chronic conditions, there is epidermal thickening with concurrent greasiness of the ear pinna and canal and of the intertriginous and interdigital areas. The ceruminous otitis that accompanies this condition is made worse by secondary bacterial and *Malassezia* infection. Without appropriate treatment, pruritus and seborrhea become progressively worse.

Diagnosis and Treatment. Diagnosis of fatty acid deficiency is based on response to therapeutic levels of fatty acid supplementation. It is mandatory to make sure that an animal's diet contains the recommended amount of fat for proper health and that an animal on a reducing diet is given follow-up and routine veterinary care. Commercially prepared and balanced veterinary omega-6 and omega-3 fatty acid supplementations are available. They contain linoleic acid and eicosapentaenoic and docosahexaenoic acid. The latter two are marine lipids that modulate arachidonic acid metabolism, thus reducing inflammatory responses in the skin through prostaglandin and leukotrienes. They also mediate epidermal proliferation. The role of linoleic acid in controlling seborrheic dermatitis in dogs is well established. The proper storage of food at room temperature and in airtight containers away from direct light is important to ensure that an adequate level of linoleic acid is present in the diet. Diets should not be stored for prolonged periods.

Supplementation with sunflower, safflower, or vegetable oil at a dose of 5 ml per cup of dry or can of dog food should elicit a response in 3 to 8 weeks. Similar results should be seen with commercially prepared veterinary supplements. Any secondary bacterial or *Malassezia* infection should be treated.

Vitamin A–Responsive Dermatosis

Epithelial cells require vitamin A to maintain their integrity. Vitamin A is necessary for the proliferation and differentiation of keratinocytes. The Cocker Spaniel has a predisposition to this condition. However, it has also been reported in the Labrador Retriever and Miniature Schnauzer. Cats lack the metabolic capability to convert carotene to vitamin A.

Clinical Signs. The effects of vitamin A deficiency on the skin include marked hyperkeratosis of the epidermis, hair follicles, and sebaceous glands. The hyperkeratosis of the sebaceous glands results in the blockage of the sebaceous secretion, giving rise to a papular-type skin eruption. In a generalized pattern, severe follicular plugging and hyperkeratotic plaques are usually secondarily infected with bacteria or *Malassezia* organisms. In the ear, ceruminous otitis is usually present, and severity depends on the chronicity of the condition. In most cases an otic secondary bacterial or *Malassezia* infection is present.

Diagnosis and Treatment. The follicular changes present in dogs with vitamin A–responsive dermatosis and the histologic findings of markedly disproportionate follicular orthokeratotic hyperkeratosis are enough to warrant treatment of this condition. The final diagnosis, however, depends on response to therapy. The condition responds to 400 to 800 IU/kg of vitamin A orally once daily with a high-fat meal. Animals on such a high level of supplementation should be monitored for signs of toxicity.

Zinc-Responsive Dermatosis

Zinc-responsive dermatosis is a chronic keratinization disorder of dogs. Predilection for the disease is observed among the Alaskan Malamutes and Siberian Huskies, with a few reports in Doberman Pinschers and Great Danes. There are two forms of this disorder: syndrome I and syndrome II.

Syndrome I. This syndrome affects mainly Siberian Huskies and Alaskan Malamutes, with reported cases in Bull Terriers. A genetic defect in the Alaskan Malamute causes a decreased ability to absorb zinc from the gastrointestinal tract.

Clinical Signs. Despite a balanced diet, clinical signs usually appear in animals between 1 and 3 years of age. Clinical signs include alopecia with crusts and scales around the eyes and on the pinnae and horizontal canals of the ears. There is erythema with some form of erosion in these areas. Excessive sebum production and secondary bacterial and *Malassezia* infections are common; this is noticeable on the pinna of the ear and in the horizontal ear canal. Secondary bacterial and *Malassezia* infections of the ear canal cause the foul odor of the otitis present in this condition.

Syndrome II. Rapidly growing puppies fed diets high in plant protein (phytate) or calcium or diets low or deficient in zinc will develop zinc-responsive dermatosis. Doberman Pinschers, Labrador Retrievers, Great Danes, Standard Poodles, and German Short-Haired Pointers are some of the breeds affected by this syndrome. Syndrome II may affect the ear canals in dogs, but hyperkeratotic plaques are the predominant lesions seen. Hyperkeratosis of the footpads and planum nasale is frequently present. Secondary bacterial infections are common.

Diagnosis. A thorough history, diet analysis, physical examination, and skin biopsy are important in the diagnosis of zinc-responsive dermatosis. A histologic finding of hyperplastic superficial perivascular dermatitis with severe epidermal and follicular parakeratosis suggests this condition.

Treatment. For dogs suffering from syndrome I, zinc supplementation is recommended (oral zinc sulfate or zinc methionine). For dogs with syndrome II, the correction of the diet usually produces a favorable response in 2 to 6 weeks. If dietary adjustment resolves the condition, there is no need for supplementation.

Allergic Dermatitis

Allergic dermatitis in the dog and cat is a dermatologic manifestation of the immune response elicited when an animal is exposed to allergens in the environment, food, insect saliva, or drugs. Allergic inhalant dermatitis (atopy), food hypersensitivity, and flea-allergy dermatitis are the three most common hypersensitivity reactions in the dog and cat.

Allergic Inhalant Dermatitis (Atopy)

Allergic inhalant dermatitis (atopy) is a type I hypersensitivity reaction to environmental allergens in dogs and cats. Predisposition to develop immunologic reactions to allergen-specific immunoglobulin E (IgE) or immunoglobulin G (IgG) is inherited. Genetic predisposition for canine atopy exists in dogs but not in cats.

Etiology and Pathogenesis. The causes of atopic dermatitis are various; they include weeds, grasses, tree pollens, molds, insect antigens, and other environmental products. The plethora of theories about the pathogenesis of atopy have in common the sensitization of animals to environmental allergens that results in a disease process.

Clinical signs are mediated by the degranulation of mast cells. When IgE fixed to mast cells reacts with specific allergens in the skin, the mast cells degranulate. When mast cells degranulate, they release vasoactive substances that cause vasodilation, edema, inflammation, smooth muscle contraction, and pruritus. Although the reaction occurs in cats, the exact pathogenesis of atopy in the cat is unknown.

Clinical Signs. Age of onset is between 1 and 3 years in the dog and between 6 and 24 months in the cat. The clinical sign of otitis externa is often the only presenting sign of atopy in the dog. Other signs of atopy include foot licking and chewing, armpit and inguinal pruritus, face rubbing with conjunctivitis, focal-to-truncal alopecia depending on chronicity, secondary seborrhea, and secondary bacterial or *Malassezia* infections.

Ceruminous otitis externa is rare in cats and when present may be an indicator of atopy. Eosinophilic granuloma complex lesions and miliary dermatitis are the most common clinical manifestations of atopy in the cat. Cats also have varying degrees of head and neck pruritus and self-induced alopecia. Chronic ceruminous otitis occurs in cases of atopy that either go untreated or fail to respond to therapy.

Diagnosis and Treatment. Identifying the offending allergens should be the focus of a diagnostic plan. However, history and physical examination findings are very important factors in the diagnosis of atopy. Every effort should be made to rule out parasitic diseases and food hypersensitivities before allergy testing is performed.

Both in vivo and in vitro allergy tests are available. The intradermal skin test (in vivo) is the most widely accepted test for atopy. The in vitro tests (radioallergosorbent test [RAST] and enzyme-linked immunosorbent assay [ELISA]) measure the level or concentration of allergen-specific IgG in the serum. The disadvantage of these tests is their high level of false-positive reactions. They do not correlate well with intradermal skin tests. More clinicians are employing these tests because of their ease of use. Nevertheless, the intradermal test is the most acceptable and preferred test for the diagnosis of atopy in the dog and cat.

The ceruminous otitis externa present in atopic dogs responds to therapy after the allergens are identified and hyposensitization is initiated. Topical and systemic therapies for the otitis should be considered in chronic cases. Therapy should be targeted to reduce inflammation and hypersecretion and hyperplasia of the ceruminous glands. Because most atopic dogs with ceruminous otitis have a secondary bacterial or *Malassezia* infection, concurrent treatment of this condition is necessary to effect a good response. Avoiding offending allergens is the ideal treatment protocol for atopic dogs; when this is not possible, hyposensitization and other medical management should be initiated. Therapy in some animals is lifelong. Avoidance of the offending allergens, medical management of clinical signs, and hyposensitization are the keys to a successful management program for atopic animals.

Some animals are subjected to surgical intervention due to chronic otitis externa because the underlying causes of this problem were not diagnosed. It must be stressed that ceruminous otitis externa with bacterial and *Malassezia* infection is sometimes the only presenting sign in an animal with an allergic dermatitis. This can either be atopy, food hypersensitivity, or a parasitic dermatosis.

In treating animals with ceruminous otitis due to atopy or any other forms of allergic dermatitis, the underlying allergic dermatosis in most cases will respond and all clinical signs will be completely controlled long before the otitis externa is cleared. Therapy for ceruminous otitis externa can be prolonged and unrewarding, depending on its chronicity.

Food Hypersensitivity

Food hypersensitivity is a type I, III, or IV hypersensitivity reaction (see Chapter 6). It is a nonseasonal, pruritic skin condition of both dogs and cats. An affected animal may have received the same diet for years or may recently have been introduced to a new diet. Dogs and cats of all breeds are susceptible.

Clinical Signs. Clinical signs of food allergy are variable. In the dog, there are atopic-like signs. Bilateral otitis externa, generalized pruritus, generalized secondary seborrhea, and signs resembling flea-allergy dermatitis are common manifestations. Although gastrointestinal signs are uncommon, vomiting, diarrhea, and excessive flatulence may be present. In the cat, miliary dermatitis, pruritic head and neck dermatitis, eosinophilic granuloma complex lesions, and induced pruritus are common presentation signs.

Diagnosis and Treatment. History and physical examination play major roles in the diagnosis of food hypersensitivity. Food elimination diets, preferably home cooked, are the best way to identify allergenic ingredients. If home cooking is not feasible, however, several commercially prepared hypoallergenic diets are available.

The aims of a diet trial are to provide foods to which the animal has had no previous exposure and to use diets that do not contain additives or preservatives. It is because of the wide range of ingredients present in commercially prepared diets that the best hypoallergenic diets are home cooked.

For proper diagnosis of food hypersensitivity, the recommended duration of the diet trial should be 10 to 13 weeks for dogs and from 9 to 13 weeks for cats. Because animals with food allergy usually have concurrent atopy or flea allergy dermatitis, these conditions should be identified and treated before attempts are made to diagnose atopy. The proper treatment and management of food hypersensitivity consist of avoiding the offending allergenic foods and controlling clinical signs with topical or systemic medications.

Flea-Allergy Dermatitis

Flea-allergy dermatitis is the most common allergic dermatosis in the dog. Flea bites can cause pruritus of the pinnal flap, but it rarely affects the ear canals of dogs and cats. The cutaneous reaction in flea-allergy dermatitis is due to the body's reaction to allergens present in the saliva of the flea. It can be a type I or type IV hypersensitivity reaction. Pyotraumatic dermatitis and fibropruritic nodules may be present in chronic flea-allergy dermatitis. This can be manifested in animals with other underlying allergies where ceruminous otitis is present.

Diagnosis and Treatment. History, physical examination, identification of fleas and "flea dirt" with flea combing, and intradermal skin testing with flea allergens allow definitive diagnosis of flea-allergy dermatitis. Response to therapy is most commonly used for the definitive diagnosis of flea-allergy dermatitis.

Various topical medications are available to kill both adults and developing larval stages. Topical medications having residual effects for up to 1 month are now routinely used to kill adult fleas. Other products available have insect growth regulators and adulticides for pet, house, and yard treatments.

Parasitic Dermatosis

Otodectes cynotis

The most common parasite affecting the ear canals of dogs and cats, *Otodectes cynotis* is transmitted by direct contact. Transmission among and between dogs and cats is extremely common. These ear mites are also present on other parts of the body. The sleeping habits of dogs and cats, where the head is in close contact with the tail, make the "tail-head region" a common site of infestation. The adult mites live on the skin surface of the horizontal ear canal, covered by a layer of debris. Mechanical irritation by these mites causes the production of a waxy, brown cerumen. The ceruminous glands become dilated with cerumen. Epidermal scales and debris combine with cerumen to form a favorable medium for the growth of secondary bacteria and *Malassezia* species. Otic discharge, complicated by secondary *Malassezia* or bacterial infection, is usually malodorous, and patients will present for the control of the odor rather than for the symptoms of otitis. Secondary bacterial and *Malassezia* infection can mask the primary underlying cause of the parasitic ceruminous otitis and thereby delay diagnosis.

Toxic and allergic substances produced by *Otodectes* mites cause hypersensitivity reactions in dogs and cats. The saliva of mites contains potent allergens that are responsible for this immune reaction. Ceruminous otitis externa can also be a result of *Otodectes* infestation.

Clinical Signs. Head shaking is common in animals with *Otodectes* infestation. The head shaking often leads to the formation of auricular hematomas. Intense pruritus of the ears is common, and animals can present with a noticeable head tilt, circling, and sometimes, in chronic untreated infestation, convulsions.

Otic examination may or may not reveal mites moving on hair shafts. Especially in dogs, the inflamed ear canal is not a hospitable environment for mites, so the migration of mites to other parts of the body is common. Ceruminous gland hyperplasia may make otic examination extremely difficult in cases of chronic *Otodectes* infestation. When there is hyperplasia of the ear canal, general anesthesia is recommended for otoscopic examination.

Histologic findings include hyperplasia of the ceruminous glands in acute cases, along with epithelial parakeratosis and hyperplasia, an increase in inflammatory infiltrate, squamous metaplasia of apocrine ducts, and atrophy of hair follicles. Similar changes are present in chronic infections.

Diagnosis and Treatment. Diagnosis is by finding mites in the ears on otoscopic examination, microscopic identification of the mites, determination of secondary bacterial or yeast identification, and response to treatment. The ears should be treated concurrently with the whole body. All animals that can come in contact with the patient should be concurrently treated. Various commercially prepared topical medications are available for the treatment of otic acariasis.

Sarcoptes scabiei

Although most commonly found on the pinnae of the ears, *Sarcoptes scabiei* mites can migrate into the external ear canal. The mechanical irritation and toxic substances produced by these mites lead to the hyperproliferation of the ceruminous glands of the horizontal ear canal. Ceruminous otitis caused by sarcoptic mites resolves when the primary problem and any secondary complications are treated.

Skin scrapes are not always positive for sarcoptic mites. If clinical signs and physical examination findings indicate sarcoptic infestation, it is best to treat the animal for the disorder and make a diagnosis by response to treatment.

Notoedres cati

The sarcoptic mite of cats, *Notoedres cati,* can also cause ceruminous otitis. Mechanical irritation, combined with the toxic substances and salivary antigens produced by the mites, results in glandular irritation and proliferation.

Diagnosis and treatment are pursued by identifying the mite and implementing proper treatment. Sarcoptic mites are not always picked up on skin scrapings in the dog; in the cat, however, skin scrapings reveal numerous mites. In some cases, however, diagnosis is confirmed by response to treatment.

Otobios megnini

Otobios megnini, the spinous ear tick, has been implicated in ceruminous otitis of dogs and cats. Although this condition is rare, the larval and nymphal stages of this mite feed on lymph and blood in the ear canal, resulting in irritation and subsequent hyperplasia of the ceruminous and sebaceous glands of the ear.

Diagnosis is made by identification of the larval or nymphal stages in the ear canal. Management of the tick population in the dog's environment is important to a successful treatment plan.

Mechanical removal of ticks with forceps is recommended. Grasping the tick on the head next to the skin is ideal. Care should be taken not to rupture the tick, to prevent exposure to disease agents that may be present. If the tick is located deep in the ear canal, a video otoscopic removal may be necessary. Environmental treatment should be initiated and routinely maintained, especially in tick-infested areas.

Demodex

Some dogs with generalized demodicosis test positive for the *Demodex canis* mite on ear swabs. In some dogs with severe ceruminous otitis, *Demodex* mites may be identified in the cerumen even before truncal lesions are found. Some cats with ceruminous otitis have also been identified as having *Demodex cati* in the secretions. Microscopic examination of the exudates from ceruminous ears suspended in mineral oil reveals the mites. Identification of mites from these animals can aid in the treatment and management of demodicosis. The physical mechanical irritation and irritation from toxins produced by these mites result in the cystic dilation of the ceruminous glands of the ear. The result is hyperplasia of the ear canal in chronic conditions. The excessive cerumen produced by these glands is irritating and predisposes to secondary bacterial and *Malassezia* infections. The treatment of generalized demodicosis with topical solution (amitraz) should involve treatment of the ear canal for complete cure and to prevent recurrence.

The use of systemic medication is now widely used, although it is not approved by the U.S. Food and Drug Administration (FDA) for demodicosis. Ivermectin and milbemycin oxime, on an extra-label basis, are the systemic agents now being used for the treatment of this disease. When these systemic medications are used, treating the ear canal is not indicated. However, infected ears should be treated for secondary infections.

Other Parasites. Other parasites implicated in ceruminous otitis are *Eutrombicula alfreddugesi* and *Cheyletiella* species. Dermatophytes are also implicated.

Tumors of the Ear Canal

Most tumors of the ceruminous glands of dogs are benign but in the cat are malignant. Ceruminous and sebaceous gland adenomas, adenocarcinomas, basal cell carcinomas, fibrosarcomas, chondrosarcomas, trichoepitheliomas, mast cell tumors, ceruminous gland hyperplasia, and inflammatory polyps have been identified in the ears of dogs and cats.

Nasopharangeal polyps have been identified in cats presented with otitis externa associated with ear masses. Tumors result in obstruction of the ear canal, with the most common ones being of ceruminous gland origin. Ceruminous gland tumors are most frequently diagnosed in older male cats; these tumors have a high malignancy rate.

Ceruminous gland adenomas (Figures 10-3 and 10-4) and carcinomas are the two most common tumors in the cat. The adenomas are smooth, nodular, or pedunculated masses with intact epithelium. If secondary infection is present, the epithelium may be ulcerated.

Histologically, adenomas are differentiated cystic or tubular growths with cuboidal eosinophilic epithelium (Figure 10-5). Cystic contents are colloidal, orange to eosinophilic secretions. The mass present in the ear canal may invade the parotid salivary gland. Inflammatory polyps in dogs and cats may be misdiagnosed clinically as neoplasia. Histopathologic diagnosis is necessary for differentiation of these masses.

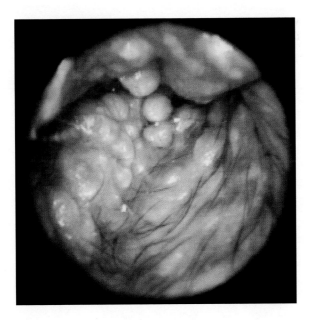

Figure 10-3

Small cerumen gland adenomas in the ear canal.

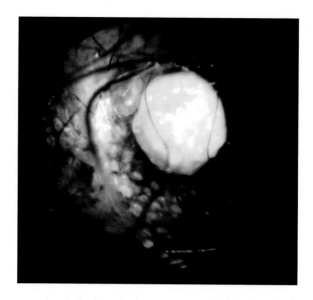

Figure 10-4

Large cerumen gland adenoma among cerumen gland hyperplasia.

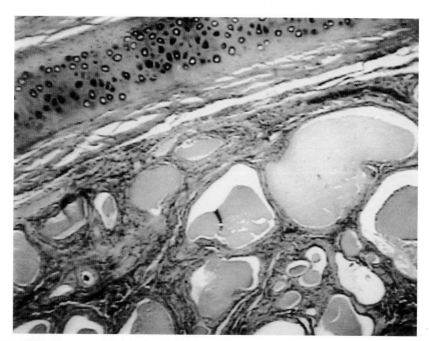

Figure 10-5

Histopathology of an ear canal, showing huge dilated cerumen glands and inflammation.

Clinical Signs. Purulent, malodorous discharges are common clinical signs associated with any type of tumor in the ear canal. Secondary bacterial and *Malassezia* infections are common. Obstructions of the canal by these masses prevent drainage and result in the accumulation of debris and cerumen. The accumulation of this debris and cerumen causes irritation to the epithelium of the canal, resulting in hyperplasia and hypersecretion of the ceruminous glands. Sinusitis and dysphagia are often present in cats with nasopharyngeal polyps.

Diagnosis and Treatment. Otoscopic examination, preferably with the patient under general anesthesia, is necessary to determine the extent of these tumors. Although it is difficult to distinguish ceruminous gland hyperplasia from a neoplastic condition, it is important to determine the extent of the condition to plan for proper diagnostic procedures. For tumors of the ear, surgical intervention is the treatment of choice. Microscopic evaluation is necessary to make a definitive diagnosis of tumors in the ears of dogs and cats.

Histologic evidence of tumors (benign or malignant) warrants surgical intervention for tumor removal and proper ear drainage.

Environmental and Conformational Causes of Ceruminous Otitis

Moisture in the ear canal due to high humidity, high ambient temperature, improper drying of the ear after cleaning, or malodorous cerumen results in the absorption of an excessive amount of water by the epithelium of the ear canal. This leads to severe maceration of the ear canal with secondary infection. This condition is complicated by the poor ventilation observed in some dogs with pendulous pinnae. Covering of the external meatus by long pendulous ears prevents proper air circulation.

Improper ear medication, harsh medications, and the inappropriate use of instruments in the ear cause irritation and abrasion, predisposing the ear canal to irritation and subsequently otitis externa with secondary infection and epithelial hyperplasia.

Proper ear drying after cleaning, avoidance of harsh medications, use of appropriate instruments for ear cleaning, and performance of routine otoscopic examination for early identification and treatment are mandatory for the successful treatment of otitis externa.

Suggested Readings

Griffin CE, Kwochka KW, MacDonald JM: *Current veterinary dermatology: the science and art of therapy,* St Louis, 1992, Mosby.

Marino DJ, MacDonald JM, Matthiesen DT, et al: Results of surgery in cats with ceruminous gland adenocarcinoma, *J Am Anim Hosp Assoc* 30, 1994.

Nesbith GH, Ackerman, LJ: *Canine and feline dermatology: diagnosis and treatment,* Trenton, NJ, 1998, Veterinary Learning Systems.

Power HT, Ihrke PJ: Use of etretinate for treatment of primary keratinization disorders in cocker spaniels, *J Am Anim Hosp Assoc* 201:419-429, 1992.

Scott DW, Miller WH, Griffin CE: *Mueller and Kirk's Small animal dermatology,* ed 6, Philadelphia, 2001, WB Saunders.

11

Failure of Epithelial Migration: Ceruminoliths

Louis N. Gotthelf, DVM

The ear canal requires a clearance mechanism to remove the accumulation of dead cells, trapped foreign debris, and wax. Without a physiologic method of debris removal, large accumulations of material would remain in the ear canal.

A number of different substances that may be found in the ear canal must be removed or they will result in significant accumulations within the canal. The ear canal is lined by stratified squamous epithelium in a constant state of growth, so desquamated surface epithelial cells must be removed. Sebaceous and apocrine glands produce ceruminous secretions, and in certain conditions, cerumen accumulation may be quite voluminous. The wax must be removed. Debris from within the ear canal such as exudates from otitis externa also must be removed, as should substances that gain access to the ear canal from outside the ear, such as plant material and accumulation of ear medications. How does the normal ear canal remove all of this accumulated debris?

Epithelial Migration

Fortunately, the ordered growth of the ear canal epithelium facilitates a clearing mechanism termed *epithelial migration.* Simply stated, the epithelium in the ear canal grows outward from the tympanic membrane toward the opening of the external ear canal. As the surface epithelial cells move, they carry along any debris on top of them. This physiologic epithelial movement process may be demonstrated by placing India ink on the eardrum and observing its dispersal along the ear canal over several weeks (Figure 11-1). The rate of epithelial movement is slow, and in older animals and people the rate becomes even slower. When the rate slows to the point of allowing accumulation of debris, the term *failure of epithelial migration* applies (Figure 11-2). When this condition causes accumulation of substances within the ear canal, ear flushes and ceruminolytic agents play important roles in its management.

A simple squamous germinal epithelium lines the lateral surface of the tympanic membrane in the external ear canal, especially in the area of the handle of the malleus (the pars tensa). It has been hypothesized that these germinal cells differentiate into epithelial cells called *basal keratinocytes,* with very loose attachments to the basement membrane.

Basal keratinocytes migrate radially on the surface of the eardrum, becoming continuous with the epithelium of the external ear canal. Evidence of this phenomenon has been gained from studying the resultant migration of squamous epithelium into the middle ear cavity following myringotomy performed at the periphery of the eardrum.

Migration of epithelium from the (pars tensa of the) tympanic membrane toward the annular region of the eardrum to the epithelium of the horizontal canal provides a clearance mechanism for the migratory keratinocytes that result from normal stratified squamous epithelial physiology in the external ear canal. Cerumen, which covers the keratinocytes, is cleared from the ear canal along with the migrating epithelium.

Besides playing a role in protecting the ear canal as a mechanical barrier to environmental substances, the keratinocytes have been shown to possess immune functions. Interleukin-1 (IL-1) is stored in keratinocytes. When these cells are damaged, IL-1 is released, stimulating other cells to release more IL-1, and a cascade of immunologic events results in the migration of granulocytes, monocytes, and macrophages into the site of damage. When an area of the ear canal has been denuded by trauma or ulcer formation, loss of this protective immune mechanism allows unchecked bacterial colonization, favoring the development of otitis externa.

Failure of Epithelial Migration

Damage to the germinal epithelium of the eardrum from infection or ear mite infestation results in damage to the keratinocytes on the surface of the tympanic membrane (Figure 11-3). During the healing process, fibrosis may cause permanent

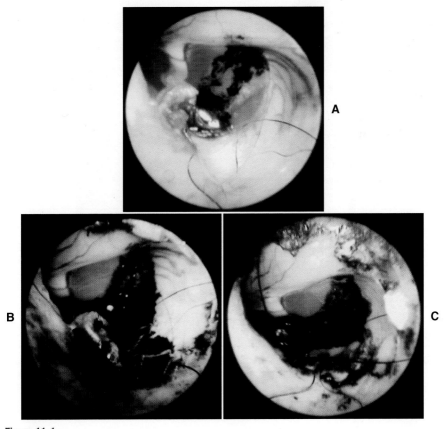

Figure 11-1

For legend, see p. 224.   *Continued*

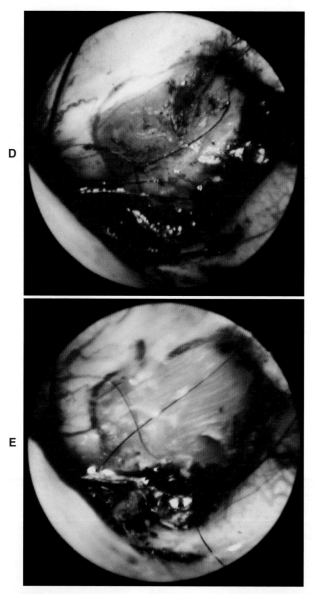

Figure 11-1—cont'd

A through **E,** Movement of India ink across the eardrum demonstrates epithelial migration. India ink was placed on the eardrum at the junction with the horizontal canal. Photos are taken at 2-week intervals. The entire series covered 2 months.

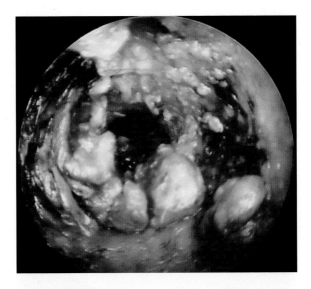

Figure 11-2

Accumulation of ceruminous exudates in the ear. Epithelial migration is not able to remove the waxy matter.

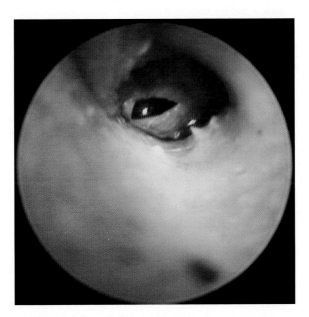

Figure 11-3

The patient, a 3-year-old cat, was presented with severe ear mite infestation. The ear canal was gently flushed with a dilute povidone-iodine solution to remove the ear mite debris. After cleaning, the eardrum can be seen to have a tear in it. It is here that epithelial cells that would migrate to the ear canal will stop their journey. This will result in waxy accumulations on the eardrum in the future.

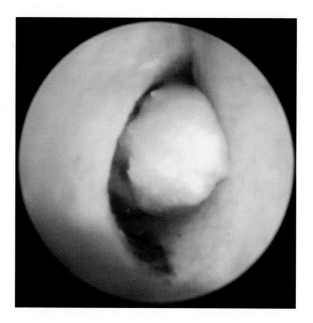

Figure 11-4

Soft wax ball seen attached to the eardrum. Part of the eardrum is visible at the ventral portion of the wax ball between it and the horizontal canal.

changes to the tympanic membrane. Normal epithelial migration may be disrupted. Failure of epithelial migration may result in the accumulation of flakes of skin in the ear canal. More often, however, wax and keratin accumulate at the base of the eardrum and form either soft wax plugs (Figure 11-4) or large, hard concretions called *ceruminoliths* (Figure 11-5). To find them when examining the ear canals with an otoscope, the veterinarian should follow the bend in the ear cartilage and look in the horizontal canal toward the eardrum. Ceruminoliths are found attached to the eardrum lying along the floor of the horizontal ear canal.

Ceruminoliths

If the dog in which a ceruminolith is developing has a large number of hairs originating from around the annulus of the tympanic membrane, the hairs are included in the matrix of the ceruminolith. As the concretion moves, in response to head movement and gravity, these hairs are pulled and may cause significant discomfort. Bristly, thick hairs, as found in some dogs, that become involved in ceruminolith formation may irritate the ear canal lining and also cause discomfort (Figure 11-6). In the author's experience, these conditions are often found in dogs and cats with histories of previously resolved ear disease. When ceruminoliths occur, they are usually seen in an ear without evidence of other disease.

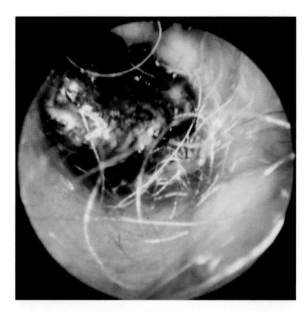

Figure 11-5

A hard concretion at the eardrum of a 15-year-old Poodle. Note the hairs included in the matrix of the ceruminolith. Also notice the normal ear canal epithelium.

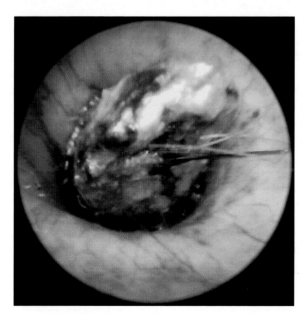

Figure 11-6

This large ceruminolith in a German Shepherd illustrates the inclusion of bristly hairs in the wax ball. In this photo, the thick hairs are touching the horizontal ear canal wall and causing discomfort. The horizontal ear canal epithelium appears normal.

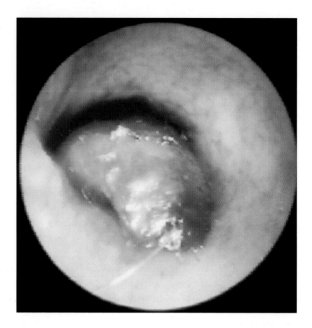

Figure 11-7

Soft wax ball. The owner of a 4-year-old cat presented the animal for diminished hearing and head tilt. The history indicated that the cat had recurrent ear mites as a kitten.

When epithelial migration is prevented from continuing, the keratinocytes on the eardrum form layers on top of each other and are pushed backward toward the eardrum. Over time, the net effect is significant accumulation of desquamation products that cannot clear away from the eardrum and out of the ear canal. Cerumen and hairs mix into the heap. Cytologic smears of these concretions will show heavy growth of *Malassezia* yeasts.

These waxy accumulations can become quite large, some of them measuring 1 or 2 inches in length. Although innocuous in appearance, ceruminoliths plugging the horizontal ear canal diminish hearing. In certain head positions, the weight of the ceruminolith pushes against the eardrum and may cause increased air pressure within the middle ear cavity, leading to signs of vestibular disease (Figure 11-7).

Otoscopic examination of a ceruminolith reveals that there is a base attached to the eardrum, with the body of the mass freely movable and unattached to the surrounding ear canal. The tips of long hairs may be seen on the surface. In many cases the peripheral portion of the pars tensa can be visualized.

Removal

The softer wax balls can be curetted or flushed out of the ear canal with fluid under pressure. If there is an eardrum present, treatment with a ceruminolytic agent such as dioctyl sodium sulfosuccinate may loosen the concretion. Warming the flush

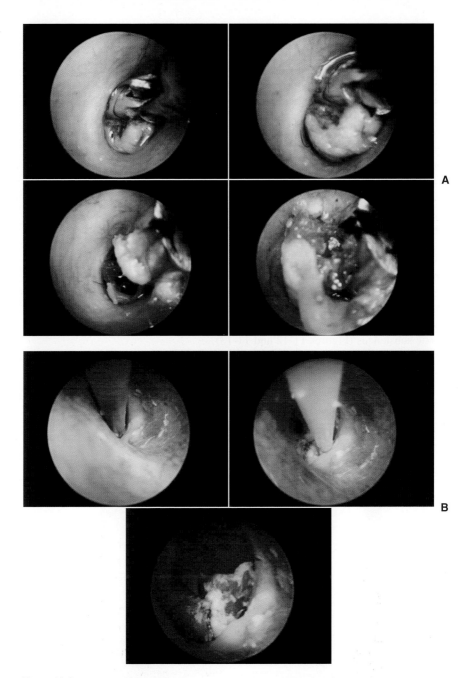

Figure 11-8

A, Removal of a wax ball from the ear canal from the cat in Figure 11-7. The mass was grasped by the endoscopic grasping forceps. Because the wax was quite soft and malleable, the endoscopic graspers were ineffective at removing the wax. **B,** The ear canal was treated with a ceruminolytic agent and flushed with warmed dilute povidone-iodine solution. The soft wax was flushed from the ear and small pieces of remaining debris were carefully suctioned off the surface of the eardrum.

solution helps to soften the waxy debris, and sometimes careful suction with a large-bore suction catheter aids in their removal (Figure 11-8).

Removing a hardened concretion type of ceruminolith requires the use of a grasping forceps. The use of a video otoscope (Video Vetscope, MedRx, Inc., Seminole, Florida) facilitates this process because the veterinarian can see the ceruminolith clearly on the video monitor. The endoscopic grasping tool, which is inserted through the biopsy channel of the video otoscope, can be carefully placed to grasp and remove the mass (Figure 11-9).

After removal of these concretions, the tympanic membrane often looks abnormal. Small holes in the tympanum may be present because the epithelium is eroded along with the concretion as it is removed (Figure 11-10). These small holes heal rapidly (Figure 11-11).

If the eardrum was previously ruptured and a ceruminolith developed as a consequence, the healing tympanic epithelium may be in the middle of a ceruminolith. When the concretion is removed, the eardrum is torn away, and a large direct communication to the tympanic bulla results. If detergent flush solutions were used for removal of the ceruminolith, copious saline flushes are used to remove these ototoxic substances (Figures 11-12 and 11-13).

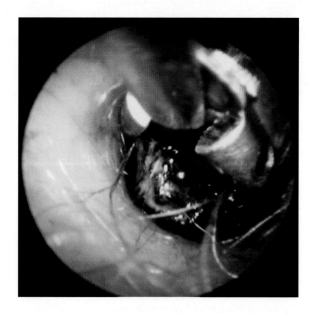

Figure 11-9

Endoscopic grasping forceps are used through the working channel of the Video Vetscope to extract the wax ball from the dog in Figure 11-5.

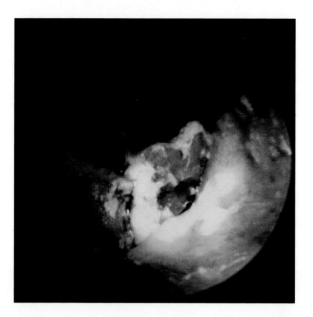

Figure 11-10

After removal of the wax plug from the cat in Figure 11-7, the eardrum was closely examined. A roughened surface and a small hole in the 5 o'clock position can be seen.

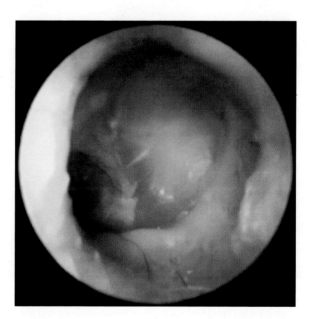

Figure 11-11

Close-up view of the eardrum from the cat in Figure 11-10 1 month after removal of the wax ball. The eardrum has healed and is almost normal in appearance. The cat was asymptomatic on this recheck visit.

Older animals may have large accumulations of waxy, cellular debris in the ear canals because the epithelial migration process is quite slow. Occasional ear flushes may be required to augment the physiologic cleaning process in these patients.

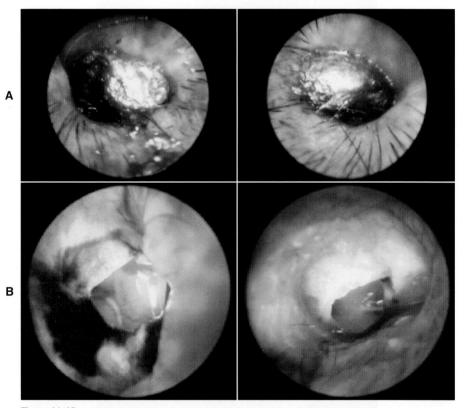

Figure 11-12

A, Bilateral ceruminoliths were identified in a 7-year-old mixed-breed dog with diminished hearing. **B,** The ceruminoliths were grasped with the endoscopic forceps and carefully removed. Both eardrums were ruptured, which may have resulted because each eardrum was involved in the matrix of the ceruminolith.

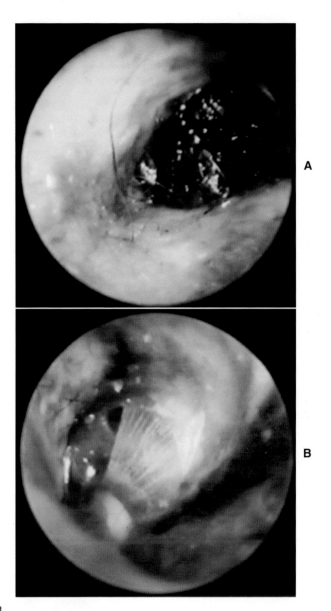

Figure 11-13

A, The patient, a 3-year-old German Shepherd, was examined because of a painful ear. The affected ear was not being carried in an erect position. Examination of the ear canal revealed a wax plug at the level of the eardrum. **B,** The wax plug was grasped with the endoscopic forceps and carefully extracted. After the ear canal was flushed and dried, a partial tear of the eardrum could be seen. Mucus and pus consistent with otitis media are present under the cerumen plug.

Suggested Readings

Michaels I, Soucek S: Development of the stratified squamous epithelium of the human tympanic membrane and external ear canal: the origin of auditory epithelial migration, *Am J Anat* 184:334-344, 1989.

Smelt G, Stoney P, Weinberger J, et al: Sequelae of experimental tympanic and inferior wall perforations: the double meaning of epithelial migration, *J Otolaryngol* 20:171-176, 1991.

12

Diseases that Affect the Pinna

Geneviève Marignac, DVM

Most skin diseases may affect the pinna in dogs and cats, but other parts of the body can also be involved. Other than neoplasia, few dermatoses are restricted to the pinnae. Dermatoses restricted to the pinnae include aural hematoma, physical dermatoses (e.g., trauma, solar dermatitis, frostbite), arthropod bites, neoplasia, vasculitis, contact dermatitis, fissure or seborrhea of the ear margin, pinnal alopecia, and psoriasiform-lichenoid dermatitis of Springer Spaniels. Many other dermatoses may induce lesions that begin or stay confined to the pinna for some time, but they usually involve other body sites at some point of their evolution (e.g., sarcoptic mange, dermatophytosis, atopic dermatitis, pemphigus complex).

This chapter focuses on these two groups of skin diseases from the point of view of their pinnal involvement. A clinical classification based on the most common and/or particular pinnal manifestation of each dermatosis has been used. However, the author is aware that most diseases mentioned here could be included under more than one heading. The reader is referred to updated specialized literature to find details on their pathogenesis, diagnostic procedures, and treatment; they are beyond the scope of this chapter.

Pinna Anatomy

The pinna, or auricle, consists of the flat part of the auricular cartilage, covered by skin on both sides. The convex surface is haired, even in some hairless breeds such as the Chinese Crested dog. Most of the concave surface is glabrous in cats and is variably haired in dogs, depending on the breed. In the most hirsute breeds such as the Cocker Spaniel the area around the ear canal opening is glabrous. The proximal part of the auricular cartilage folds into different tubercles and ridges and forms the ear canal opening, which includes the anthelix (medial), tragus (lateral), and antitragus (caudal) (Figure 12-1). (See also Chapter 1.)

Nineteen muscles attached on the skull and the auricular, annular, and scutiform cartilages allow the independent and complex pinnal movements observed in dogs and cats. The evolutionary role of pinnae is not clear. It may be related to sound collection (mobility of the pinna) or to prevention against foreign bodies (pendulous ears); it may even play an ornamental role.

Aural Hematoma

Aural hematomas can form within (intrachondrally) or along (subparachondrally) the cartilage of the pinna. They are considered more common in pendulous-eared breeds, but any dog or cat can be affected. There is no sex predilection, but affected dogs are usually middle-aged or older.

Clinically, aural hematomas result in large fluctuant swellings of various sizes, but usually they affect most of the ear pinna above the anthelix. During the first days, the swelling is warm to hot to the touch, and the overlying skin is erythematous. The animal is greatly bothered by the increased weight of the ear and sometimes seems

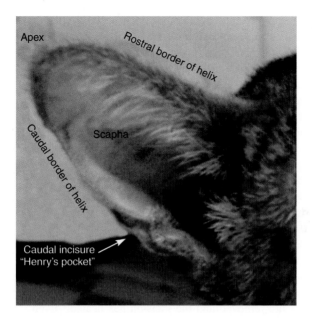

Figure 12-1

Right pinna of a cat, concave surface.

to experience pain. Aspiration fluid obtained within hours of hematoma formation is sero-hemorrhagic and usually rich in fibrin. The presence of fibrin can prevent aspiration of any fluid later in the disease. The normal evolution of a hematoma is resorption of the fluid and healing. Fibrosis is always a major feature of the aural hematoma healing process, especially if left untreated. The pinna becomes thick, hard, and permanently distorted as the fibrosis in the wound contracts. Because aural hematoma is rarely seen in dogs and cats with major trauma to their pinna, minor ear trauma and/or pruritus is more likely a precipitating factor than a primary cause. Most studies reveal the following:[1]

- Trauma seems a precipitating factor rather than an underlying factor in aural hematoma.
- Aural hematoma is an uncommon finding in chronic skin diseases.
- Many dogs affected with aural hematoma do not have signs of any concurrent auricular, cutaneous, or systemic disease.

In one study, results were in favor of an autoimmune cause.[2] Joyce and Day could not confirm these results, even though they did find histopathologic evidence of cartilage degeneration associated with fibrovascular granulation tissue filling the cartilage defect.[1] They presumed that their samples (incisional biopsies of affected pinna) reflected the end process of cartilage degeneration that might have been caused by the mediators released by macrophages earlier in the process. These considerations are in favor of a process, most probably immune-mediated, that began several weeks before the aural hematoma was observed by the owner. Diagnosis of aural hematoma is usually straightforward and is based on history, clinical presentation, and fluid collection. Because the disease is self-limiting and heals spontaneously, some owners may choose not to treat their animal. Nevertheless, the hematoma greatly bothers the animal. Cosmetic considerations are also in favor of surgical treatment.

Several surgical techniques have been described. Fluid drainage (aspiration, indwelling drain, partial or whole-length incision) and flushing are effective in relieving the animal but usually result in post-treatment deformity of the ear pinna. Griffin found that surgical procedures aiming at prevention of immediate relapse by compression (without necrosis) and at restoration of the pinna's initial shape and carriage are the most cosmetically effective and have the least recurrences.[3] This can be achieved by several techniques. The most commonly used are multiple mattress sutures placed after incision or multiple punch holes made through the skin (see Chapter 19). Mattress sutures may also be placed through a soft but rigid device (several types are marketed that usually contain foam).

Because the healing of aural hematomas is highly fibrotic, glucosteroids are flushed into the hematoma cavity. They are also given orally with antibiotics, at least until the sutures are removed and the incision has healed.[2] Even though trauma is probably only a precipitating factor, it should be avoided as much as possible to prevent relapses. It is mandatory to identify and correct the cause. Otitis externa and pinnal skin diseases are most commonly encountered (Figure 12-2).[6]

Pinnal Trauma

The most common causes of pinnal trauma are pruritus or fight wounds; they also may be related to common dog habits such as earth digging and chasing other animals (Figure 12-3). Complications at the surgery site, including infection and tearing of the stitches, are common where ear cropping is still allowed. Pinnal trauma is usually associated with prolific bleeding. Routine wound cleaning and topical hemostatic application (peroxide, epinephrine, or collagen) are usually sufficient treatment. In severe cases, cauterization under anesthesia and/or compressive bandage might be necessary. Due to the thin edges of the pinna, laceration of the ear margin can be a permanent sequel.

Dermatophytosis is another possible consequence, which is often associated with a history of cat fighting or soil digging. Both cat claws and soil can be a source of various dermatophytes. The trauma associated with contact facilitates the inoculation of the fungi. This may happen during a fight or if the pinna is scratched with a soil-covered paw during digging or shortly after.

Blood sampling from the ears of dogs and cats has been recently developed in order to monitor blood glucose. Pinnal lesions may result from frequent sampling. The local ischemia associated with the vascular problems commonly associated with diabetes mellitus probably predisposes diabetic patients to pinnal complications.

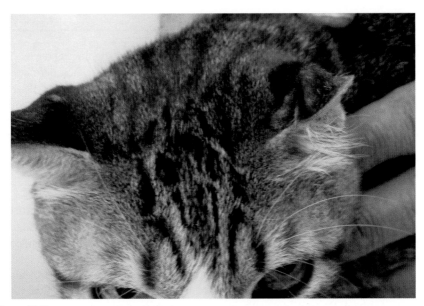

Figure 12-2

Fibrosis and folding of the pinna of a 13-year-old cat with a history of aural hematoma that was left untreated.

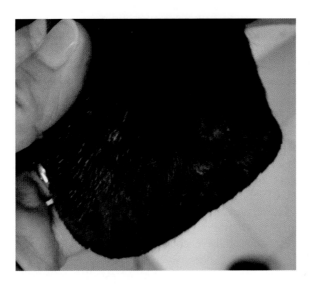

Figure 12-3

Hypothrichosis due to intense ear scratching caused by otitis externa.

Pruritic Dermatoses

Pruritus is probably the most common cause of pinnal lesions in dogs and cats. The origin of the pruritus can be the pinna itself, as in arthropod-related dermatoses, atopic dermatitis, or contact dermatitis.[4] Nevertheless, pinnal pruritus is most commonly caused by otitis externa (e.g., otodectic mange, foreign body, *Malassezia* otitis externa, atopic dermatitis) or facial diseases (e.g., intertrigo, food allergy, atopic dermatitis, conjunctivitis).[4] Pruritus results in pinnal alopecia, excoriation, and crusting.

Sarcoptic Mange

Sarcoptic mange is a cosmopolitan, transmissible, nonseasonal, highly pruritic, generalized dermatosis of dogs caused by *Sarcoptes scabiei* var *cani*. It is contagious among dogs and can cause transient lesions on humans because sarcoptic mange is a zoonosis. Other variants of *Sarcoptes scabiei* are found on most mammalian species.

The pinna is one of the favorite habitats of the mite. Early pinnal lesions are abundant, with yellowish crusts that adhere between hairs. The entire border of the pinna may be involved. Pruritus is usually intense and results in pinnal trauma, hair loss, excoriation, and erythema. Because the pathogenesis of scabies involves a hypersensitivity reaction, some dogs may experience only mild pruritus. An anergic form is described where affected animals are almost nonpruritic in spite of the presence of hundreds of mites.[5] More commonly, clinical signs of scabies can be more subtle or have a different localization in dogs treated for fleas and ticks with drugs used against acarids (permethrin, other pyrethroids, fipronil, amitraz) that are not completely efficient due to their spectrum, the formulation used (spot-on, collars, shampoo), the amount used, or the frequency of application.

Differential diagnosis includes otodectic dermatitis, trombiculosis, pediculosis, cheyletiellosis, contact dermatitis, *Malassezia* dermatitis, and atopic dermatitis. Definitive diagnosis is based on finding *Sarcoptes scabiei* mites. Multiple skin scrapings are sometimes necessary and should involve at least both pinnae and both elbows. Pinnae should be sampled preferentially in areas where thin crusts are present. They feel like sand when the pinnal margins are palpated between the fingers. Nevertheless, mites can be difficult to find. If sarcoptic mange is suspected, a complete treatment should be instituted regardless of skin scraping results.

The pinnal-pedal reflex is often positive. When the pinnal margin is scratched with a fingernail, a reflexive rear leg scratch is initiated. Most pruritic conditions of the pinna and even pruritic otitis externa can also induce a positive response. False-negative reactions are also encountered.

Treatment for scabies should involve the whole body, even if lesions are localized. Systemic treatments (selamectin, ivermectin) are usually preferred because they are easy to use, have minimal side effects, and are environmentally safe. In case of treatment failure or for cost considerations, especially in kennels, acaricidal rinses are a good alternative (lime sulfur, amitraz, rotenone, phosmet). Hair clipping is mandatory if the hair coat is thick and/or long. Lime sulfur rinses can be used on young dogs.

Notoedric Mange

Notoedric mange is a nonseasonal, transmissible, pruritic dermatosis of cats caused by *Notoedres cati*. It can cause transient lesions on most mammals, including dogs and humans. All in-contact cats, especially littermates, are more or less affected. The incidence is reported to have greatly decreased, and notoedric mange is considered rare in most countries. The distribution is epizootic; in a given country, it can be seen commonly in one region and rarely in another.

The medial borders of both pinnae are affected first, then the whole pinna is affected; the lesions then spread all over the face, eyelids, neck, and, infrequently, the perineum and feet. Generalization is unusual. Papules are early transient lesions. The skin rapidly becomes thickened and forms large wrinkles covered with thick, adherent, yellowish to silvery crusts. Pruritus is intense and results in alopecia. Severe excoriation leads to infected wounds. Lymphadenopathy is a common feature.

Differential diagnosis includes otodectic dermatitis, cheyletiellosis, food allergy, atopic dermatitis, contact dermatitis, and pemphigus foliaceus or erythematosus. Mites are more readily found on skin scrapings than *Sarcoptes scabiei*. Nevertheless, due to their small size, the scraping should be scrutinized under 10× objective, closed diaphragm, medium light, and after good clearing of the sample.

Many acaricidal drugs are toxic in cats, particularly organochlorates, organophosphates, permethrin, and amitraz. Avermectins (selamectin, ivermectin) and lime sulfur are effective.

Treatment of the premises is mandatory because the mite can survive for more than 2 weeks in the environment.[5]

Trombiculiasis

The six-legged larvae of the genera *Trombicula* (chigger mite, harvest mite) cause a seasonal (in temperate or continental climates) and pruritic papular dermatosis both in dogs and cats. Numerous species of *Trombicula* are associated with the disease in various countries. The more commonly recognized are *Neotrombicula automnalis* (Europe) and *Eutrombicula alfreddugesi* (America).

Mites are often found on and around the pinna. The legs, interdigital areas, ventrum, and face are often involved, too. Pruritus is almost always present. Crusts, alopecia, and erosion are present on affected areas.

The diagnosis is usually easy because the larvae are visible to the naked eye (0.5 mm), have a bright orange to red color, and are tightly adherent to the skin, usually in clusters.

Treatment should aim at killing the mites present on the animal, relieving the pruritus, and preventing subsequent infestation. If infestation is localized, topical application of an otic ointment containing steroids and an insecticide is sufficient. Otherwise, an acaricidal spray should be associated with a 5- to 8-day course of oral prednisolone (1 mg/kg). If free roaming cannot be prevented, the prevention of reinfestation is difficult. An acaricidal spray with a strong repellent effect such as permethrin is an option for dogs but is toxic in cats. In one study on a small number of animals, fipronil spray applications seemed to achieve a more effective and lasting result in dogs than in cats.[6] *Trombicula autumnalis* adults are found in the outside environment. Compost areas should be enclosed so that the pet cannot access them. Treatment of other favorable areas (under trees, under the house, in bushes) with insecticides should be discouraged because of the toxicity to invertebrates (pollinating insects, honeybees) and children and the presence of residue on fruits or vegetables grown in the garden.

Louse Infestations

Pediculosis can be caused by sucking lice (*Anoploura,* such as *Linognathus setosus* in dogs) or chewing lice (*Mallophaga,* such as *Felicola subrostrata* in cats and *Trichodectes canis* or, in warm climates, *Heterodoxus spiniger* in dogs). Lice are dorsoventrally flattened wingless insects. They cause few direct lesions but usually cause intense pruritus. The whole body is often involved, but they particularly accumulate on the concave surface and base of the pinna.

Nits (louse egg cases) are usually visible, adherent to the hair. The hair coat is often matted and dirty. Lice infestation is associated with neglect (overcrowding, poor sanitation), and affected animals are often debilitated. Anemia can be associated with heavy *Linognathus setosus* infestation because sucking lice feed on blood. Asymptomatic carriers exhibit only mild pruritus and seborrhea sicca.

Differential diagnosis includes flea-allergy dermatitis, scabies, cheyletiellosis, *Dermanyssus* or *Trombicula* infestation, *Malassezia* dermatitis, allergic skin diseases, and seborrheic disorders. Acetate tape allows lice immobilization and identification by microscopic observation. Hair coat observation with the video otoscope is another possibility. Nits are visible both on macroscopic and microscopic examination. They are larger and more tightly attached to the hair than *Cheyletiella* eggs.

In dogs and cats, most routine insecticides are active on adult lice (spray, shampoo, powder, dips), which might explain the observed decrease in pediculosis prevalence. Nevertheless, treatments are usually ineffective on eggs and have to be applied repeatedly.

Insect Bite Dermatitis

Insect bite dermatitis can be caused by various hematophagous insects due to the mediators or toxic products present in their saliva; it is sometimes associated with hypersensitivity reactions. Cats are more commonly affected than dogs, perhaps because they roam more and because of their "lie and wait" way of hunting. Papules, erythema, erosion, and alopecia are seen mainly on the thickened tip of the pinna. The border and the dorsal side can also be affected. In dog breeds with pendulous or broken ears, lesions are seen on the surface of the pinna where the ear folds down. In severe cases, multiple small ulcers covered with hemorrhagic crusts are present.

The causative insects vary with the season, environment, and climate.

The rabbit flea *(Spilopsyllus cuniculi)* can infest dogs and cats that are in contact with infected rabbits *(*pet, hutch, hunting*)*. Transmission is reported to occur mainly at the time of rabbit parturition. This flea is found mainly in Europe and Australia. It stays tightly attached to its host's skin, usually at the tip of the pinna, and should not be confused with a tick.

Mosquitoes (*Aedes* spp., *Culex* spp.), stable flies (*Stomoxys calcitrans*), and blackflies (*Simulium* spp.) may cause lesions on the pinna. The bridge of the nose and/or the periocular area can also be affected. Their presence is seasonal in endemic areas. Because they do not stay on their host, the diagnosis is often putative.

Differential diagnosis includes actinic dermatitis, trauma, canine eosinophilic pinnal folliculitis, and eosinophilic furunculosis of the face. Diagnosis is based on history and clinical signs. Lesions are often infiltrated with eosinophils and show secondary infection.

Treatment should be aimed at the lesions and at reinfestation prevention. Lesions are cleaned and topical antibiotics are applied. Steroids are often used because of the common hypersensitivity component of the disease. Steroids are not indicated if ulceration is present because they slow the healing process. Elimination of the animal's exposure to the insects is the only effective prevention but is usually difficult to achieve. Measures include treatment of farmed or pet rabbits, prevention of free roaming, and application of a repellent. Permethrins and pyrethroids have good repellent activity, as shown with a deltamethrin-containing collar against phlebotomes, but they are toxic in cats. Vaseline mixed with citronella, DEET, or N,N-diethylmetatoluamide allows the product to stay longer on the ear tip.

Atopic Dermatitis

Erythema of the concave pinna is seen in more than 50% of atopic dermatitis cases in dogs and is the only symptom for a year or more before the development of other symptoms in at least 3% of canine cases.[10-12] Associated pruritus is intense (Figure 12-4).

Lichenification and thickening of the concave pinna usually occur. Seborrhea and *Malassezia* dermatitis are common complications. This frequent feature might be explained in part by the observation made on 10 normal dogs, where mast cell counts were found to be highest in the medial and lateral pinna.[7] Otitis externa, cheilitis, and conjunctivitis are also frequently encountered in canine atopic dermatitis and also cause pinnal pruritus and trauma.

The clinical presentation of atopic dermatitis is very different in cats. Otitis externa and the related pinnal trauma caused by pruritus are uncommon, even rare. Atopic dermatitis is a common underlying cause of the initially non-lesional pruritus of the face, neck and pinna, even though *Otodectes cynotis* and food allergy are the main differential diagnosis for this condition in cats.

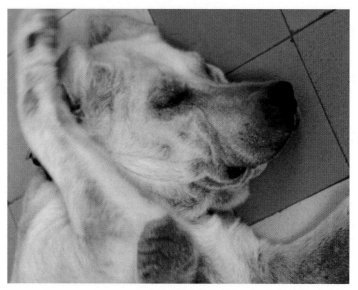

Figure 12-4

Intense pruritus of the inner pinnae in a 5-year-old female atopic Labrador with secondary *Malassezia* dermatitis and otitis externa.

Food Allergy

Food allergy is commonly associated with auricular disease both in dogs and cats (see Chapter 6). The pathogenesis of cutaneous nontoxic adverse reaction to food can involve immune-mediated or non–immune-mediated mechanisms. They are respectively called *food allergy/hypersensitivity* and *food intolerance.* The precise mechanisms are not elucidated in animals and are a point of controversy in humans.

In cats, facial pruritus is probably the most common presentation of food allergy. Excoriations caused by the intense self-mutilation are usually not restricted to the pinna but also affect the preauricular area, face, and neck. As opposed to canine cases of food allergy, otitis externa is rare in cats.

In one study of 51 food-allergic dogs, Rosser[8] stated that 80% of cases had otitis externa and that it was the only symptom in 20%. Pinnal lesions mainly result from otitis externa–related pruritus (Figure 12-5). Improvements in pruritus and skin lesions during the food trial may not be obvious if the perpetuating factors of the otitis externa are not treated initially (bacteria or yeast proliferation, inflammation associated ear canal or pinna changes).

Contact Dermatitis

Contact dermatitis is a common cause of skin lesions on the concave surface of the pinna, probably because it is hairless.[9] Topical ear treatments are a common cause.

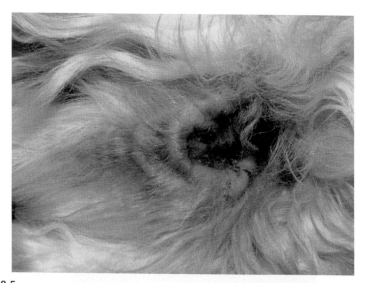

Figure 12-5

Erythema and lichenification on the inner pinnae of a female Bichon Frisé with food allergy.

Typically, the animal is treated topically for otitis externa; 1 to 3 days after the start of treatment, the condition worsens. Almost any treatment can cause an allergic reaction. In humans and animals, neomycin has been most commonly involved.[9,10] Propylene glycol is a very common vehicle of topical auricular medications. It is considered by Griffin to be the most common cause of contact dermatitis of the pinna.[11]

Some ointments can be applied on the skin for transdermal absorption such as vasodilators for cardiac disease (e.g., nitroglycerine). The concave pinna is the usual site because it is glabrous and vascular and the animal cannot lick the product easily. The drug and its vehicle are potential causes of contact dermatitis. Erythema is often observed after repeated application of medications, especially if applied on the same pinna.[12] Recently, ear pinna transdermal methimazole application for hyperthyroidism has been evaluated in cats.[13] Contact dermatitis is also possible, so it is recommended that pinnal application be alternated.

In contact dermatitis associated with topical ear ointments, the concave surface of the pinna is erythematous and swollen. Erosion or even ulceration can be present, especially if an irritant product (diethyl ether, toluene, essential oil) has been applied. Pruritus is usually more severe, and ear scratching and rubbing cause alopecia and excoriation. In some cases the ear is painful. A definite diagnosis can rarely be achieved because drug challenge is usually not performed due to a possible worsening of the symptoms.

When symptomatic treatment is opted for, two points should be considered:
1. Steroids can be the cause of the adverse reaction.
2. The drug vehicle can also be implicated. Because it is identical in most ointments, change of drug does not always resolve the symptoms.

Ear flushing and pinna cleaning with saline (with or without systemic antiinflammatory treatment) is a possible option.

Cutaneous Adverse Drug Reaction

Any drug, drug vehicle, or food product can cause an adverse reaction in the skin (toxiderma) (Figure 12-6). Most authors agree that toxiderma can mimic any skin disease. Some specific drugs preferentially induce pinna lesions.

Self-induced mutilation of the head and neck has been reported in hyperthyroid cats treated with carbimazole. The same symptoms have been observed less

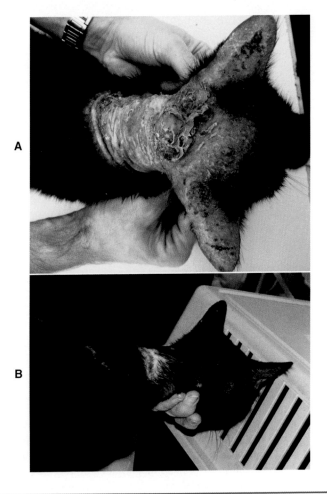

Figure 12-6

A, Sudden onset of ear and neck excoriation in an 8-year-old male domestic short-hair cat associated with treatment. No other lesions could be seen on the body. **B,** The same cat 2 months later.

commonly in cats treated with the carbimazole metabolite, methimazole.[14,15] Facial pruritus has also been associated with propylthiouracil and clavulanic acid and amoxicillin.[16] Cephalexin-induced pemphigus foliaceus lesions on the whole ear pinna and extending to the face have been observed in one cat.[16] Vasculitis, causing necrotic pinnal lesions and onychomadesis, was associated with penicillin injections.[16]

Dermatoses of the Ear Margin

Vasculitis

Extremities (pinna, digits, tail) have a vasculature that lacks anastomosis and is particularly susceptible to environmental injuries (trauma, temperature). Clinical manifestations of diseases causing vascular lesions such as inflammation (vasculitis) and thrombosis often involve the extremities, particularly the pinna borders (Figure 12-7). Nevertheless, some specific types of vasculitis induce local lesions such as rabies vaccine–related vasculitis (lesions at the injection site) or lesions resulting from perivenous injection of irritant substances.

Clinical manifestations of pinna vasculitis are quite stereotypic, regardless of the cause of the vasculitis. The pinna borders are preferential sites, especially the apex and its concave surface. Primary lesions include purpura, plaques, papules, pustules, and in severe cases, hemorrhagic bullae. Purpura can be distinguished from erythema because it does not blanch on diascopy (looking through a glass slide firmly applied on the lesion). Punched-out ulcers and necrosis quickly result from

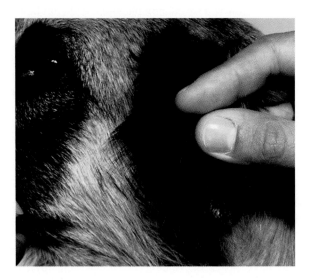

Figure 12-7

Crusts and scales on the apex of a female Malinois Shepherd dog. The cause of the vasculitis was not identified.

the lack of perfusion. The shape and disposition of the lesions clearly correlate with the vascular pathways. As the disease evolves, the whole pinna border can become involved. Differential diagnosis includes arthropod bite, fight wounds, cold agglutinin diseases, frostbite, and coagulopathies.

Because necrosis occurs within hours of the infarct, biopsy should be taken preferably on the most recent lesions. The biopsy should involve both diseased tissue and the border of the lesions because the vascular event is situated there. The owner should be aware that biopsy of the pinna can cause lifelong and visible deformation and tissue defects. If the submitted sample includes the area where vascular injury occurred, dermatopathology allows the diagnosis of vasculitis, but it usually does not permit precise identification of the cause. This part of the diagnosis is mandatory if an appropriate treatment regimen is to be chosen and relapse is to be prevented.

Underlying causes of vasculitis are divided into the following:
• *Precipitating factors:* Infection, drugs, low temperatures. Vaccines are reported to cause injection site vasculitis as well as lesions on the apex of the pinna and often on the concave surface. Other extremities, the face (periocular area), and bony prominences can also be affected.
• *Concurrent diseases:* Infection, insect bite, neoplasia, food-related causes, connective tissue disorders (e.g., lupus erythematosus), cold agglutinin diseases.

In one study, no underlying cause for vasculitis could be found in about 50% of cases.[14] Two idiopathic conditions have been described that can affect the pinna: familial cutaneous vasculopathy of German Shepherd dogs and proliferative thrombovascular necrosis of the pinna. They are described in the following sections. Cold agglutinin diseases are described under *Frostbite*.

The outcome and treatment depend on the suspected or diagnosed underlying cause(s). Because vasculitis is a severe complication, it should be treated while the underlying cause is being explored or at the beginning of its correction. Pentoxyfylline has many effects, including increased red blood cell pliability and immunomodulation. It is considered the first-line treatment in vasculitis and other ischemic diseases. Propentoxyfylline is licensed in many countries for geriatric dogs with behavioral problems related to microvascularization disorders in the brain. Pentoxyfylline itself remains in the peripheral circulation. This latter drug has not been thoroughly evaluated in dogs, but the proposed dosage is 10 mg/kg q8h to q24h. Side effects appear to be minimal and are considered to regress after treatment cessation. They include vomiting and diarrhea; the author has also observed a few cases of rectal bleeding. An anecdotal report of thrombocytopenia indicates that care should be taken when prescribing pentoxyfylline in affected dogs.

Steroids can be added to pentoxifylline. Topical treatment is usually suficient. Systemic prednisolone (2 to 4 mg/kg, q24h, by mouth) can be necessary in the most severe cases (especially in cases of neutrophilic vasculitis), if no underlying infectious process has been identified. Other possible treatments that have been proposed include large doses of vitamin E (adjunct therapy), dapsone (to be used with caution in cats), cyclophosphamide, azathioprine, and the association tetracycline/niacinamide.

Familial Cutaneous Vasculopathy of German Shepherd Dogs

In German Shepherd puppies, a familial cutaneous vasculopathy has been recognized with an autosomal, recessive mode of inheritance.[17] Initial lesions include depigmented and swollen footpads. The pinnae, tail, and nasal planum are usually also affected, displaying alopecia, crusts, and ulceration. Dermatopathology demonstrates vascular degeneration and vasculitis, as well as other dermal changes: nodular dermatitis, collagenolysis, and cell-poor interface dermatitis with basal cell apoptosis.

Proliferative Thrombovascular Necrosis of the Pinna

This condition is recognized in the dog and differs from other types of vasculitis affecting the ear by its histopathologic features—arterioles initially develop into folds in the lumen. Sclerosis and hyaline degeneration are also observed, and eventually thrombosis. Clinical features are similar to those of other types of vasculitis affecting the pinna border. Pentoxyfylline is usually partially to 100% effective.[14,18] Topical steroids are an option. Because this condition is restricted to the pinna, more potent immunosuppressive treatments with potential systemic side effects should be avoided. If medical treatment is unrewarding, surgical removal of diseased tissue is effective. Relapses are reported following excisions with a narrow margin.[3]

Solar Dermatitis and Actinic Keratosis of the Ear

Repeated exposure to direct or reflected sunlight (especially ultraviolet B [UVB] and ultraviolet C [UVC]) on white skin causes actinic reactions (from the Greek *actin,* ray) that can vary from the so-called sunburn (solar dermatitis) to actinic keratosis and eventually squamous cell carcinoma. Animals with white ears or white spots that include the pinna are at risk if they live in a sunny region; these include white cats, Dalmatians, American Staffordshire Terriers, Bull Terriers, and white Bulldogs.

In animals with erect ears, especially cats, the pinna borders are seldom protected from sunlight by the fine pinnal hair coat. In white animals, erythema and fine scaling (solar dermatitis) can appear as early as 3 months of age. As the lesions aggravate, the erythema is more pronounced and associated with crust formation. The lesions bother the animal and are usually painful; self-trauma aggravates the condition. Careful observation shows that the border of the pinna is finely curled. The nasal planum is usually also affected, especially in dogs, where it can be the only involved area. The lower eyelids and the lips may also be involved. Differential diagnosis includes insect bites, fight wounds, vasculitis, and early sarcoptic or notoedric mange. At this stage, keeping the animal indoors (including the prevention of lying in the sunlight) from 10 AM to 4 PM should be sufficient.

In the summer, lesions recur and worsen (Figure 12-8). The ear margins become thickened, indurated, and hyperkeratotic. Atypia and dysplasia of the epidermis, as well as follicular keratinocytes and solar elastosis, are observed on dermatopathologic examination. Sun avoidance is sufficient only in early cases. Systemic retinoids

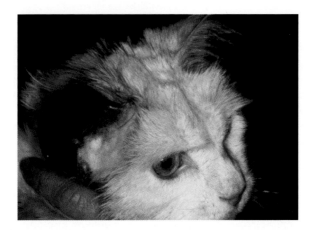

Figure 12-8

Squamous cell carcinoma on the right ear of a white domestic short-hair cat. The right ear apex is finely curled, an almost pathognomonic early symptom of sun-related injury.

or surgical excision of damaged tissue is usually necessary. If the lesions are pruritic and/or painful, topical or systemic glucocorticoids are indicated.

Squamous cell carcinoma can result, especially if the disease is neglected or the animal cannot be kept inside. The neoplasm can be proliferative or ulcerative, but usually bleeds easily. Squamous cell carcinoma is considered to be mainly locally invasive and slow to metastasize, so amputation of the pinna is effective in many cases.

Frostbite

Frostbite is caused by prolonged exposure to temperatures below freezing (cold climate, contact with cold objects). All extremities are predisposed to frostbite, but especially the pinnae, which are very thin but have a large surface area (Figure 12-9). Other predisposing factors include previous frostbite, vasculopathy, internal illness, insufficient acclimatization to cold weather, lack of shelter, freezing wind, and wetting. All these factors decrease the time needed for lesions to appear. Frozen skin is pale and cold, with reduced sensitivity. The skin should be thawed as soon as possible to prevent necrosis. Warm water is gently applied on affected areas. Thawing of the skin may be painful. In areas that are not necrotic, erythema and edema are usually present.

In mild cases, frostbite may induce no lesions besides mild ear-border curling, whitening of the hair, alopecia, and in more severe cases, necrosis. It may take some time for the skin to reveal the total extent of the damage, so the affected tissue can take some weeks to heal. Pentoxyfylline associated with aspirin has been shown to improve tissue viability in rats.[14]

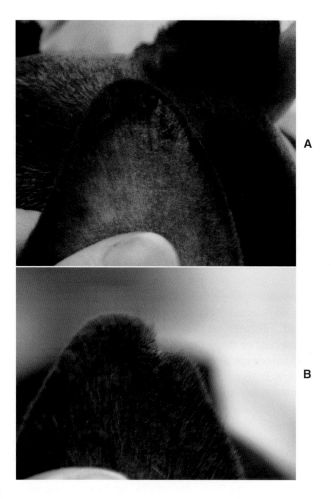

Figure 12-9

A, Early lesions of cold agglutinin–related pinnal vasculitis (December) in a 1-year-old male Pinscher cross: crusts and hyperpigmentation are present on the concave surface of the apex of the auricle. **B,** In February, crusted, punched-out lesions are present on the same dog. Two episodes of bleeding were associated with temperatures below 0°C.

Cryoglobulinemia and Cryofibrinogenemia

Different components of the serum (cryoglobulins) or the plasma (cryofibrinogens) may precipitate under cold temperature. The process is usually reversed when the temperature rises again. These diseases were formerly termed *cold agglutinin diseases.* At least three types of cryoglobulinemia have been identified. Symptoms result from the anemia and/or hemagglutination associated with the process.

Because of the lack of anastomoses on their margins, the ear pinnae are more commonly affected.

Ear-Margin Seborrhea

Ear-margin seborrhea or dermatosis is most commonly observed in pendulous-eared breeds such as the Dachshund, Springer and Cocker Spaniels, Beagles, Basset Hounds, and Dobermans with uncropped ears.[3] The pathogenesis of this condition is not established, even though predisposing factors have been proposed.

On both sides of the pinna but restricted to the margins, numerous follicular casts ("waxy plugs") can be seen adhering to the skin and hair. As the disease evolves, lesions become confluent and involve the whole ear margin. Partial alopecia is observed. Later on, the debris remains tightly adherent but becomes hard and thick. Fissuring of both the aggregate and underlying skin results. This is painful and bothers the dog so that it shakes its head even more and aggravates the process.

History and careful clinical observation are usually diagnostic early in the course of the disease. As the lesions become fissured and crusty, the differential diagnosis includes most other causes of ear margin lesions such as sarcoptic mange, vasculitis, and some insect-bite dermatoses, especially stick-tight flea infestation. Severe hyperkeratosis and follicular keratosis that may lead to a pseudopapillomatous appearance are observed on dermatopathologic examination.

No underlying causes are usually associated, and the treatment is symptomatic: removing the seborrheic aggregates and decreasing further production. Ceruminolytic shampoos containing salicylic acid as well as sulfur are used regularly. Because tar has been shown to be carcinogenic in humans (squamous cell carcinoma[19]), it might be preferable to avoid dispensing tar-containing products; most clients do not wear gloves when applying products to their animals. To initiate the dissolution of the waxy aggregates, the lesions can be soaked 15 minutes before the shampoo with warm water or a ceruminolytic ear solution. These solutions can be irritating, especially those that contain toluene derivatives, but they are removed by the shampoo shortly after their application. Peroxide, vitamin A, or retinoids can be applied topically between shampoos to slow down the buildup of the waxy material. Gel formulations are preferred because they penetrate the coat better and do not build up as much as do ointments. Because these treatments are symptomatic, their frequency is based on the clinical appearance of lesions. When fissuring is extensive, surgical ear cropping is indicated.

Acquired Folding of the Pinna

This benign condition is reported in adult cats. The apexes of both pinnae suddenly fold rostrally and, usually, somewhat laterally (Figure 12-10). On palpation, the cartilage is usually lacking in the folded apex. Most affected cats have a history of long-term steroid treatment; when performed, adrenocorticotropic hormone (ACTH) stimulation test results are depressed. Stopping the glucocorticoid treatment may improve the condition.

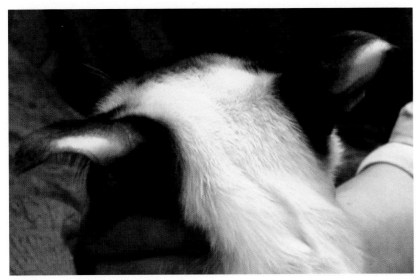

Figure 12-10

Acquired folding associated with partial alopecia on both pinnae of a Siamese cat. No history of steroid treatment could be found. One year later, the ears were back to normal without treatment.

Crusty and Scaly Dermatoses

Crusts and scales are frequently associated with trauma, either caused by fights or self-inflicted, as in pruritic dermatoses. Most dermatoses of the ear margin are also associated with crusting. Scales are a common feature of dermatophytosis. In some dermatoses that usually involve the whole pinna, including dermatophytosis, pemphigus, and zinc-responsive dermatitis, these symptoms can be a main feature (Figure 12-11).

Dermatophytosis

Dermatophytes live on keratin, and the most common dermatophyte found in dogs and cats, *Microsporum canis,* invades mainly the hair; the primary lesions of dermatophytosis are follicular casts and scales. Infected hairs are abnormal and fragile; they break easily, and alopecia quickly results. The classical presentation of dermatophytosis in dogs and cats is annular alopecia associated with fine silvery scales, central healing, and peripheral follicular papules and crust. This lesion is commonly observed on the pinnae.[4] In cats, pinnal lesions caused by dermatophytes are more common than they are in dogs. In both species, lesions usually are not symmetrical, as opposed to other causes of pinnal alopecia.

Dermatophytosis is a complex disease and its clinical manifestations are variable. They include seborrhea, localized folliculitis or furunculosis (especially on the face),

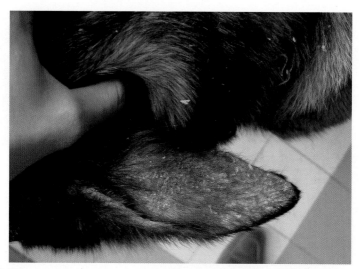

Figure 12-11

Generalized and severe scaling in a 5-year-old German Shepherd dog with advanced leishmaniasis. The pinnae are also involved. The dog goes to Portugal each summer.

kerion or other granulomatous reactions, papular dermatitis, erythematous dermatitis, pruritus, and even subcutaneous nodules (termed *dermatophytic pseudomycetoma*). Lesions with both macroscopic and dermatopathologic features of pemphigus foliaceous or pemphigus erythematosus have been reported that are caused by a dermatophyte (usually *T. mentagrophytes* or *M. persicolor*).

The clinician should consider dermatophytosis as a possible differential diagnosis if the clinical features and the history are compatible:

- *Age:* Dermatophytosis is most commonly seen in young animals. Adults (more commonly cats) can be asymptomatic carriers, especially Persian cats. Sylvatic dermatophytosis (i.e., acquired from wild mammals) is usually seen in older animals. In these cases the causative dermatophyte is not *M. canis,* and the clinical signs can vary greatly.
- *Breed:* Persian cats in particular but also exotic short-haired cats, Yorkshire Terriers, and Pekingese are predisposed to *M. canis* infection. Yorkshire Terriers may be susceptible to develop severe forms. Dogs and breeds used for hunting or with hunting habits are predisposed to sylvatic dermatophytosis because of their more frequent contact with wild mammals.
- *Contagion:* Dermatophytes are transmitted by contact with fungal elements (infected hair or scales, soil); they also may be present on infected animals, in the environment, or on fomites. Contact with infected animals is the most common source for the most prevalent dermatophytes. Exact identification usually allows identification of the source of infection.

Experimental diagnosis is mainly based on positive fungal culture. A recent study has confirmed the importance of daily observation if dermatophyte test medium (DTM) is used because contaminants can also cause the color to change from yellow to red. Most dermatophytes do not develop fully on this medium, and they can be difficult to identify precisely unless cultured again on Sabouraud's medium.

Microscopic observation of infected hair or scales in skin scrapings can be sufficient if the clinician is experienced. Because infected hairs are fragile and break easily and dermatophytes can infect the stratum corneum, skin scraping is probably more favorable than trichography for sample collection (both microscopic examination and fungal culture). Trichography can be performed under the Wood's lamp to collect fluorescent hair (Figure 12-12). *M. canis* is the only commonly encountered dermatophyte that fluoresces. In order to reduce false positives, the clinician should make sure that the fluorescence involves the hair shaft and/or the follicular ostia. A diffuse positive reaction over the skin is probably caused by topical drug application. False negatives are also encountered. Some cases of dermatophytosis, especially atypical clinical presentations, can be detected on dermatopathologic examination.

Treatment of dermatophytosis should always involve the whole body surface even if the pinna is the only site with macroscopic lesions. Systemic and/or topical treatments

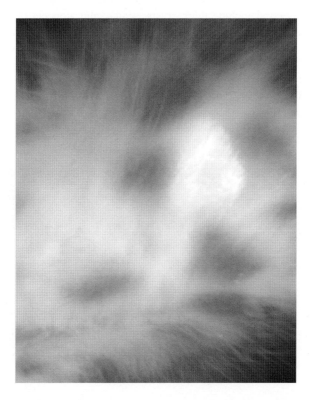

Figure 12-12

Positive Wood's lamp examination of a cat with dermatophytosis caused by *Microsporum canis*.

are widely available (griseofulvin, ketoconazole, itraconazole, econazole, terbinafine). Dermatophytosis is zoonotic, and the practitioner has the responsibility to inform owners to seek medical attention if they develop lesions.

Pemphigus Complex

The classification of the pemphigus group of diseases is still controversial. They are the most frequent autoimmune skin diseases in dogs and cats, the most common being pemphigus foliaceus (PF) and then pemphigus erythematosus (PE). In the pemphigus group, these two diseases have a characteristic facial and aural involvement.

Pemphigus complex diseases are primarily pustular in dogs and cats. Most pustular dermatoses involve the hair follicle. PF and PE are almost the only diseases to cause numerous pustules and crusts in the concave surface of the pinna (Figure 12-13). They can be restricted to the inner pinna but commonly also affect the dorsal pinna.

In PF, lesions usually also affect other areas of the skin: face (periocular area, nasal planum), feet, clawbed, footpads, and inguinal area. General involvement is not uncommon. In PE, lesions are almost always restricted to the face and ears. Because pustules are transient in dogs and cats, observed lesions in PF and PE are usually secondary and include thick crusts, scales, and alopecia overlying oozing and erosive skin bordered by epidermal collarettes. Pain and/or pruritus can be present but are not primary features. Depigmentation is common in PE but occurs rarely or late in the course of the disease in PF (Figure 12-14).

Differential diagnosis should include contact dermatitis, cutaneous adverse drug reaction, dermatophytosis, demodicosis, bacterial folliculitis, discoid and systemic lupus erythematosus, leishmaniasis, and zinc-responsive dermatitis. Both dermatophytosis and drug reactions can cause pustular acantholytic dermatoses.

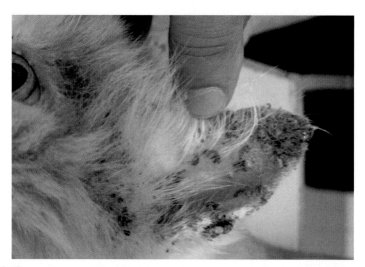

Figure 12-13

Erosive and crusted lesions on the concave surface on the pinna of a cat with PF.

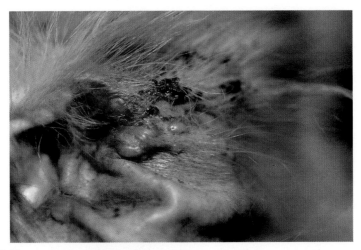

Figure 12-14

Erythema and large, fluctuant, fragile pustules on the inner pinna of an 8-month-old Golden Retriever with PF. These lesions are seldom seen.

Diagnosis is based on the elimination of other differential diagnoses, compatible histologic examination of biopsy samples, and positive immunofluorescence and/or immunochemistry results. Most pemphigus cases are considered spontaneous, but some anecdotally reported cases have been identified or suspected to be paraneoplastic or food related.[16]

Treatment includes mainly immunosuppressive drugs such as prednisolone, azathioprin (dogs), or chlorambucil.

Zinc-Responsive Dermatosis

Zinc-responsive dermatosis causes hyperkeratotic or crusty skin lesions on the pinna. Other parts of the body are also usually involved, especially the face.

Two syndromes are recognized. A strong breed predisposition is observed in syndrome I for Siberian Huskies and Alaskan Malamutes. Other breeds such as the Bull Terrier have been mentioned. The early lesions occur at 1 to 3 years of age. Erythema affects the ears, mouth, chin, eyes, and pressure points (elbows, hocks). Alopecia, crusting, and scaling (with or without underlying suppuration) quickly occur, often associated with secondary pruritic bacterial and/or *Malassezia* infection. Otherwise, pruritus is variable. The hair coat is usually dull with a generalized seborrhea. Other signs are less common (onychomalacia, modifications in the sense of taste or smell). Stress of any kind could be a precipitating factor. The pathogenesis of this syndrome is controversial, considering that in these dogs the zinc intake is usually normal, but the condition responds to zinc supplementation.

Syndrome II is seen in rapidly growing dogs (mainly of large or giant breeds) with insufficient zinc intake resulting from inappropriate food formulation or the presence of elements in the diet that interfere with zinc such as phytates (zinc chelation)

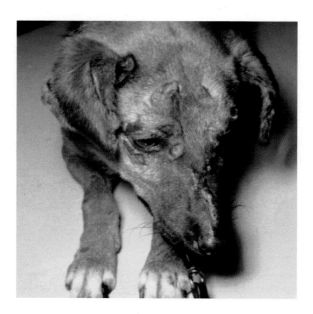

Figure 12-15

Areas of alopecia, hyperkeratosis, and hyperpigmentation of both pinnae and the face of a dog with generic food dermatosis.

and calcium (modification of zinc absorption). Oversupplementation with minerals and vitamins can be sufficient to cause zinc-responsive dermatosis. Hyperkeratotic plaques are seen on areas of repeated trauma on pressure points, including the pinna, footpads, and nasal planum. Treatment should be aimed at correction of the diet.

Generic Food Dermatitis

Generic food dermatosis is often difficult to differentiate from zinc-responsive dermatosis syndrome II because the causes, predisposed animals, clinical signs, and treatment are similar (Figure 12-15).

Dermatoses of the Concave Pinna

Atopic dermatitis and contact dermatitis are the most common dermatoses affecting the concave pinna. Severe diseases affecting the ear canal, whether they are primary or secondary, can result in lesions of the concave pinna around the ear canal opening, such as the following:
- Pain, erythema, erosion, ulceration and crusting in cases of bacterial otitis externa
- Pruritus, seborrhea, and lichenification in cases of *Malassezia* otitis externa (Figure 12-16)
- Skin hyperplasia and lichenification in cases of hyperplastic changes secondary to chronic ear inflammation

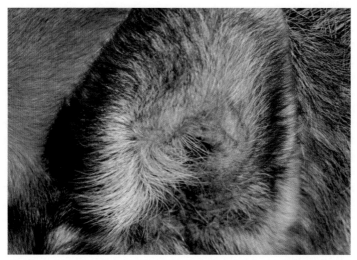

Figure 12-16

Malassezia dermatitis in the inner pinna of a German Shepherd with hypothyroidism.

Symmetrical Pinnal Alopecia

Alopecia can be a primary or secondary lesion. Secondary alopecia caused by trauma is the most common cause of alopecia of the pinna. Trauma includes fight wounds, physical or chemical trauma, and self-inflicted trauma as in the pruritic dermatoses detailed earlier.

The new classification of primary canine alopecia proposed by Mecklenburg (personal communication, 2002) can be applied to the ear pinnae:
- Inflammatory alopecias, such as the immune-mediated (vasculitis, dermatomyositis) and infectious causes (dermatophytosis, bacterial folliculitis, demodicosis). The infectious causes are usually not symmetrical.
- Noninflammatory alopecias, such as disorders of the hair-follicle cycle (pattern alopecia, cyclic alopecia, postclipping alopecia, endocrinopathy, telogen/anagen defluxion), dystrophic alopecia (traction alopecia), and alopecia caused by structural defects of the hair shaft (color dilution alopecia and other follicular dysplasias, congenital alopecia)

The noninflammatory causes of primary alopecia affecting the ear pinna are described together because symmetrical alopecia is the main feature of these diseases. Other causes are described previously.

Pattern Baldness

A type of pattern baldness restricted to the pinnae is described primarily in male Dachshunds, but also in other breeds of dogs (Chihuahuas, Boston Terriers,

Whippets, Italian Greyhounds, Staffordshire Bull Terriers); it has been reported in cats as well.

Bilateral symmetrical hypotrichosis begins when the dog is about 1 year old and can remain unnoticed for some years. As the alopecia evolves, the underlying skin becomes hypopigmented. According to Scott,[14] pattern baldness restricted to the ear results in complete baldness as the dog ages (8 to 9 years). In canine pinnal alopecia, a small vellus hair usually remains. In both cases the dermatopathologic features are similar: normal epidermis and dermis, hair follicles in any phase of the cycle, normal number but reduced size of hair (both length and diameter). The adnexae are normal also. These features allow differentiation from other causes of bilateral alopecia such as endocrine disease, follicular dysplasia, and alopecia areata.

Treatment is not necessary because the condition is purely cosmetic. If the owner requires a treatment, melatonin or topical minoxidil can be tried; they are not reported to cause any major side effects in dogs.

Periodic Alopecias

Griffin reports a periodic alopecia affecting adult Miniature Poodles. Alopecia of one or both ears is followed by spontaneous hair regrowth within several months.[3] The author advises ruling out telogen effluvium, drug reaction, and endocrine diseases. Dermatopathologic features are unknown. No treatment is advised because the condition is purely cosmetic and spontaneously resolves.[20]

In cats, a spontaneous periodic alopecia restricted to the pinna was described by Scott in Siamese cats. Both ears are affected. The skin is normal, and the alopecia affects the whole pinna or is patchy. Dermatopathologic features are unknown. Spontaneous regression is observed without treatment after several months.

Melanoderma and Alopecia in Yorkshire Terriers

Melanoderma and alopecia are quite common in Yorkshire Terriers and occasionally recognized in other breeds such as the Doberman Pinscher.[4] The alopecia begins between 6 months to 3 years of age on the bridge of the nose and both pinnae. The tail and feet may also be affected. Affected areas are markedly hyperpigmented ("melanoderma"), alopecic, smooth, and shiny, giving a leathery appearance ("leather ears").

Diagnosis is based on history, clinical features, and elimination of other diagnoses. Dermatopathologic features are not specific. Carlotti[21] demonstrated decreased dermal elastin in eight cases and abnormal growth hormone response to clonidine administration.

The disease slowly worsens as the dog ages; spontaneous recovery is rare in the author's experience. In three Yorkshire Terriers, growth hormone supplementation resulted in transient hair regrowth and relapse subsequent to treatment cessation. Due to the severe systemic side effects of growth hormone in dogs, such a treatment is not advisable because alopecia and melanoderma are purely cosmetic problems.

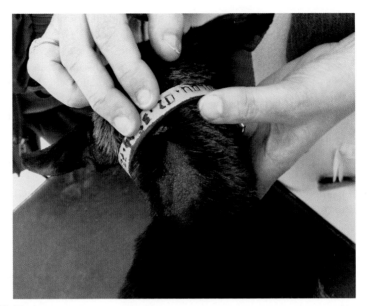

Figure 12-17

Compared with the rest of the body, pinnal alopecia is moderate in this male Pinscher with testicular tumor and elevated estradiolemia.

Endocrinopathy

Endocrine diseases are the most common cause of noninflammatory primary alopecia in the dog (Figure 12-17). But in a stereotypic manner, the extremities, including the pinna, are usually spared. In the cat, endocrine diseases usually cause nonspecific cutaneous signs (seborrhea, dull hair coat). Alopecia is a very rare feature of feline endocrinopathy, except for the secondary alopecia associated with the overgrooming behavior observed in some cases of hyperthyroidism.

Nodules and Plaques

Neoplasia is a common cause of cutaneous or subcutaneous nodular (>1 cm), papular (<1 cm), or plaquelike (flat) lesions. The aspect of neoplastic lesions can mimic most other causes; they cannot be distinguished with sufficient confidence on clinical grounds solely. Cytologic evaluation may confirm the diagnosis. A positive Wood's lamp test favors dermatophytosis (kerion) if no topical medication interfering with the method has been applied (e.g., iodine). Nevertheless, histopathologic examination of a biopsy or the excised nodule is strongly indicated in most cases. Any tumor type can cause nodular lesions on the pinna, but papilloma, canine cutaneous histiocytoma, and mastocytoma are probably the most common.

Other diseases causing one or more papular to nodular lesions on the pinna include granulomas and arthropod bites. Ticks and horseflies (*Tabanus* spp.) often leave papules 1- to 5-mm wide at the sites of their bites; they can become ulcerated. The same kind of lesion can be seen at the site of transmission of an insect-borne disease such as leishmaniasis. This reaction at the inoculation site is often called *chancre of inoculation.*

Because its anatomic location makes it prone to trauma, the pinna is prone to granulomatous lesions. Causes are numerous and include the following:
• Foreign bodies
• Bacterial infection: Staphylococci, *Nocardia,* actinomycetes, mycobacteria (both tuberculous and atypical)
• Fungal infection: Dermatophytosis, phaeohyphomycosis, cryptococcosis
• Algae: *Prototheca*
• Leishmaniasis

Granulomas may be multiple and are often exudative, if not ulcerative. Pruritus is not a primary feature but can be observed if the animal is bothered by the lesion. The clinical approach is the same as proposed previously for neoplasia. Apart from cleaning and antiseptic applications on opened lesions, treatment should be specific to each etiology.

References

1. Joyce J, Day M: Immunopathogenesis of canine aural haematoma, *J Sm Anim Pract* 38:152-158, 1997.
2. Kuwahara J: Canine and feline aural hematoma: clinical, experimental and clinicopathological observations, *Am J Vet Res* 47:2300-2308, 1986.
3. Griffin C: Pinnal diseases, *Vet Clin North Am Sm Anim Pract* 24(5):897-904, 1994.
4. Harvey R, Harari J, Delauche A: *Ear diseases of the dog and cat,* Ames, IA, 2001, Iowa State University Press.
5. Bussiéras J, Chermette R: *Parasitologie vétérinaire, entomologie,* Maisons-Alfort, France, 1991, Service de Parasitologie, ENVA.
6. Nuttal T, et al: Treatment of *Trombicula automnalis* infestation in dogs and cats with a 0.25% fipronil pump spray, *J Sm Anim Pract* 39(5):237-238, 1998.
7. Auxilia S, Hill P: Mast cell distribution, epidermal thickness and hair follicle density in normal canine skin: possible explanations for the predilection sites of atopic dermatitis? *Vet Dermatol* 11(4):247-254, 2000.
8. Rosser E: *Food allergy in the dog: a prospective study of 51 dogs.* In: Proceedings of the AAVD/ACVD meeting, 1990.
9. August J: Otitis externa, a disease of multifactorial etiology, *Vet Clin North Am Sm Anim Pract* 18(4):731-742, 1988.
10. Devos S, Mulder J, V.d.V. PGM: The relevance of positive patch test reactions in chronic otitis externa, *Contact Dermatitis* 42:342-355, 2000.
11. Griffin C, Kwochka K, MacDonald JM: *Current veterinary dermatology, the science and art of therapy,* St Louis, 1993, Mosby.
12. Chetboul V: Personal communication, 2003.
13. Hoffmann G, et al: Transdermal methimazole treatment in cats with hyperthyroidism, *J Feline Med Surg* 5(2):77-82, 2003.

14. Scott D, Miller W, Griffin CE: *Mueller and Kirk's Small animal dermatology,* ed 6, Philadelphia, 2001, Saunders.
15. Mooney C, Thoday K: Medical treatment of hyperthyroidism in cats. In Bonagura J, Kirk R, eds: *Kirk's Current veterinary therapy,* Philadelphia, 2000, Saunders.
16. Scott D, Miller M: Idiosyncratic cutaneous adverse drug reactions in the cat: literature review and report of 14 cases, *Feline Pract* 26(4):10-16, 1998.
17. Weir J: Familial cutaneous vasculopathy of German Shepherds: clinical, genetic and preliminary pathologic and immunological studies, *Can Vet J* 35:763-766, 1994.
18. Marignac G: *Atlas des otites chez les carnivores domestiques,* Paris, 2000, Med'Com.
19. Dlugosz A, Yuspa S: Carcinogenesis: chemical. In Freedberg IEA, ed: *Fitzpatrick's Dermatology in general medicine,* New York, 2003, McGraw-Hill.
20. Scott D: Observation on canine atopy, *J Am Anim Hosp Assoc* 17:91-100, 1981.
21. Carlotti D: A propos des alopécies auriculaires, *Point Vétérinaire* 25:8-13, 1993.

Suggested Readings

Casella M, Wess G, Reusch CE: Measurement of capillary blood glucose concentrations by pet owners: a new tool in the management of diabetes mellitus, *J Am Anim Hosp Assoc* 38(3):239-245, 2002.
Chermette R, Bussiéras J: *Parasitologie vétérinaire, mycologie,* Maisons-Alfort, France, 1993, Service de Parasitologie, ENVA.
Scott D: Canine sterile eosinophilic pinnal folliculitis, *Companion Anim Pract* 2(6):19-22, 1988.
Scott D: Sterile eosinophilic pustulosis in the dog, *J Am Anim Hosp Assoc* 20(4):585-589, 1984.
Scott D, et al: Pemphigus erythematosus in the dog and cat, *J Am Anim Hosp Assoc* 16(6):815-823, 1980.
Scott D, Miller M, Shanley KJ: Sterile eosinophilic folliculitis in the cat: an unusual manifestation of feline allergic skin diseases, *Companion Anim Pract* 19(8-9):6-11, 1989.

13

Simple Diagnosis and Treatment of Pruritic Otitis

Steven A. Melman, VMD

Most cases of acute otitis externa are pruritic. The pet is presented to the veterinarian for scratching at the ear, erythematous pinnae, head shaking, or pain when the ears are manipulated. The differential diagnosis for pruritus is extensive and is dealt with in other textbooks on dermatology.

This chapter contains a "rapid-fire" clinical approach to the treatment of the itchy pet with or without otitis externa. Using this approach, treatment for several different etiologic causes of pruritus are addressed at once. Not only does this regimen promise the best chance at fast and lasting relief from pruritus, but it also allows the veterinarian to make a rapid clinical diagnosis based on the response to the various elements involved in the trial. Protocols to treat most known types of ear problems, including *Malassezia* and bacterial (e.g., *Pseudomonas*) otitis, follow the discussion of treating pruritus.

Perhaps the most common etiology for acute otitis externa is hypersensitivity. The most common hypersensitivities encountered in small animal practice are flea allergy, food allergy, and atopy. Dogs with atopic dermatitis are presented to the veterinarian with a clinical history of pruritus of the feet, face, axilla, and ears. It has been estimated that as many as 80% of dogs with atopy have otitis externa and pruritic ears. In dogs and cats with food hypersensitivity, otic pruritus may be the only clinical sign. Flea allergy may contribute to overall pruritus, but rarely causes otic pruritus singularly.

If the clinician suspects atopy, then prior to starting this pruritic clinical trial, which involves the use of some corticosteroids, a pretreatment blood sample for in vitro allergy testing should be drawn. The blood should be spun and the serum frozen. Frozen serum can be submitted for in vitro allergy testing for as long as 60 to 90 days without affecting the results. Testing and therapy for atopy is both tedious and expensive. The treatment is lifelong. The following clinical trial affords clients proof that their pet is suffering from hypersensitivity, making the decision to test and hyposensitize easier.

Of course, a good physical examination and observational skills are not to be neglected in attempting to sort out the etiology of dermatologic disease. It is prudent to do skin scrapings, fecal analysis, heartworm testing, fungal culture, skin and ear cytology, and other tests as indicated by clinical common sense during the initial examination.

In addition, recheck visits and the observational skills of the client are crucial to securing an accurate diagnosis. Have the client keep a daily diary of the pet's response using a scale of 1 to 10 to quantify the intensity of pruritus, erythema, pain, any discharge from the ear, and head shaking.

Clinical Treatment Trial for Pruritus

Here is an outline for the pruritic clinical trial. This clinical trial should be done in conjunction with topical ear treatment. Start all steps on day 1.

Before starting the trial, which involves the use of corticosteroids, take serum and freeze it. Allergy testing is variably adversely affected by the effects of prednisone.

Step 1: Shampoo Therapy

Of the approximately 116 million dogs and cats in the United States, 12% to 20% have allergy-induced skin problems that require frequent bathing, preferably with "hypoallergenic" shampoos.

Shampoo therapy has moved to the forefront as a component in the treatment of all but the rarest skin disorders. It involves the use of cleansing, moisturizing, antiseborrheic, degreasing, antiparasitic, antibacterial, antifungal, and antipruritic shampoos. Specific products and protocols usually are selected on the basis of the presenting morphologic characteristics such as dryness, oiliness, scaling, inflammation, and associated pyoderma.

Generally, the use of a milder, more elegant product before a coarser, more potent one increases compliance on the part of the pet owner and reduces the risk of side effects such as irritation. Under the circumstances of a short-term clinical trial, where concurrent infections with *Staphylococcus* and *Malassezia* may be present, use a shampoo that is strong enough to treat both yet mild enough to use for frequent bathing.

Various issues should be considered when selecting therapeutic shampoos to relieve pets' specific symptoms.

Cleansers and Moisturizers. Cleansing and moisturizing shampoos are designed to do just what their names say. The mechanical process of bathing (even with water alone) helps remove scales, crusts, organisms, dander, loose hair, and other debris. All such shampoos should be pH-adjusted for dogs, which, despite breed variation, have the highest skin pH of any mammal (6.2 to 7.2), including humans.

Oils and Conditioners. Moisturizing agents such as bath oils, conditioners, emollients, and humectants may be applied after bathing and rinsing to soften, lubricate, and rehydrate the skin. They can be used on a more regular basis on dry animals. When the patient has a concurrent infection, a "medicated" conditioner may add moisture as well as medication to the coat. One such example is MalAcetic Conditioner (DermaPet, 2% acetic acid and 2% boric acid), used after a shampoo.

Antiseborrheic Treatments. *Seborrhea* is the term used for any skin disease involving dry (sicca) or greasy (oleosa) scaling. The term also encompasses disorders in the formation of keratin, a complex protein unique to the skin, hair follicles, and nails. Today, many experts prefer the term *disorders of keratinization.* This subject is covered in detail in a separate section of this book.

The epidermis turns over every 22 days in the normal dog. Epidermal turnover time in dogs suffering from idiopathic seborrhea, more common among Cocker Spaniels, may be as little as 3 to 6 days. This fast turnover creates a defect in the normal protective barrier, which may result in dry or greasy scales, comedones, alopecia, inflammation, crusts, pyoderma, and pruritus. Any of these conditions, in turn, may lead to skin damage. In these cases, it is important to slow the turnover process and treat the secondary problems.

Bathing Procedure. Bathe the pet daily in a hypoallergenic or medicated shampoo, as described previously. If the pet remains itchy after these baths, an oatmeal shampoo or conditioner may help resolve mild pruritus. If pyoderma, *Malassezia,* or seborrhea oleosa is present, the owner may also use a shampoo that is degreasing and antiseptic every 2 or 3 days. The author prefers an acetic acid/boric acid shampoo (MalAcetic, DermaPet) followed by an acetic acid/boric acid conditioner. This unique combination kills bacteria and yeasts on the skin. Shampoo therapy should be used as a component of the plan for 3 weeks. If the pet improves symptomatically, the owner should continue bathing.

Step 2: Food Elimination Diet

Follow a strict food elimination diet for a minimum of 30 days (some food-allergic dogs may require 60 to 90 days to see a beneficial effect). Many diets that can be used for the food elimination trial are commercially available. They contain either uncommon, novel protein sources (venison, rabbit, duck, fish) or purified low–molecular-weight polypeptides. The author prefers to use a home-cooked vegetarian diet.

Step 3: Fatty Acid Supplementation

Supplement the pet's diet with a high-quality fish oil supplement (omega-3 fatty acids) to help reduce the inflammation associated with pruritus. Antioxidants such as vitamin E should be included in the supplement because they are depleted more rapidly when there is fish oil (omega-3) in the diet. Because fish oil does *not* contain any protein, it will not interfere with the hypoallergenic diet. The current recommended dose is 1000 mg of fish oil containing 180 mg of eicosapentaenoic acid (EPA) per 10 lb per day as found in EicosaDerm (DermaPet) or generic fish oil

---

ALL-VEGETABLE HYPOALLERGENIC DIET

1. Vegetable puree (multiple batch)
   Three undrained #1 cans of carrots, peas, green beans, and tomatoes, and greens (kale, dock, spinach, or mustard).
   One 10 oz. package of chopped, frozen, broccoli.
   Boil the broccoli in 2 cups of water until tender. Combine with other vegetables in a large kettle, mix, and puree until smooth. Fill 18 1-pint plastic containers and freeze.
2. Rice (prepare as required)
   2½ cups rice
   5 cups water
   ½ cup sunflower oil
   1 tsp salt
   Mix ingredients, bring to boil, reduce heat, and simmer until water is absorbed. Allow to cool.
3. Thaw 1 pint of vegetable puree and add to rice; mix thoroughly.
4. Feed ½ to ¾ cup per 10 lb body weight twice daily. Monitor weight weekly. Do not add meat supplements.

From Byrne K: Food allergy. In Melman SA, editor: *Skin diseases of dogs and cats,* Potomac, MD, 1994, DermaPet, Inc.

capsules. Most fish oils and all flaxseed oil do not contain the necessary EPA content.

Step 4: Corticosteroids

Administer a low-dose corticosteroid for 12 days (e.g., prednisone at 0.5 mg/lb twice a day). Use a declining dosing regimen that ends with 0.5 mg/lb every other day. The rationale is to break the pruritic cycle and observe whether the case is corticosteroid responsive.

Step 4a

A topical corticosteroid spray (Genesis, 0.015% triamcinolone, Virbac) has been helpful in reducing the pruritic cycle. Some cases require less to no further systemic corticosteroid supplementation.

Step 5

If the pet has pyoderma, use an antibiotic such as cephalexin at 10 to 15 mg/lb twice a day for a minimum of 21 days. If the ear is also infected with bacteria, use a fluoroquinolone such as enrofloxacin at 5 mg/lb twice a day or 10 mg/lb once daily. If *Malassezia* dermatitis is present, bathe with the acetic acid/boric acid shampoo as outlined in Step 1; antibiotic therapy usually controls the pruritus. On rare occasions, or when there is very severe involvement of the skin with *Malassezia,* oral ketoconazole at 10 mg/kg once daily or itraconazole at 5 mg/kg once daily may be used. Duration of treatment varies, but treat for at least 2 weeks. Systemics such as itraconazole and ketoconazole do not work as effectively in the ear as they do in the skin. When treating *Malassezia* dermatitis that does not respond to topical and systemic antibiotic therapy, itraconazole is my preference because of its low level of toxicity and ability to persist in the epithelium.

Step 6: Ectoparasites

Treat scabies, other ectoparasites, and some endoparasites with a trial of ivermectin. In all breeds except Collies or their mixes, use ivermectin (Bovine Ivomec, MSD/AgVet), 0.1 to 0.2 ml per 10 pounds of body weight. Use every 7 to 10 days for four treatments. The extralabel use of this drug requires the informed consent of the client. Other methods of flea control are reported to control scabies. However, for the purpose of this trial, in order to be sure scabies is eliminated from the differential diagnosis, the author prefers ivermectin.

Step 7: Endoparasites

Treat phantom endoparasites with a dewormer that kills whipworms.

Step 8: Flea Control

If not already on flea control, begin flea control program.

Analyzing the Results of the Trial

If the clinical signs stop during the time that the prednisone and ivermectin are given and never return, diagnose ectoparasites (most likely scabies) or ear mite hypersensitivity. The ivermectin killed the parasites, and the prednisone reduced the pruritus.

If the response is more gradual and the pruritus does not return after bathing with the acetic acid/boric acid shampoo and ketoconazole or itraconazole, cutaneous *Malassezia* is the likely cause. Unfortunately, *Malassezia* is often a secondary complication that perpetuates otic pruritus in many atopic dogs. An acetic acid/boric acid ear cleaner (Malacetic Otic, DermaPet) may need to be used on a maintenance basis once or twice a week to control otic *Malassezia* yeasts.

If the pruritus returns between days 12 and 21, a cortisone-responsive hypersensitivity is most likely and allergy testing should be done. The frozen pretreatment serum can then be submitted for in vitro allergy testing.

If itching remains controlled comfortably after the original pretreatment diet is reinstituted, the possibility that this is a fatty acid/shampoo therapy–responsive atopy is high. Suspect primary food allergy if the itching returns within 72 hours after the hypoallergenic diet is withdrawn and the pet is returned to the pretreatment diet.

Unresponsive allergy cases have recently been described to respond favorably to cyclosporine at 5 mg/kg. This may account for why some researchers have treated unresponsive end-stage ear cases with cyclosporine, allowing dogs to become comfortable while not reversing the progressive pathology.

Bacterial hypersensitivity is a disease entity that may be suspected if the itching returns within 30 days of stopping the antibiotic, provided that the pruritus was controlled during antibiotic therapy. If the itching disappears after a second course of antibiotic therapy, the diagnosis is confirmed.

Keratinization disorders, including hypothyroidism, skin neoplasia, and other less common primary skin diseases, will prevent the itch from fully resolving. Incomplete treatment of *Malassezia* dermatitis or failure to treat all in-contact animals for scabies may cause persistent pruritus. Biopsy of the skin may be helpful in many circumstances to identify the etiology of pruritic skin diseases.

In many cases of acute otitis externa without progressive pathologic changes, resolution of pruritic skin disease also decreases otic pruritus. However, the skin of the ear is treated differently than the skin of the trunk, primarily with concentrated topical medications.

Ear Therapy

Here is a simple, logical, progressive method of providing ear therapy. Before initiating these steps, appropriate cytology and/or culture samples should be retrieved. Use each step and continue to the next step if necessary.

Step 1: Ear Cleaning

Clean the ear thoroughly using a non-ototoxic ear cleaner in the hospital so that a thorough otic examination can be performed, including assessment of the tympanic membrane. The author prefers an acetic acid/boric acid ear cleaner (MalAcetic Otic). Problems may arise when detergents and alcohols are used as ear cleaners in situations where the eardrum may be ruptured. Use anesthesia when appropriate.

Acetic acid and boric acid in combination has been shown to be an effective combination in vivo to treat *Malassezia* otitis.[1] In many cases, continued daily ear cleansing by the owner at home for 1 week is all that is needed to treat the ear. Maintenance cleaning twice weekly may prevent recurrence of *Malassezia*. Cleaning the ear is important for removal of surface debris from the affected ear canal epithelium. Apply medications, if needed, after cleaning.

How to Clean an Ear

1. Apply approximately 5 ml (1 teaspoon) of the ear cleaner into the ear canal and massage thoroughly. A cotton ball may be inserted into the canal to protect against drenching should the pet shake its head.
2. For maximum benefit, allow the ear cleaner to remain in the ear canal for at least 5 minutes before attempting to clean manually.
3. Clean the ear by using a cotton ball at the opening of the ear canal to absorb liquid and dislodged debris. As days of treatment go by, less debris will be removed.
4. Stop daily cleaning when the cotton ball remains free of debris after cleaning.

In dry and/or irritated ears with little debris and/or wax, the cotton ball may be irritating. In these cases, a tiny bulb syringe or Water Pik can be helpful. Warmed solutions seem to soften waxy debris. In problem ears, the frequency of cleaning may need to be increased to one to three times daily.

It is important to remember that infected ears are very acidic, which inactivates some antibiotics commonly used in the ear such as gentamycin and amikacin. Many ear cleaners are also acidic. In those cases, waiting 4 hours after cleaning to apply these antibiotics may be warranted.

Cleaning with Tris-EDTA. One non-ototoxic alkalinizing agent that the literature reports to have primary antimicrobial properties is tris-ethylenediaminetetraacetic (tris-EDTA [TrizEDTA, DermaPet]). To use tris-EDTA, one should follow the previous instructions on how to clean an ear, substituting the alkalinizing tris-EDTA for the acidic ear cleaner MalAcetic Otic. It appears that tris-EDTA pretreatment allows increased antimicrobial activity for many antibiotics used to treat ear disease. It is especially useful in stubborn *Pseudomonas* otitis cases. Gentamycin or enrofloxacin may be added to the tris-EDTA solution.

Step 2: Topical Therapy

Logical otic therapy is based on the results of otic examination and cytology. In bacterial infections, use antibiotics. In yeast infection, use an anti-yeast therapy.

TOPICAL EAR FORMULA (GEMISH)

MALASSEZIA GEMISH

12 ml acetic acid/boric acid ear cleaner
6 mg dexamethasone sodium phosphate (for increased solubility)
Also add as appropriate:
0.5 to 1 ml medical-grade dimethyl sulfoxide (DMSO)
0.5 ml ivermectin

BACTERIAL GEMISH

12 ml tris-EDTA
60 mg Baytril injectable
6 mg dexamethasone sodium phosphate (for increased solubility)
Also add as appropriate:
0.5 to 1 ml medical-grade DMSO

TRIS-EDTA GEMISH

Add 600 mg Baytril LA to a 4-ounce bottle of tris-EDTA. This creates a 5% Baytril/tris-EDTA solution. The increased emphasis on topical therapy versus systemic therapy has led to the popularization of this formula. This better affords the recommended usage of 0.5 to 2 ml per ear twice daily, allowing sufficient volume for effective topical therapy. If sufficient volume is not used, the infected surface area cannot be thoroughly reached.

In inflammation (neutrophils on the cytology) or erythema, use topical corticosteroids. If ear mites are present, use a topical insecticide or topical ivermectin. After the ear has been cleaned, apply the topical formula.

The use of these gemishes has many advantages over all current commercial products. The application of oils tends to have adverse consequences, including not reaching the affected sites, not covering the surface area, and ototoxicity. The fact that these products often only come in 7.5- to 15-ml packaging should not be overlooked.

Step 3: Systemic Therapy

Continue Steps 1 and 2 and, if there is inflammation or purulent material present, use a systemic antibiotic and/or a short-acting systemic corticosteroid.

Step 4: Further Complications

When Steps 1 through 3 do not cause remission of signs after 2 weeks, reexamine the ears. If there is stenosis and strangulation of the canal, using a 1.5-inch 20-gauge needle, inject approximately 0.5 ml of methylprednisolone acetate (Depo-Medrol, Pharmacia-Upjohn) between the epithelium and cartilage as distal in the canal as possible.

If the eardrum is bulging, a myringotomy may be done to relieve the pressure and pain, and a culture of the middle ear can be obtained. If the eardrum is ruptured, infuse a combination of 0.5 ml of dexamethasone sodium phosphate and 0.5 cc of enrofloxacin directly into the tympanic bulla.

Myringotomy may reveal pathology in the middle ear that, once removed and treated, will reduce cervical, head, or neck pain. An example is primary secretory otitis media (PSOM) of Cavalier King Charles Spaniels.

The use of corticosteroids is multifunctional. Although we are most familiar with their antiinflammatory properties, in cases of otitis media the reduction of viscosity of the secretions and exudate are also noteworthy goals. The tympanic bulla is covered with pseudostratified squamous epithelial cells with mucus-secreting goblet cells that need to be toned down by 2 mg/kg daily of prednisone for as long as 2 weeks.

Step 5: Step 4 and Culture and Sensitivity

Many dermatologists recommend a culture from each ear in difficult cases to assess the bacterial microflora. It is possible to have different bacteria in each ear, and it is also possible to have bacteria complicating otitis media that are not normally found in the external ear. Topical treatment (see tris-EDTA gemish) with antibiotics achieves much higher topical levels than the mean inhibitory concentration (MIC) reported by the laboratory, so bacteria resistant on the culture results may be susceptible to the higher topical doses.

Step 6: Tris-EDTA

In stubborn bacterial otitis externa or media, use tris-EDTA (TrizEDTA, DermaPet) before instilling the antimicrobial. Clean the ear thoroughly for 7 to 21 days. Tris-EDTA is an alkaline solution with a pH of 8.0. There are reports in the literature of the primary microbiocidal properties of tris-EDTA, particularly to *Pseudomonas.* Those reports also indicate the evidence for potentiation with antibiotics that otherwise are inactivated by other acidifiying ear cleansers. If *Pseudomonas* is suspected from cytology or cultured, use the appropriate systemic and topical antibiotics after a 15-minute pretreatment with tris-EDTA. Others recommend using the tris-EDTA gemish, allowing both cleansing, pretreatment, and treatment simultaneously.

The mechanism of action of tris-EDTA is discussed elsewhere in this book.

Step 7: Surgery

If corticosteroid injection into the ear canal epithelium fails to open up an inflamed, swollen, occluded ear canal (Step 4), if permanent pathologic changes are evident, or if there is severe calcification of the ear canal, surgery of the ear canal is indicated for relief of pain and to allow for drainage.

Reference

1. Gotthelf L, Young S: A new treatment for canine otitis externa, *Vet Forum* 14(8):46-53, 1997.

14

Diagnosis and Treatment of Otitis Media

Louis N. Gotthelf, DVM

Otitis media is a common disease process that often goes unrecognized in most veterinary practices. The fact that otitis media is present in more than half of all canine patients with chronic otitis externa should stimulate a reformulation of the diagnostic process when faced with these cases. Just the common history that the patient has been treated repeatedly for ear infections should alert the veterinarian to think about otitis media as a possibility.

The diagnosis of otitis media in dogs can be quite difficult to make, owing to the long, bent, funnel-shaped conformation of the dog's ear canal, which makes visualizing the tympanic membrane (TM) difficult. In addition, many patients with otitis media have an intact TM, giving the clinician the impression that there is nothing wrong in the middle ear. Most canine patients with otitis media also have a chronic otitis externa with pathologic changes to the ear canal that cause stenosis, making visual examination of the TM impossible. It is often theorized that otitis media is an extension of otitis externa that was either not treated, improperly treated, or resistant to treatment. The result is significant damage, resulting in porosity to the eardrum over time.

Otitis media in cats most often results as a sequela to respiratory disease, so a history of sneezing, ocular discharge, and/or nasal discharge may provide a clue. Some cats with otitis media also have a visible polyp in the ear canal after the ear is cleaned of the dried exudates and mucus. Many feline otitis media cases have a dark, dried, crumbly exudate in the ear canal that mimics an ear mite infestation. The diagnosis of otitis media in cats may be easier to determine with the otoscope because of their relatively short ear canals.

Otitis media should be considered when the clinician is presented with a patient showing any neurologic disease affecting the head, including vestibular disease, Horner's syndrome, or facial nerve damage.

By definition, *otitis media* refers to the extension of an inflammatory disease into the middle ear cavity. This may or may not be infectious. The inflammatory reaction of the mucous membrane lining the tympanic bulla is different than the reaction of the skin of the external ear, so the symptomatology and treatment of otitis media are different from those for otitis externa. The mucous membrane lining the tympanic bulla reacts to foreign substances, including infectious organisms, hair, cells, cerumen from the external ear canal, chemicals, and pharmaceuticals used in the external ear canal. It produces a purulent exudate and increases its secretion of protective mucus from activated goblet cells.

If the eardrum has a hole in it during active otitis media, copious mucoid exudate is often seen along the floor of the horizontal canal. Although this material is usually in liquid form, the mucus and pus may be inspissated and dry. Mucus is not produced anywhere along the external ear, but oozes from the tympanic bulla into the horizontal canal through any rent in the TM. The presence of mucus indicates a hole in the eardrum; precautions should be taken not to introduce ototoxic substances into the ear canal.

Otitis media in dogs is much more prevalent than previously thought. In dogs, secondary otitis media occurs in approximately 16% of acute otitis externa cases and as many as 50% to 80% of chronic otitis externa cases.[1,2] Many cases of otitis media are well hidden from visual detection by the significant exudates present in the ear canal and the severe pathologic changes that have occurred in the ear canal as a result

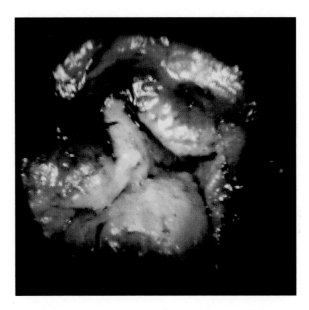

Figure 14-1

Stenotic ear. Extensive fibrosis in the horizontal ear canal prevents visual examination of the TM.

of chronic otitis externa. These changes include stenosis, fibrosis, tumors, polyps, epithelial hyperplasia, and glandular hyperplasia (Figure 14-1). Chronic changes in the external ear canal prevent adequate visualization beyond these blockages, so determining the integrity of the eardrum is not always possible.

Some dogs with otitis media have intact eardrums but also have significant bacterial and yeast populations that can be isolated from the middle ear.[2] These dogs may have had a ruptured eardrum that healed, trapping bacteria and yeast in the tympanic bulla. Therefore the presence of an eardrum does not rule out otitis media. Healed eardrums trap infectious organisms in the middle ear, and suppurative otitis media results (Figure 14-2). Secretions and exudates are trapped behind the healed eardrum, causing it to bulge outward under pressure, which in turn causes severe pain. Myringotomy may be necessary to investigate the contents of the bulla in suspected cases of otitis media where the eardrum is intact.

Signalment and History

It is uncommon for a patient to present to the veterinarian with a history of acute otitis media. However, iatrogenic rupture of the eardrum during ear cleaning can lead to an inflammatory acute otitis media. A foreign body that has become lodged in the ear canal can cause acute otitis media. Often plant awns and foxtails work their way through the eardrum and cause a considerable bacterial infection and inflammatory reaction in the ear canal.

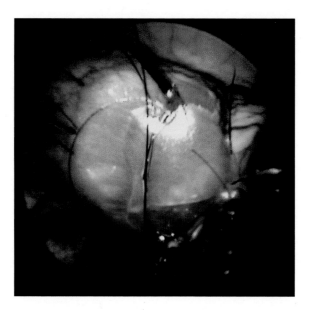

Figure 14-2

The TM is opaque and cystic. Serous fluid behind the eardrum causes increased pressure on the eardrum.

More commonly, a dog with otitis media will have a history of recurrent or chronic bacterial external ear infections. Perhaps the pet owner will present all the external ear medications already tried on the pet; that is a signal for the veterinarian to look deeper in the ear canal for middle ear disease. Chronic otitis media is almost always suppurative, with large amounts of fluid draining into the ear canal. The presence of liquid in the ear canal may signal otitis media (Figure 14-3).

In dogs and cats with otitis media where the eardrum is open, a copious, malodorous liquid discharge is often present when the ear canal is examined with the otoscope. Some patients produce so much exudate that it overflows onto the periaural region of the face; in a floppy-ear dog, there will be dried exudate on the ear flap adjacent to the external opening of the auditory canal. Head shaking to relieve the pain and tickle associated with liquid exudate is very common in otitis media. It may be wise to check for otitis media in cases of aural hematoma. Pain on palpation of the base of the ear canal or pain on manipulation of the pinna should also alert the clinician to otitis media.

Some patients with otitis media are reluctant to have their mouth opened and may have histories of reluctance to chew hard food. This is due to inflammation, swelling, and pain within the bulla, which is located adjacent to the temporomandibular joint.

When otitis media affects the nerves that course around the base of the ear or through the tympanic bulla, the patient may show signs as subtle as keratoconjunctivitis sicca on the ipsilateral side. This results from damage to the palpebral branch of the facial nerve. When otitis media affects the sympathetic nerves from the facial and trigeminal nerves coursing through the middle ear, the patient may show mild signs of Horner's syndrome (enophthalmos, ptosis, and miosis) (Figure 14-4). Some patients

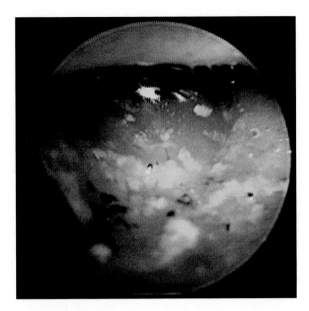

Figure 14-3

Otitis media in a cat. Liquid discharge filling the horizontal canal. Flecks of thick, inspissated mucus can be visualized floating in the fluid.

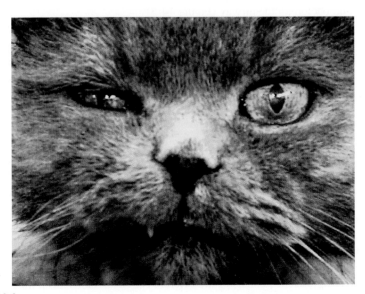

Figure 14-4

Horner's syndrome in a cat with cerumen gland adenocarcinoma extending into the tympanic bulla. The eyelid opening is small, the pupil is pinpoint, and the eyeball rolls inward (not pictured).

may show pain, head tilt, or, with facial nerve palsy, a drooped lip, drooped ear, or loss of the ability to close the eyelid, leading to exposure keratitis.[3] Since the facial nerve courses in and around the ear canal, it is easily affected by swelling, inflammation, and trauma from the dog scratching at the base of the ear. Facial neuropathy should be suspected if there is drooping of the facial muscles and skin or drooling of saliva because the lips and facial muscles cannot create an oral seal. Peripheral vestibular disease with nystagmus and circling may be evident if the infection and inflammation have affected the inner ear.

An owner may present a patient for a hearing deficit. These cases should be evaluated for otitis media. Fluid in the middle ear dampens hearing. If this fluid is the result of previous flushing, it is usually absorbed within 7 to 10 days, and the patient regains the hearing. When the eardrum is ruptured or when the ossicles of the middle ear have sclerosed, air-conduction hearing is reduced. High-pitched sound waves cannot be effectively transmitted from the ear canal to the cochlea. If a tumor or a polyp has filled the middle ear, air-conduction hearing is eliminated. Bone-conduction hearing is usually still present in these patients, but the pet can only hear the lower range of tones. (Bone-conduction hearing can be demonstrated by placing your fingers in your ears and listening to the sounds around you.) If there is hearing loss detected, this is usually as a result of bilateral ear disease. Unilateral hearing loss is difficult to assess in animals.

If there is pharyngeal drainage of mucus and exudates resulting from otitis media, the patient may be presented for inspiratory stridor. In these cases, a pharyngeal examination may reveal a nasopharyngeal polyp interfering with breathing or thick mucus draining from the auditory osteum in the nasopharynx, covering the caudal pharynx, and occluding the airway (Figure 14-5).

Otitis media with an intact, bulging eardrum may be very painful for the patient. Simply manipulating the pinna can lead to behavioral changes consistent with pain. Many dogs with otitis media cry out when the base of the skull is palpated at the junction of the ear cartilage and the skull. Some dogs even bite their owners while they are trying to administer medication because of the intense pain. Strong pain relievers are indicated in these patients. After the eardrum ruptures or is intentionally perforated by myringotomy, the pressure decreases and the pain significantly diminishes.

Evaluation of the Patient

Careful examination of the TM in the dog or cat with otitis media requires general anesthesia. It is recommended that the patient have an endotracheal tube placed in case there is a ruptured eardrum. Manipulation or flushing can cause material to drain through the eustachian tube into the nasopharynx, resulting in aspiration.

If there is significant stenosis of the external ear canal, either from inflammation or from permanent pathologic changes to the ear canal, the eardrum may not be adequately visualized. Patient preparation using potent topical and/or systemic corticosteroids (prednisone, 1 mg/lb daily for 10 to 14 days, then taper or dexamethasone

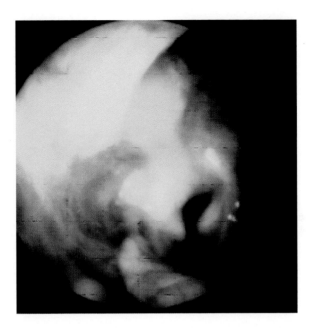

Figure 14-5

Pharyngeal drainage of mucus from a 12-year-old cat with mucoid otitis media. The mucus drainage is coming from under the soft palate. No organisms were cultured from this cat's middle ear, but both bullae were sclerotic.

2 mg/ml at a dose of 0.1 mg/lb intramuscularly [IM] once) may be needed to reduce otic inflammation and allow examination of the TM on a subsequent visit. If permanent changes to the ear canal prevent visual determination of the integrity of the eardrum, other techniques are used to identify disease proximal to the stenosis.

Recently, with the introduction of video otoscopes, it is possible to get a very detailed, magnified examination of the ear canal and eardrum. The video otoscope provides excellent lighting at the tip of the tapered probe by transmitting light through the probe by a fiberoptic cable attached to a high-output light source.

After the veterinarian is comfortable looking at normal eardrums—the location, color, clarity, and the normal tension on it—using the TM to diagnose otitis media becomes much easier. If the eardrum remains translucent, the middle ear can be transilluminated with the bright light from the video otoscope and the contents of the middle ear can be visualized (Figure 14-6).

In obvious cases of canine otitis media, there is no eardrum present. The ear canal is filled with a liquid secretion, often with flecks of material mixed with it. A mucus-filled ear canal may alert the clinician to otitis media. Most patients with chronic otitis externa that has been present for 45 to 60 days will have a coexisting otitis media. In otitis externa, purulent exudates and proteolytic enzymes elaborated by inflammatory cells have a caustic effect on the thin epithelium of the eardrum, causing it to become necrotic, weaken, and eventually rupture. When this happens, hairs,

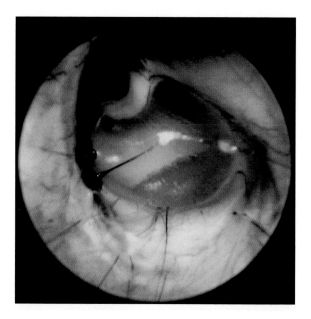

Figure 14-6

Transillumination of the TM with high-intensity light allows examination of the middle ear. Air fills the normal middle ear, and a bony prominence called the *promontory* (behind which is the cochlea) can be seen on the medial wall of the bulla.

ceruminous secretions, exudates, and infectious bacteria or yeast organisms in the external ear move into the middle ear. In these patients it is difficult to visualize any part of the eardrum, since it may not be present at all. Sometimes only a small ring of granulation tissue may be seen at the annulus fibrosus, where the eardrum attaches to the ear canal. With the otoscope, an otitis media case without suppuration looks like a deep, dark hole. The mucosa becomes dark as it becomes hyperemic, and brownish ceruminous exudates fill the bulla.

There is a condition described in dogs called a "false middle ear." Obstructions along the horizontal ear canal from hypertrophic or cystic glands, neoplasia, inflammation, or ceruminous plugs increase pressure on the TM, causing it to stretch and bulge into the middle ear cavity. Coupled with poor air movement through the eustachian tube, negative pressure inside the bulla pulls the eardrum even farther into the middle ear cavity. A false middle ear may develop as a result of the distended membrane ballooning into the bulla. Examination of this ear also reveals the absence of an eardrum at the end of the horizontal canal. Computed tomography (CT) scans of these ears reveal a "finger" lesion protruding into the bulla. The invaginating eardrum may collect large amounts of debris from the external canal such as keratin, wax, and desquamated epithelial cells. The invaginated eardrum forms a cavity that needs to be flushed out thoroughly. Often misdiagnosed as having otitis media, these patients can be retrospectively diagnosed when on 2-week recheck the previously unseen eardrum is back in the normal location.

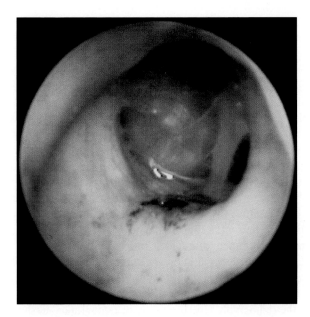

Figure 14-7

The middle ear of this cat contains a fleshy mass that can be seen by transillumination.

In some cases of otitis media the eardrum is intact, but it may look abnormal. It may change color in response to inflammation on the medial side, becoming opaque and gray in color rather than pearly and translucent. Sometimes there is fluid behind the eardrum, and examination of the intact TM may indicate that it is bulging into the external ear. Purulent material in the middle ear may be seen as yellow fluid behind the eardrum. Early polyps and tumors in the middle ear may be seen as fleshy masses through the eardrum (Figure 14-7).

Imaging of the Tympanic Bulla

Radiographic assessment of the bullae can be very helpful in determining the extent of bony involvement and the presence of increased tissue or fluid filling the bullae (see Chapter 2). However, the absence of radiographic changes in the bullae does not rule out otitis media, especially the more acute cases.

The first radiograph is taken using an open-mouth, rostrocaudal view with the x-ray beam directed through the pharynx. The tongue should be pulled rostrally to remove soft tissue that overlies the bullae. If an endotracheal tube is in place, it should be temporarily removed for this view. The procedure requires angling the mandible and maxilla to an angle of 10 to 15 degrees away from perpendicular while maintaining symmetry of the skull.

In a dog with minimal bony changes, the bullae appear as normal, eggshell-thin circular structures medial to the mandibular rami on the rostrocaudal view. The cortical outline is thin and the middle of the bullae radiolucent because the bullae are filled with air. The cat has an air-filled, two-chambered tympanic bulla separated by a bony septum.

When the bulla is chronically affected, either the intraluminal or extraluminal bone shows new bone production or remodeling. Bone lysis may be evident. The cartilage of the external canal may also be calcified and easily visible on a radiograph. Dystrophic mineralization of soft tissue surrounding the ear canal may be present. Often an entire bulla appears radiopaque because of large volumes of thick exudate or tissue growths (neoplasm, polyp, or choleasteatoma) filling the air space. If lytic lesions are present, there may be radiolucent areas or the bone constituting the bulla may be absent, as in squamous cell carcinoma or osteomyelitis. Dogs or cats with recent ventral bulla osteotomy may be identified by the absence of a segment of bone; however, bone may regrow after bulla osteotomy. One or both bullae may be affected. If unilateral disease is present, a comparison between the normal and abnormal bulla makes radiographic assessment of middle ear disease easier.

If large volumes of flushing solution are infused into the ear canal of a dog with a ruptured eardrum before radiographic assessment, a misreading of the radiograph can occur because the bullae become filled with the flushing fluid and appear radiopaque on the radiograph. One limitation of radiographic evaluation is that old sclerotic lesions in the bulla of aged animals cannot be differentiated from a more current proliferative otitis media lesion.

Computed axial tomography (CAT scan) of the tympanic bullae, where available, may aid in differentiating bony lesions in the bulla from soft tissue reactions. Many universities and teaching hospitals have access to CAT scanners. In the United States, specialty referral centers are acquiring older CAT scanners from human hospitals and may be able to provide this type of radiographic examination.

These radiographs provide views in the horizontal, vertical, and sagittal planes. CAT scans provide a number of views in these planes taken at various distance intervals, each successive view slightly farther from the previous. Each successive view may be considered as one slice of bread removed from an entire loaf, with each slice being derived from a different part of the whole.

Even when the ear canal is stenotic and otoscopic examination is impossible, CAT scans are able to give clear impressions of the status of the ear canal distal to the stenosis as well as clues to the pathology in the middle ear. Bony lesions of the bulla can be differentiated from soft tissue lesions using CAT scans. Three-dimensional measurement of the size of a lesion may be estimated by calculating the distance between successive views in different planes.

Magnetic resonance imaging (MRI) of the ear is also being done to visualize the middle and inner ears. MRI can use such fluids as the endolymph within the cochlea and semicircular canals to provide contrast to the examination. Patients with neurologic signs relating to middle- or inner-ear disease can be seen. Extension of infection into the cerebrospinal fluid space and meninges can be detected by MRI. The computer-generated images can be viewed in three planes, as with the CAT scan. At the present time, this technology is available to veterinary medicine on a very limited basis.

Is the Eardrum Ruptured?

Several techniques have been described to determine the integrity of the TM when it cannot be visualized in an ear with a stenotic external ear canal.[4] A small-diameter (3½ to 5 Fr) catheter can be inserted into the ear canal until it stops. It is then extended and retracted to get a feel for the rigidity of the "stop." If there is a spongy feel, the eardrum is intact. If there is a definite hard feel to the "stop," the eardrum is ruptured and the catheter is hitting the medial wall of the tympanic bulla. This technique should be practiced on cadaver specimens to acquire the necessary sensitivity.

Tympanometry uses a sensor that measures the compliance of the eardrum in response to sound waves. It is not practical to perform this test in the veterinary clinic, however, because it is still a research tool in animals.

An easy, indirect method for determining the integrity of the eardrum is to infuse warmed, very dilute povidone-iodine solution (or dilute fluorescein solution) into the ear canal with the anesthetized dog or cat in lateral recumbency. If the orange or yellow-green flushing fluid comes out of the nose or if the patient snorts out this solution through the oropharynx when pressure is applied by the flushing fluid, the eardrum is ruptured (Figure 14-8). The fluid has flowed from the external ear canal through the ruptured eardrum, into the tympanic bulla, and through the auditory tube into the nasopharynx.

Another technique used by some is to fill the ear canal of a patient in lateral recumbency with the suspected ruptured eardrum up with warmed saline and to insert the tip of the video otscope into the ear canal. By looking through the clear

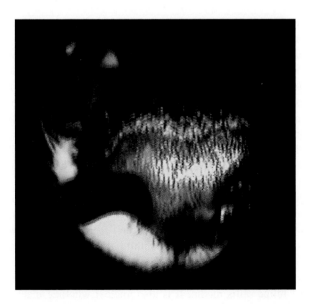

Figure 14-8

Nasal drainage of dilute povidone iodine flushed from the middle ear during ear cleaning.

fluid, if air bubbles rise from the ear canal while the animal breathes, the eardrum is ruptured. Air from the nasopharynx rises through the auditory tube into the tympanic bulla to escape from the middle ear through a ruptured eardrum.

Positive contrast canalography has been described as a method for detecting a ruptured TM in dogs with otitis media.[5] Two to 5 ml of dilute iodinated contrast agent is instilled into the ear canals of these anesthetized patients while in lateral recumbency with the affected ear up. The author uses 0.3 ml of Hypaque 50% or similar contrast agent in 2.7 ml of saline. In a stenotic ear canal, a $3\frac{1}{2}$- or 5-Fr catheter is threaded into the stenosis if possible. Contrast agent is then infused beyond the stenosis. An open-mouth view of the bullae is then taken, using a horizontal x-ray beam. If the eardrum is intact, there will be a distinct contrast/air interface at the eardrum. If the eardrum is not intact, the contrast material will enter the bulla, and a continuous column of contrast will extend into the bulla.

In a study of this technique, eardrums of cadaver dogs with normal ear canals and intact eardrums were intentionally ruptured and contrast material was introduced into the external ear canal. In every case, contrast media entered the tympanic bulla and was detected by a radiograph. In clinical otitis media cases, positive-contrast canalography was positive in most of the cases where the eardrum was determined to be ruptured otoscopically, and it was positive for other cases in which the eardrum appeared to be intact otoscopically. In normal ears, canalography was more accurate for detecting iatrogenic TM perforation than otoscopy.[5]

Primary Otitis Media in Cats

In the cat, primary otitis media occurs as a result of infection ascending through the eustachian tube to the middle ear. The cat can also have a secondary otitis media as a result of eardrum damage from ear mites or extension of a polyp through the TM.

An exact mechanism for the development of otitis media in the cat has not been reported, although the bacterial isolates from the bullae of cats with middle ear disease are consistent with respiratory pathogens. It has been hypothesized that chronic viral upper respiratory infection early in life may play a role in initiating otitis media in cats because these infections and polyps occur in younger cats. However, this has not been documented with virus isolation studies. The presence of these viruses, however, may affect the ability of the auditory tube to protect the bulla from infection with other agents.

In many species, including humans, rats, pigs, and cattle, *Mycoplasma* has been reported as an inducing agent in middle ear disease.[6] In addition to the more common streptococci and staphylococci isolated from clinical feline otitis media cases, organisms much more difficult to culture and identify, such as *Mycoplasma* and *Bordetella,* have also been cultured from the middle ear of cats with otitis media.[7,12] It is unclear what role these upper respiratory bacteria may play in the pathogenesis of feline otitis media. It is also unclear whether anaerobic organisms may be involved when the eardrum is intact and the auditory tube swells, thus sealing these bacteria within the bulla. In the author's experience, treatment of cats with otitis media using azithromycin (Zithromax Oral Suspension, Pfizer), which has excellent activity against both *Mycoplasma* and *Bordetella,* at a dose of 5 mg/lb every 48 hours for two or three treatments, hastens recovery from otitis media. Often, culture and/or cytology do not reveal an infectious organism. This raises the question of whether allergy, viruses, and/or fungi have a role in middle ear disease in dogs and cats.

Secondary Otitis Media in Dogs

Exudates and infectious organisms draining into the middle ear from the external ear canal through an eroded or ruptured eardrum get trapped in the ventral portion of the bulla. (Samples for cytology or culture should be taken from the ventral bulla before flushing and suctioning.) After the medications, chemicals in ear flushing products, and/or debris contained within the external ear canal enter the middle ear through an eroded eardrum, tissue reaction of the respiratory epithelial lining of the middle ear begins.[8] This is called *secondary otitis media.*

Pathogenesis of Secondary Otitis Media

Due to the L-shaped configuration of the canine external ear canal, proteolytic enzymes within exudates produced as the result of otitis externa accumulate against the thinnest portion of the eardrum. The resulting inflammation and enzymatic destruction lead to necrosis of the epithelium and supporting collagen, which results in thinning of the tympanic membrane, causing it to weaken.

Ulceration along the ear canal can extend to the eardrum (Figure 14-9). The ulcerated tissue leaks serum, which can cause maceration and excoriation of the epithelium. The reaction is similar to a "hot spot" on the skin of the trunk of the dog. Liberation of bacterial proteases, collagenases, elastases, and lysozymes from phagocytic cells and epidermal maceration resulting from the excessive amount of serum in the ear canal disrupt the epithelial layers of the ear canal and can lead to either erosion or rupture of the eardrum.

Many cases of acute otitis media can be prevented. Special care in cleaning and attention to fluid pressure, especially with the use of bulb syringes used to flush the external ear canal, can prevent the high pressure from causing an iatrogenic rupture. Removal of exudates by careful flushing and suctioning of the ear canal eliminates the source of destructive enzymes acting on the eardrum. Specific therapy for infectious organisms based on cytology or culture results can shorten the course of the bacterial or fungal disease. Treatment of underlying skin disease such as atopy, food allergy, and hypothyroidism may remove or improve primary causes of otitis externa. Proper client education concerning the chronic nature of ear diseases increases compliance in allowing frequent rechecks to follow the progress of treatment. Recheck visits allow the veterinarian to examine the eardrum and to make changes in the treatment protocol when therapeutic response is inadequate.

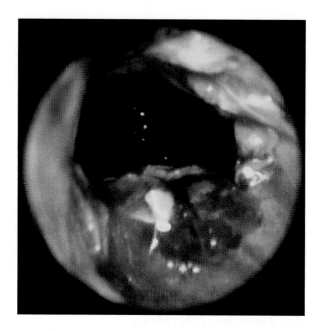

Figure 14-9

Otitis media with no eardrum present in an ulcerated ear canal. *Pseudomonas* was cultured from both the external ear canal and from the bulla. A slight ring of tissue (annulus fibrosus) can be seen where the eardrum was attached to the ear canal.

Whether primary or secondary, the resulting inflammation causes the lining epithelium, called the *mucoperiosteum,* in the bulla to change from cuboidal to pseudostratified columnar ciliated, leading to an increase in the number of secretory cells and glands, further adding to the quantity of exudate. Chronic inflammation leads to mucosal ulceration and breakdown of the epithelial lining.

The lamina propria thickens in response to inflammation, and as vascularity increases, edema and granulation tissue form. As otitis media becomes more chronic, the lamina propria changes to dense connective tissue, and bone spicules may develop within it.[1]

The cycle of inflammation, ulceration, infection, and granulation tissue formation may continue, destroying the surrounding bone. For example, septic arthritis of the ossicles may cause pain and decreased hearing owing to the fusion of these joints. The normal air conduction of sound waves is prevented, and the patient may suffer decreased ability to detect high-pitched sounds. With time, the ossicles are dissolved from osteomyelitis, and irreversible hearing deficit occurs.

The exudates and secretions thus formed in the bulla escape into the external ear through the ruptured eardrum and contribute to the exudate already present in the external ear canal. This large amount of liquid fills the ear canal and overflows onto the pinna when the patient shakes its head. If a polyp or tumor is blocking the outflow of secretions and exudates from the middle ear, significant quantities of inspissated material can be present when the obstruction is removed.

The fluid pressure gradient created by suppurative otitis media and increased mucus secretion prevents the eardrum from completely sealing. As the fluid pressure increases within the bulla, it pushes against a healing eardrum with a very thin, tenuous covering. The pressure allows fluid to escape through the path of least resistance, and a small hole remains in the TM. As long as there is a hole in the eardrum, this condition remains in a state of flux—that is, fluid can enter or leave the bulla, carrying infectious materials and exudates in both directions.

When the amount of middle ear secretion and exudate is decreased, when the infection is controlled by therapy, and when the fluid pressure is decreased, the eardrum can heal and otitis media resolves. Sometimes, however, the eardrum seals but the infection is not completely resolved. If the trapped organisms lead to a return of inflammation and secretion, the eardrum can once again bulge and/or rupture. Patients with otitis media may have had histories of repeated episodes because of this alternating rupture of the TM and subsequent healing. A report by Cole et al demonstrated that 70% of eardrums in documented cases of canine otitis media were intact.[2]

Microbiology of Otitis Media

The most common microbes recovered from chronic otitis media in the dog include *Pseudomonas aeruginosa* and *Staphylococcus intermedius.*[9,13] In one study, one or the other of these two bacteria was isolated in over 70% of the cases.[2] Other isolates include streptococci, *Proteus, Klebsiella, E. coli,* and some anaerobes.

When microbiologic samples from the middle ear were compared with the same bacterial isolates found in the horizontal canal, the antibiotic sensitivity of organisms isolated from the horizontal ear canal was different from the antibiotic sensitivity of organisms from the middle ear. This occurred in almost 80% of these cases.[2] This supports the notion that different strains of the same bacteria may be better suited to survive on different tissue types.

Bacterial sensitivity reports are based on the amount of antibiotic *in serum* required to kill the organism. So an antibiotic reported capable of treating an external or middle ear infection may be useless if the antibiotic cannot get to the bacteria. Due to the poor blood supply in the external ear canal and middle ear, there is limited diffusion of antibiotic from the serum into the lumen of the ear canal or tympanic bulla. In some inflammatory conditions, blood supply increases and may slightly increase antibiotic levels. For example, enrofloxacin (Baytril, Bayer) has been shown to produce poor skin levels in the normal skin. When tissue levels were measured in inflamed skin, the tissue level doubled. However, even with the doubling effect, the levels were much lower than the MIC for many resistant bacteria.

It is not uncommon for a number of different isolates of the same bacteria to be found in a microbiologic sample from the middle ear. This further confounds interpretation of culture and sensitivity results. The laboratory may report that the organism was *Pseudomonas aeruginosa*. Was the antibiotic sensitivity pattern representative of all the different strains in the sample or from only one isolate? If the report indicated that the bacteria were sensitive to an antibiotic, would there be other strains in the same sample that were resistant?

In ear disease, laboratory assessment based on culture and sensitivity does not usually correlate to clinical response. Antibiotic resistance mechanisms differ markedly, so even though the organism may be reported as resistant to an antibiotic, alterations in the use of the antibiotic may render it sensitive. In dogs that have been repeatedly treated for chronic otitis externa with a variety of topical antibiotics or suboptimal doses of systemic antibiotics, the bacteria adapt readily and become resistant to further antibiotic therapy.

Three mechanisms of antibiotic resistance are recognized. The first relates to the organisms producing substances that inactivate or modify the antibiotic. The second relates to the ability of the bacterium to provide a membrane barrier to antibiotic diffusion. Often resistant bacteria have undergone mutation and a gene expression of "efflux pumps" functions to extrude absorbed antibiotic actively from the bacteria through the cell membrane. The third mechanism of resistance involves the bacteria altering the sites at which antibiotics bind to them, rendering the antibiotic incapable of acting on the bacteria.[8] The challenge to the veterinarian treating dogs with resistant external and middle ear infections is to provide different therapeutic options to outwit the bacteria.

Examples of the first mechanism of resistance include penicillinase-producing bacteria and β-lactamase enzyme–producing bacteria. These enzymes either bind to penicillins or cleave the penicillins and prevent them from interfering with bacterial wall synthesis. Semisynthetic penicillins such as methicillin fool the penicillinase enzyme by having a modified ring structure. Strategies for treating β-lactamase enzyme producers include formulating the antibiotic with compounds that inactivate the enzyme such as clavulanic acid. Both amoxicillin–clavulanic acid (Clavamox, Pfizer) and ticarcillin–clavulanic acid (Timentin, Smith Kline, Beecham) are used in dogs.

When there is an efflux pump mechanism involved in bacterial resistance, increasing the extracellular concentration of the drug to overwhelm the pumps increases the intracellular concentration of the drug. In the middle ear, this can be achieved by using topically infused antibiotics with 100 to 1000 times the concentrations in the tympanic bulla compared with their parenteral administration. Much current research is underway to identify substances that act as efflux pump inhibitors that can inactivate the pumps and allow antibiotics to concentrate in the bacteria. Increased antibiotic concentrations can also be achieved in the middle ear by using certain antibiotics that concentrate in inflammatory cells. However, there is a limit to the concentrations of these drugs that can be achieved in tissue, ranging from 5 to 15 times serum levels.

By chelating metal ions (magnesium, calcium [Ca^{++}], and zinc) from the gram-negative bacterial cell membrane, tris-EDTA (TrizEDTA, DermaPet, Inc.) makes the bacterial cell membrane more porous so concentrated antibiotic solutions can diffuse more easily into the bacteria.[10] Tris-EDTA may indirectly interfere with the efflux pump mechanism by chelating the Ca^{++} ions required for the active pump mechanism. Future drug formulations may contain a mixture of an antibiotic and an efflux pump inhibitor.

When the bacteria become resistant by preventing the antibiotic from binding to it, another antibiotic with a different mechanism of action is required. For example, certain bacteria can add a methyl group to their ribosomal ribonucleic acid (RNA), inhibiting the binding of macrolide drugs such as erythromycin and lincomycin to the 50S ribosome, so they become resistant to these drugs. Cross-resistance among the lincosamides and the macrolides is common because all of these drugs bind to the same site. Changing to an antibiotic that does not bind to the ribosome may be a more effective choice for therapy than using another macrolide.

In cats with otitis media and polyps, the most common bacterial organism isolated was *Staphylococcus intermedius.* Other bacteria have been isolated from cat middle ears, including *Pseudomonas, Bordetella, Bacteroides, Fusobacterium, and Mycoplasma.*[11] Fortunately, bacterial resistance problems are not usually a feature of feline otitis media.

Antibiotic sensitivity patterns are important in treating otitis media because systemic antibiotics alone are often used to achieve levels within the bulla. If a bacterium is reported as sensitive to an antibiotic, and that antibiotic can get to the site of infection, systemic therapy may help. Unlike treating otitis externa, where topical antibiotics can achieve many times the blood MIC, systemic antibacterial therapy for otitis media relies on lower levels of antibiotics arriving in the middle ear hematogenously or through inflammatory cells.

Certain antibiotics can achieve therapeutic levels in the tympanic bulla when administered parenterally. Both clindamycin and the fluoroquinolones concentrate in inflammatory cells. They may be carried into areas of inflammation by these cells. Suppurative otitis media with purulent exudation provides the pathway for increasing the amount of antibiotic within the bulla. Azithromycin (Zithromax, Pfizer) also concentrates in inflammatory cells, but this erythromycin analogue also tends to concentrate in respiratory tissues at many times the level in serum.[9] Due to its intracellular accumulation, azithromycin has a long half-life of 48 hours in cats and 72 hours in dogs.[12] Its spectrum in cats includes those upper respiratory bacteria that are commonly isolated from the middle ear (staphylococci, *Mycoplasma,* and *Bordetella*). Clindamycin and azithromycin can be used in dogs and cats for nonpseudomonal otitis media. Development of resistance to clindamycin is common, so its use should be limited to the first occurrence. Certain oral fluoroquinolones such as enrofloxacin and marbofloxacin are effective for treating some *Pseudomonas* infections in the middle ear, but even at maximal oral doses the levels within the bulla may not be high enough for resistant *Pseudomonas.*

Topical antibiotic treatment of otitis media has gained recent favor in veterinary medicine. The use of topical antibiotics is based on the high levels of antibiotic that can be placed into the bulla, coupled with the poor drainage of the tympanic bulla. Aqueous solutions of non-ototoxic antibiotics can be placed directly onto the infected mucoperiosteum. Infused antibiotics can remain in contact with the inflamed, granulating middle ear mucosa much longer because the fluid filling the bulla cannot readily escape. Antibiotics for infusion should have a spectrum of activity against gram-negative organisms, which include *Pseudomonas,* and gram-positive organisms, which include *Staphylococcus.*

The dilemma facing the clinician treating otitis media is that systemic drug levels may not reach a sufficient MIC in the bulla and topical treatment requires frequent applications. Using maximal doses of oral antibiotics along with weekly bulla infusions of a fresh supply of antibiotic increases therapeutic successes.

Many infections are polymicrobial, including mixed infections of bacteria and yeasts. Cytology of a middle ear specimen may reveal *Malassezia,* which would not be reported if only bacterial culture was submitted to the laboratory. Cytology may not reveal bacteria because they are often protected from the cytology stains by mucus. Many cytology-negative specimens have been reported as culture positive.

Malassezia yeasts found in the middle ear may cause disease, but their presence there is the result of cellular and ceruminous debris falling into the middle ear through a perforation or rupture. This condition responds to systemic antifungal therapy.

Myringotomy

To diagnose and treat patients with otitis media, it is sometimes necessary to perform a myringotomy to get a cytology specimen and allow for culture and antibiotic sensitivity testing on the material trapped behind the eardrum. If there is fluid pressure pushing on the eardrum or negative pressure retracting it, perforation of the eardrum using a controlled myringotomy incision immediately relieves the intense pain associated with these pressure changes.

To perform a myringotomy, the patient is anesthetized and the external ear canal is thoroughly cleaned with a disinfectant such as dilute povidone iodine. The ear canal is then dried using suction. A sterile, rigid polypropylene catheter is cut to a 60-degree angle with a surgery blade to provide a sharp point. A long spinal needle can also be used to puncture the eardrum. The tip of the cut catheter is advanced under good visualization, and the pars tensa is punctured at either the 5 or 7 o'clock position in order to remain away from the germinal epithelium and blood vessels overlying the manubrium of the malleus (Figure 14-10).

Alternatively, a small Buck curette (2 mm) can be used to make a hole in the eardrum. This instrument makes a larger hole in the eardrum and is more difficult to direct accurately to the proper site for puncture. This technique may be used to create a large hole in the eardrum to allow middle ear exudates to drain into the horizontal canal and to prevent pressure gradients from recurring. Larger instruments should not be used for myringotomy because they cause tearing of the eardrum.

Many veterinary practices are using CO_2 lasers to make the myringotomy incision. A 0.8 mm × 180 mm rigid tip or a long, flexible Teflon tip can be inserted through the working channel of the video otoscope and can be advanced to the eardrum. Applying a pulsed, low wattage (3 or 4 watts) laser impulse melts the eardrum. The advantage of laser myringotomy is that the tip does not have to touch the eardrum, so there is less chance of contamination of the bulla with external ear canal material.

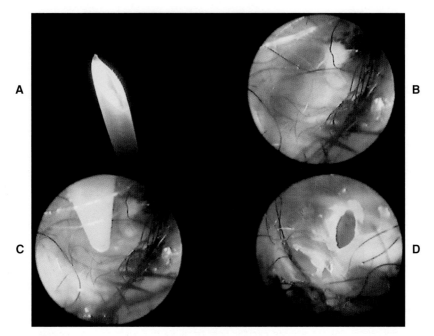

Figure 14-10

Myringotomy. **A,** A 5-Fr polypropylene catheter cut to a 45-degree angle with a scalpel blade. **B,** Surgical landmarks are identified. Blood vessels identify the pars flaccida and the hooked bone is the malleus. These structures should be avoided. **C,** The sharp pointed catheter is advanced along the floor of the horizontal canal with the bevel up. In the dog the tympanic membrane is at a 45-degree angle to the horizontal canal. **D,** Advancing the catheter and pushing it through the eardrum creates a "smiler" type of incision.

In addition, the hole made by the laser is circular and takes longer to heal, which is sometimes beneficial in providing drainage (Figure 14-11).

Fluid under pressure may freely flow into the horizontal canal as the perforation begins, and it should be suctioned to ensure that the myringotomy incision is large enough to accommodate a 3½- or 5-Fr catheter. In the case of suppurative otitis media, myringotomy serves to decrease the fluid pressure behind the eardrum. The fluid escapes into the external ear canal and may continue to drain for several days, so during therapy the ear canals need to be flushed to remove this debris. The catheter is advanced through the incised TM and directed ventrally into the bulla; gentle suction is then used to retrieve any material within the bulla. If a spinal needle was used, the stylet is withdrawn before suctioning. If the bulla is dry, 1 or 2 cc of normal saline can be infused into the bulla and then immediately retrieved. This material is submitted for cytology, bacterial culture, and antibiotic sensitivity.

Certain antibiotics or corticosteroids can be infused directly into the tympanic bulla through the myringotomy incision, providing high topical levels within the tympanic bulla.

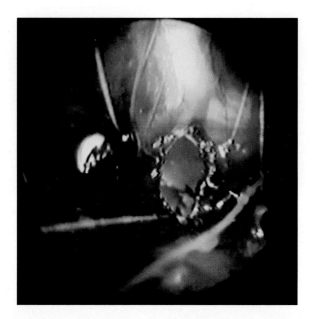

Figure 14-11

Laser myringotomy creates a more circular hole because the eardrum is vaporized. Laser myringotomy heals slower than catheter myringotomy, which may be an advantage for repeated treatments.

Treatment of Otitis Media

Planning treatment of otitis media requires a stepwise protocol for maximal effect. An organized approach allows the clinician to formulate treatment or change existing treatment based on observations. The steps outlined below provide a framework for treating otitis media.

1. Access middle ear—myringotomy
2. Bacterial culture or cytology (not always helpful)
3. Flush bulla—suction until clean
4. Infuse topical medication into the bulla
5. Reduce inflammation with corticosteroids
6. Systemic antimicrobials
7. Recheck weekly—re-treat two or three times
8. Surgery

Sample Collection

Accessing the middle ear by myringotomy has been previously discussed. In order to get a culture or cytology sample from the bulla in an ear without an eardrum, a sheathed catheter is used. A sterile 3½-Fr polypropylene urinary catheter is

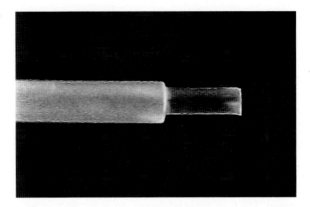

Figure 14-12

A 5-Fr polypropylene urinary catheter with the closed end cut off acts as a shroud for a 3½-Fr catheter, which is used for sampling the middle ear without contamination from the external ear canal.

threaded into a 5-Fr polypropylene urinary catheter (Figure 14-12). With the closed irrigating ends removed, the 5-Fr catheter is first threaded through the external ear canal until it reaches the bulla. This acts as a shroud to prevent contamination of the sample with debris from the external ear canal. It should be inserted into the bulla along the floor of the horizontal canal and directed ventrally into the bulla. After this catheter is placed, the 3½-Fr catheter is threaded into the 5-Fr catheter and extended beyond the cut end. The sample is aspirated with a syringe or suction apparatus using the flanged end of the 3½-Fr catheter. If no liquid is in the bulla, 1 cc of sterile saline can be infused and suctioned back. Any fluid or mucus that enters the lumen of the 3½-Fr catheter is submitted to the laboratory for cytology and culture and sensitivity.

If a myringotomy incision is made with a sharp-pointed 5-Fr catheter, as the incision is made the catheter is extended into the bulla and the contents aspirated. The lumen contents are submitted to the laboratory. If a laser myringotomy was made, a sterile catheter is inserted through the hole and a sample is taken.

Flushing and Suctioning the Bulla

Probably the most important technique for treating otitis media is flushing the bulla. Topical otic medications cannot penetrate through the thick exudate that fills the middle ear during otitis media, so this exudate and secretory material must be removed. In the bulla, many destructive enzymes that are trapped in the mucoid secretions remain in contact with the mucoperiosteum, which prolongs the disease. Hydrating the mucus with the water in flushing solutions makes it less dense and easier to suction.

Using fluid under pressure to irrigate the bulla loosens mucus from the tissue. This material does not stick to the mucous membrane as cerumen sticks to the epithelium in the external ear canal.

The fluid the author uses for flushing the bulla is warmed, very dilute povidone-iodine solution in warm tap water. If there is an identifiable bacterial infection, warmed tris-EDTA is also infused into the bulla. Acidic solutions should be avoided in the middle ear to prevent pain and irritation. Using a device that delivers the fluid under high pressure allows the mucus and pus to flush out of the bulla either into the external ear canal, where it can be suctioned out, or through the auditory tube into the throat. The MedRx Earigator (MedRx, Inc., Seminole, Florida) makes flushing and suctioning the tympanic bulla a simple, efficient procedure. A 5-Fr or smaller polypropylene catheter connected to the irrigation/suction unit is placed into the 2-mm working channel built into the Video Vetscope. The entire cleaning process is observed on the video monitor. The veterinarian positions the Video Vetscope in the proper location in the horizontal canal, and the assistant manipulates the catheter under direction from the veterinarian. The catheter is advanced along the floor of the horizontal canal and is directed ventrally into the bulla (Figure 14-13). A less rigid red rubber feeding tube can be used for flushing, but it may collapse when used for suctioning.

Use of a flush/suction instrument allows small pieces of wax, mucus, pus, blood clots, and other material in the bulla to be removed quite easily without the need for an assistant to manipulate a suction syringe. Repeated infusion-suction cycles are done to ensure that the bulla is as clean as possible. Without this equipment, catheter placement and evaluation of the efficiency of cleaning are hard to determine, but that should not deter the attempt to flush the bulla.

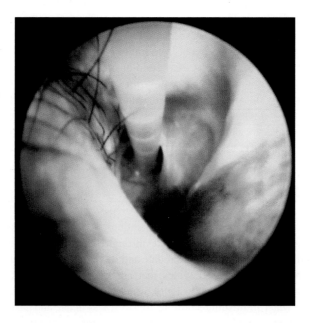

Figure 14-13

A catheter attached to a flush/suction device is used to clean and dry the tympanic bulla before infusing medication into the bulla.

A recent retrospective analysis from a major university looking at the effect of flushing the bulla on the outcome of otitis media showed that high-pressure bulla flushing resulted in an 82% resolution of otitis media.

Topical Ototoxicity

When the eardrum is perforated or totally absent, topical medications and the chemicals used in ear cleaners can gain access to the inner ear via the round and oval windows, resulting in neurologic ototoxicity. The ingredients of an ear cleaner should be carefully considered before use. Many manufacturers of otic products are now putting warnings on the labels of these products stating that their use should be avoided if the eardrum is not intact. In addition to topical ototoxicity, many pharmacologic agents are ototoxic when administered parenterally.

The aminoglycosides, polymyxins, detergents, and most alcohols routinely used in the treatment of the external ear canal are known to be toxic to the nervous structures of the inner ear.[13] Potentially ototoxic antimicrobial pharmaceuticals are present in most topical formulations for treatment of otitis externa. Many ear-cleaning solutions contain a mixture of ototoxic substances that may gain access to the inner ear, resulting in alterations of vestibular and cochlear function. Of these compounds, chlorhexidine is probably the most toxic, especially in cats. Severe, prolonged vestibular signs can be caused by chlorhexidine, and its use in ears is strongly discouraged.

An assessment of the risks of topical use of a drug or ear flush solution that may cause ototoxicity versus the therapeutic benefit must be considered when using these formulations to treat otitis media. For example, the aminoglycoside tobramycin has shown to be an effective antibiotic for many multidrug resistant *Pseudomonas* organisms. Although it is an aminoglycoside with potential ototoxic side effects, it is often infused into the bulla to treat the bacterial infection because of its efficacy.

In acute otitis media, the thin, permeable membranes of the round and oval windows provide easy access into the inner ear for many compounds. Access of ototoxins to the inner ear structures may be enhanced by inflammatory damage to the round window. Enzymes contained in otic exudates can cause maceration of the epithelium covering the round window, increasing its permeability. It is also possible for the round window to become hyperplastic and thickened after longstanding otitis media, providing a barrier to prevent these ototoxins from reaching the inner ear. Because the round and oval windows cannot be visually examined, it is difficult to know whether the membrane is thinned or thickened. By using non-ototoxic products, this issue can be made less important. If there is thick mucus within the bulla, it may act as a barrier covering the round window, effectively shielding the toxic material from contact.

Ototoxicity results from damage to the hair cells either in the cochlea and/or in the vestibular apparatus. This results in hearing deficits, vestibular disease, or both. Overt deafness or severe clinical vestibular disease (nystagmus, head tilt, and circling) may be obvious. However, subtle changes in either hearing or balance may not be detected by the owner or the veterinarian. Many common topical antibiotics can cause ototoxicity. Gentamycin, for example, concentrates in the hair cells of the organ of Corti in the cochlea when administered parenterally. However, it may also cause vestibular signs when administered topically in the middle ear. The cell permeability is altered so the hair cells swell and become deformed. They are rendered rigid and are unable to respond to movements of the endolymph within the semicircular canals. Ataxia, head tilt, and circling can result. A similar situation occurs in the cochlea when neomycin or kanamycin concentrates there. The cochlear nerve cells are damaged and cannot respond to vibrations, leading to hearing loss.

Safe Drugs for the Tympanic Bulla

There is a very short list of products that can be infused into the tympanic bulla without the risk of ototoxicity. These products are generally recognized as safe. Before selecting a product for use in the bulla, the ingredients contained in the preparation should be evaluated to determine the ototoxic potential.

For antibiotics, the fluoroquinolones (ciprofloxacin, enrofloxacin, and ofloxacin), aqueous penicillin G, some semisynthetic penicillins (carbenicillin and ticarcillin), and some cephalosporins (ceftazidime and cefmenoxime) are safe to use in middle ear disease.[14]

The antifungals clotrimazole, miconazole, nystatin, and tolnaftate can be safely infused.

The aqueous forms of the antiinflammatories dexamethasone and fluocinolone are safe in the middle ear.

Most ceruminolytics cannot be used in the bulla. The exception is Squalene (Cerumene, Evsco), which has been shown to be safe. Tris-EDTA as a flushing agent is safe.

Bulla Infusion and Topical Therapy

Removal of the mucus and pus within the tympanic bulla during the treatment of otitis media allows topical medications to penetrate in and around the thickened, folded mucoperiosteum. The use of aqueous formulations of *non-ototoxic* topical antibiotics, steroids, or antifungals placed on the mucoperiosteum hastens recovery from otitis media. Topical levels of these drugs may be many times the level that can be achieved using parenteral therapy, even when there is severe hyperemia of the mucoperiosteum. Antibiotic concentrations are high in inflamed tissues because the increased blood flow allows increased serum levels of antibiotic to perfuse the inflamed tissue. But even these levels may not achieve the MIC necessary to kill the bacterial target.

Infusing drugs into the bulla is an effective method of providing long-acting high-concentration effects. The tympanic bulla in the dog and cat is a deep, blind pouch. When the bulla is filled with antibiotic, the fluid cannot escape easily. Because of the small diameter of the swollen auditory tube and its location high on the medial wall of the bulla, drainage from the auditory tube is unlikely. Depending on the amount of eardrum present, fluid has to traverse a jut in the petrous temporal bone, which forms the floor of the horizontal ear canal and extends into the bulla. Fluid escape from the bulla is difficult and requires severe changes in head position to allow drainage through the eardrum. If a myringotomy incision was made, it would be difficult for fluid to escape the middle ear because of the surface tension across the incision. There may be a small movement of the infused antibiotic solution into the external ear canal, which actually may be beneficial, but the majority of the topical antibiotic solution can remain within the bulla for several days after infusion.

The antibiotic, antifungal, or corticosteroid solution is infused into the bulla through a small catheter placed into the bulla until the fluid overflows into the external ear canal. During the first bulla infusion, less than 1 cc of solution can be infused into the inflamed bulla. The entire procedure of flushing, suctioning, and bulla infusion should be repeated weekly during therapy. With each successive treatment, the mucoperiosteum should retract slightly, increasing the volume of fluid the bulla can accommodate.

With successive recheck visits, the eardrum and the horizontal canal should be examined for fluid, mucus, and pus. If there is fluid within the bulla, it should be flushed out and the bulla suctioned to prepare it for reinfusion. When the weekly examination reveals a dry canal and little liquid within the bulla, the inflammation and infection within the bulla has subsided (Figure 14-14).

At this point, bulla infusion treatments can be discontinued. Subsequent 2-week rechecks should reveal a healing eardrum.

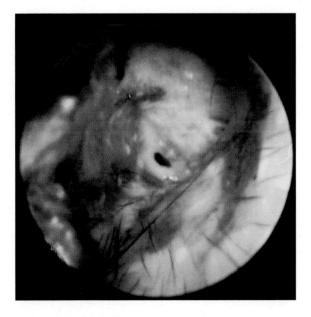

Figure 14-14

When otitis media resolves, the mucoperiosteum stops mucus and pus production and the ear canal is dry on subsequent examinations.

Topical therapy of otitis media in the author's practice is 75% successful. A small number of chronic otitis media cases require total ear canal ablation and bulla osteotomy in spite of proper medical therapy.

The basis for topical therapy is that oral antibiotic levels in the bulla cannot approach topical levels. Even resistant organisms cannot survive the extremely high topical levels that can be achieved in the middle ear. For example, oral enrofloxacin at high levels (20 mg/lb daily) may achieve no more than 4 to 6 μg/ml in the bulla, but infusing 1 ml of injectable enrofloxacin provides 22,700 μg/ml. Even recommended off-label dilutions of injectable enrofloxacin of 1:1, 1:2, and 1:4 provide extremely high concentrations within the bulla. The limitation of topical therapy is that bulla infusion must be repeated at intervals frequent enough to maintain peak antibiotic levels. Daily infusion would be ideal,[15] but weekly treatment seems adequate.

Much has been made of the use of the inhibitory quotient (IQ) for determining the efficacy of parenteral antibiotic therapy. The IQ is determined by dividing the tissue level of the antibiotic (Cmax) by the MIC of the bacteria.[16] The tissue level is determined by the drug insert supplied with the antibiotic. The MIC is provided by the laboratory. High IQ values have been associated with a lower development of resistant bacteria. By definition, if the IQ is greater than 8 to 10, the antibiotic dose is optimal. For ciprofloxacin and marbofloxacin, resistant *Pseudomonas* organisms have an MIC greater than 2 μg/ml, so to achieve the proper IQ, a middle-ear tissue level of 16 μg/ml is necessary. For enrofloxacin, the laboratories usually consider greater than 4 μg/ml "resistant," so a 32-μg/ml concentration would be necessary. It is doubtful whether oral doses of these medications can achieve these levels in the middle ear. Sensitive bacteria with low MICs may be adequately treated with systemic drugs that can reach the bulla.

If there is a resistant infection, the veterinarian should try to determine whether oral therapy alone is appropriate. For example, in a resistant *Pseudomonas* middle ear infection, if the MIC of the bacteria is reported as 3 μg/ml (resistant) for enrofloxacin and the tissue level within the bulla using very–high-dose oral enrofloxacin (20 mg/kg once daily) is 6 μg/ml, the IQ is only 2. This indicates a suboptimal dose of oral antibiotic, although it is being administered at the highest recommended dose. Resistant organisms result from suboptimal antibiotic doses.

The Use of Corticosteroids in Otitis Media

When the character of the middle ear secretions is mucoid and cultures do not reveal a bacterial infection, aqueous topical corticosteroids such as dexamethasone sodium phosphate (DMSO, 4 mg/ml) or a DMSO/fluocinolone combination (Synotic, Ft. Dodge) may be infused through a catheter placed in the cleaned and dried bulla. These potent topical antiinflammatories are not ototoxic. Other potent injectable topical corticosteroids are formulated with such ototoxins as benzyl alcohol or propylene glycol, or they are in suspension. These should not be used in the bulla.

Corticosteroids slow the intense inflammation and exudation found in middle ear disease. As described earlier, the mucoperiosteum undergoes severe pathologic changes in response to inflammation. Corticosteroids can reverse some of the extensive granulation that forms in the bulla, enhancing the ability of topically applied antibiotics to penetrate into the infected tissue. The tympanic cavity is crowded out by this hyperemia and proliferating granulation tissue, so the amount of free space within the bulla decreases. Reducing the inflammation helps this lining membrane retract back toward the bone, increasing the volume within the bulla. When the eardrum heals, this space should refill with air.

Corticosteroids reduce the amount of mucus produced in the bulla and decrease the viscosity of the secretions from the inflamed mucous membrane in the bulla. Changing the character of the mucus aids in its removal. Thickened, tenacious, inspissated material is more difficult to remove than thin mucus. Corticosteroids may also reduce the swelling in the auditory tube, increasing lumen diameter, which has the beneficial effect of offering limited drainage of mucus into the nasopharynx.

If there is bacterial or fungal disease and the space in the bulla is needed for antibiotic or antifungal topical therapy, decreasing doses of systemic corticosteroids may be used for a few weeks during the recovery phase of otitis media. The high initial doses of corticosteroid required mirror the doses used for such other diseases as inflammatory bowel disease. Patients should be screened for diabetes, Cushing's disease, demodicosis, and potential pregnancy before using high doses of corticosteroids. Prednisone or prednisolone at 1 to 2 mg/lb daily for 2 weeks then decreasing to ½ mg/lb every other day provides high enough levels to decrease inflammation within the bulla. Owners of these animals need to be warned that there will be side effects of prednisone at such a high dose. Many owners discontinue the medication when the side effects occur. The author prefers to use a 0.1 mg/lb intravenous dose of dexamethasone (2 mg/ml) at the time of treatment and then repeat this injection weekly at the recheck appointment if there is significant exudate that needs to be suctioned from the bulla. (The presence of exudate indicates continuing inflammation in the membrane.) This prevents the owners from having the choice to stop the medication. Dexamethasone has a higher degree of antiinflammatory activity than prednisone and has no mineralocorticoid activity, which minimizes the undesirable side effects (polyuria/polydypsia) seen with prednisone. Dexamethasone, however, depresses the pituitary-adrenal axis.

Because many dogs with otitis media also have concurrent otitis externa, systemic corticosteroids aid in reducing the swelling and pain from otitis externa. In addition, they reduce the signs associated with atopic disease, which is a primary cause of otitis externa in the dog.

Systemic Antimicrobials

Systemic antibiotic therapy is appropriate when topical therapy is impossible, such as in a Cocker Spaniel with stenotic ear canals. When topical therapy of otitis media fails, it is usually the result of inability of the antibiotic to get to the bacteria.[17] There may be sequestration of bacteria within folds or pockets of granulation tissue, which therefore remain unexposed to the topical antibiotic. In infections where the bacteria are sensitive, even the lower concentrations of systemic antibiotics may be sufficient to treat the infection.

Oral fluoroquinolones often are sufficient for non-pseudomonal gram-negative middle ear infections.[16] Because fluoroquinolone efficacy is based on a peak blood level, what level can be achieved and for what period should be determined. This is a dose-dependent antibiotic. Other antibiotics are time dependent. Their levels need to be constant to treat a bacterial infection, so the dose and the interval of dosing are crucial. When systemic time-dependent antibiotic therapy is required to treat resistant infections, it often requires the use of intravenous drugs. Ticarcillin–clavulanic acid (Timentin, Smith Kline, Beecham) has been reported as effective in treating multidrug resistant *Pseudomonas* otitis media in dogs when used as an intravenous injection of 15 to 25 mg/kg given three times daily.[18] In human medicine, intravenous ceftazidime has been used successfully for resistant *Pseudomonas* infections of the middle ear.

Summary

Otitis externa/media is commonly found in dogs with chronic ear diseases and in cats with upper respiratory disease and polyps. Diagnosis of otitis media requires attention to history and clinical signs, but it also requires other methods of determining disease within the bulla. If the integrity of the eardrum cannot be determined, assume that there is middle ear disease and proceed accordingly. It is prudent to take necessary precautions to avoid the use of potentially ototoxic ear cleaners or topical medications in suspected otitis media cases. Therapeutic success is possible using systemic and topical treatment within the cleaned bulla. Referral to a dermatology specialist or a radiologist for CT scan may be indicated in some refractory cases. Surgical intervention may be required to cure these difficult cases.

References

1. Little CJL, Lane JG, Pearson GR: Inflammatory middle ear disease of the dog: the pathology of otitis media, *Vet Rec* 128:293-296, 1991.
2. Cole LK, Kwochka KW, Kowalski JJ, et al: Microbial flora and sensitivity patterns of isolated pathogens from the horizontal ear canal and middle ear in dogs with otitis media, *JAVMA* 212(4): 534-548, 1998.
3. Kern TJ, Erb HN: Facial neuropathy in dogs and cats: 95 cases (1975-1985), *JAVMA* 191(12):1604-1609, 1987.
4. Little CJL, Lane JG: An evaluation of tympanometry, otoscopy, and palpation for assessment of the canine tympanic membrane, *Vet Rec* 124:5-8, 1989.
5. Tower ND, Gregory SP, Renfrew H, et al: Evaluation of the canine tympanic membrane by positive contrast ear canalography, *Vet Rec* 142(4):78-81, 1998.
6. Walz PH, Mullaney TP, Redner JA, et al: Otitis media in pre-weaned Holstein dairy calves in Michigan due to *Mycoplasma bovis, J Vet Diagn Invest* 9(3):250-254, 1997.

7. Trevor PB, Martin RA: Tympanic bulla osteotomy for treatment of middle ear diseases in cats, *JAVMA* 202(1):123-128, 1993.
8. Gotthelf LN: Otitis media. In Gotthelf LN, ed: *Small animal ear diseases: an illustrated guide,* Philadelphia, 2000, Saunders.
9. Jordan DG: Azithromycin, *Comp Cont Ed Vet Pract Vet* 21(3):242, 2001.
10. MedScape Today: *Antibiotic resistance varies with underlying biologic mechanism,* www.medscape. com/viewarticle/417558_3.
11. Foster AP, DeBoer DJ: The role of *Pseudomonas* in canine ear disease, *Comp Cont Ed* 20(8):909-918, 1998.
12. Faulkner JE, Budsberg SC: Results of ventral bulla osteotomy for treatment of middle ear polyps in cats, *JAAHA* 26(5):496-499, 1990.
13. Colombini S, Merchant SR, Hosgood G: Microbial flora and antimicrobial susceptible patterns from dogs with otitis media, *Vet Dermatol* 11:235-239, 2000.
14. Martin Barrasa JL, Lupiola JL, Gomez P, et al: Antibacterial susceptibility patterns of *Pseudomonas* strains insolated from chronic canine otitis externa, *J Vet Med B Infect Dis Vet Public Health* 47(3):191-196, 2000.
15. Mansfield PD, Miller SC: Ototoxicity of topical preparations. In Gotthelf LN, ed: *Small animal diseases: an illustrated guide,* Philadelphia, 2000, Saunders.
16. Dohar JE, et al: Treatment of chronic suppurative otitis media with topical ciprofloxacin, *Ann Otot Rhinol Laryngol* 107(10, Pt 1):865-871, 1998.
17. Ihrke PJ, Paqpich MG, DeManuelle TC: The use of fluoroquinolones in veterinary dermatology, *Vet Dermatol* 10:193-204, 1999.
18. Parry D, et al: *Middle ear, chronic suppurative otitis, medical treatment,* http:/www.e-medicine.com/ ent/topic214.htm, April 18, 2002.

Suggested Readings

Anderson DM, Robinson RK, White RAS: Management of inflammatory polyps in 37 cats, *Vet Rec* 147:684-687, 2000.
Dunn CJ, Barradell LB: Azithromycin. A review of its pharmacological properties and use as 3 day therapy in respiratory tract infections, *Drugs* 51(3):483-505, 1996.
Nuttall TJ: Use of ticarcillin in the management of canine otitis externa complicated by *Pseudomonas aeruginosa, J Sm Anim Pract* 39(4):165-168, 1998.
Schachern PA, et al: The permeability of the round window membrane during otitis media, *Arch Otolaryngol Head Neck Surg* 113(6):625-629, 1987.
Stanley BJ: *Management of nasopharyngeal polyps in cats,* Walham Feline Medicine Symposium, North American Veterinary Conference, January 14, 1998.
Tos M, Wiederhold M, Larsen P: Experimental long term tubal occlusion in cats. A quantitative histopathological study, *Acta Otolaryngol* 97(5-6):580-592, 1984.
VanHeerbeek N, et al: Effect of exogenous surfactant on ventilatory and clearance function of the rat's eustachian tube, *Otol Neurotol* 24(1):6-10, 2003.
Veir JK, Lappin MR, Foley JE, et al: Feline inflammatory polyps: historical, clinical and PCR findings for feline calici virus and feline herpes virus—1 in 28 cases, *J Feline Med Surg* 4(4):95-199, 2002.

15

Healing of the Ruptured Eardrum

Louis N. Gotthelf, DVM

Veterinarians are often faced with the problem of ruptured eardrums. It is difficult to assess the eardrum in a small animal because most otoscopes do not provide good lighting or adequate magnification. Many cases of otitis externa result in an ear canal that is inflamed, stenotic, and full of exudates that impede the visual determination of the integrity of the eardrum (Figure 15-1).

Causes of Rupture

Tympanic membrane perforation occurs in dogs and cats for a variety of reasons, the most common being chronic otitis externa. Otitis media results from the destructive effects of proteolytic enzymes on the thin epithelial layers of the membrane. These enzymes are released from bacteria, inflammatory cell degradation, and ulcerations along the ear canal produced as a result of otitis externa; the enzymes then gain access to the sensitive respiratory lining of the tympanic bulla through the perforation.

Traumatic perforations of the tympanic membrane also occur as the result of either excessive fluid pressure achieved during flushing of the ear canal or traumatic

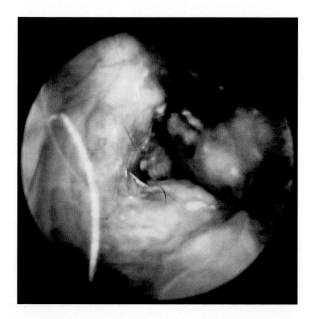

Figure 15-1

The eardrum of a 10-year-old German Shepherd is ruptured. Copious mucoid debris filled the ear canal. This ear canal is edematous and the eardrum cannot be visualized. Flush solution drained from the dog's nose and throat during the flushing process, confirming that the eardrum was ruptured and the eustachian tube was open.

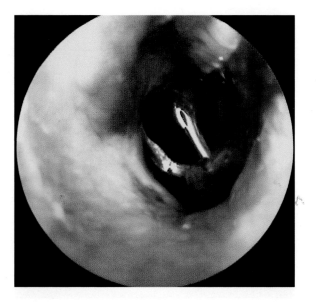

Figure 15-2

Traumatic myringotomy created by using a cotton-tipped applicator that was pushed too far into the horizontal canal.

use of instruments during cleaning of the ear canal (Figure 15-2). Myringotomy, a traumatic perforation of the eardrum, may be iatrogenic or may be intentionally induced in therapy for otitis media.

Cats with respiratory disease may rupture their eardrums through sneezing. Increased air pressure builds within the eustachian tube during the violent act of sneezing, and that air pressure is transmitted through the eustachian tube to the middle ear cavity. When the pressure in the tympanic bulla exceeds 300 mm Hg, the eardrum ruptures (Figures 15-3 and 15-4).

Rarely, ascending respiratory infections in dogs and cats resulting in suppurative otitis media may cause fluid pressure buildup inside the tympanic bulla. Without an exit point for the fluid, the increasing pressure within the tympanic cavity weakens the tympanic membrane, resulting in perforation. Children often suffer from this painful condition and require insertion of ventilation tubes in the eardrum to equalize the pressures between the tympanic bulla and the ear canal. In dogs and cats, myringotomy is indicated to relieve the pressure.

Nasopharyngeal polyps found in dogs and cats either grow along the eustachian tube toward the oropharynx or enlarge into the tympanic bulla. A large polyp within the tympanic bulla pushes against the eardrum, creating pressure necrosis, and its continued growth results in the ultimate destruction of the tympanic membrane (Figure 15-5).

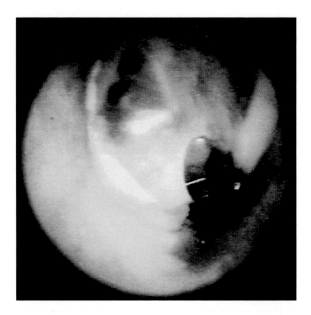

Figure 15-3

The patient, a young kitten with upper respiratory disease, was presented with the complaint of sneezing and blood in the ear. Close examination of the eardrum revealed an acute perforation caused by increased air pressure in the bulla created by sneezing.

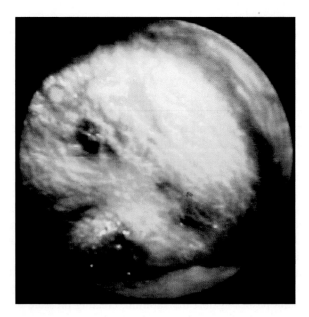

Figure 15-4

Another example of an eardrum with a small peripheral perforation caused by sneezing. The eardrum in this patient is thickened, perhaps as a result of herpesvirus infection.

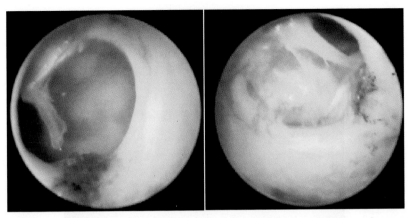

Figure 15-5

Left, Normal eardrum and tympanic bulla in a cat. *Right,* A polyp mass growing within the bulla pushing against the eardrum.

Healing Process

Unless the structures associated with the eardrum are completely destroyed, the eardrum attempts to heal. The mechanism for healing of a ruptured eardrum requires the presence of an adequate blood supply and a viable germinal epithelium. Regrowth of the eardrum depends on these vital structures, so the ability of the eardrum to heal is determined by the extent of the damage to them.

As discussed elsewhere, the germinal epithelium for the epidermal layer of the tympanic membrane is located in the area of the manubrium of the malleus and grows radially toward the annulus of the tympanic membrane from that location. Vascular supply to the germinal epithelium is derived from the blood vessels branching from the pars flaccida along the "vascular strip." If the malleus is preserved and the vascular strip is not compromised, the process of healing can continue (Figure 15-6).

The mechanism of healing in experimentally induced acute perforations of the eardrum has been studied in the dog. Tympanic membranes were perforated using a technique of subtotal myringectomy or by electrocautery. In these experiments the attachment of the malleus to the tympanic membrane and vascular strip were preserved. Tympanic membrane healing was observed in all dogs otoscopically. The time required for complete regeneration of the ruptured eardrum ranged from 3 weeks to 4 months.

Cytologic studies of the way the tympanic membrane heals reveal that around the perforation border, keratinocytes on the external surface of the eardrum begin to proliferate. At the same time, fibrous connective tissue cells from the middle layer proliferate. The inner mucosal epithelial layer differentiates into ciliated and secretory cells only at the perforation border and cooperates with the proliferated

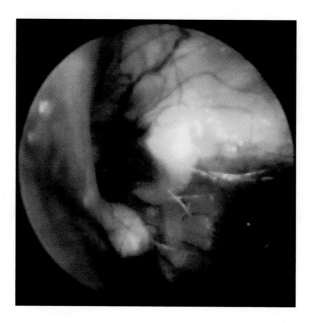

Figure 15-6

Prominent blood vessels demonstrated along the pars flaccida. This is the major blood supply to the eardrum.

keratinocytes to close the perforation. The superficial epithelial layers of the eardrum appear to be effective at rapidly moving toward the tympanic membrane perforation to form a temporary patch, but it is the slower-moving basal epithelial cells that are involved in permanent closure of the perforation (Figure 15-7).

The intensity of this process may be directly proportional to the oxygenation provided to the cells by the intact vasculature. Vascular compromise or ischemia may impede tympanic membrane healing. Experimentally, in rats, aeration of the ruptured eardrum with increased oxygen concentrations resulted in acceleration of the healing process. This finding may have clinical implications in a patient in which the ear canal is stenotic and the eardrum is ruptured. Decreased ventilation of the ear canal may slow the healing rate.

The effects of naturally occurring otitis externa or otitis media on the tympanic membrane are different from those of experimentally produced perforations of the tympanic membrane. Progressive pathologic changes interfere with the natural healing ability of the tympanic membrane. Inflammation, excessive fibrosis, tympanosclerosis, and hyperkeratosis are frequently found in and around the eardrum. Keratinized epithelial proliferation at the edge of the perforation often grows inward and localizes on the medial side of the tympanic membrane. A thick keratin layer protrudes into the middle ear at the periphery of a permanent perforation.

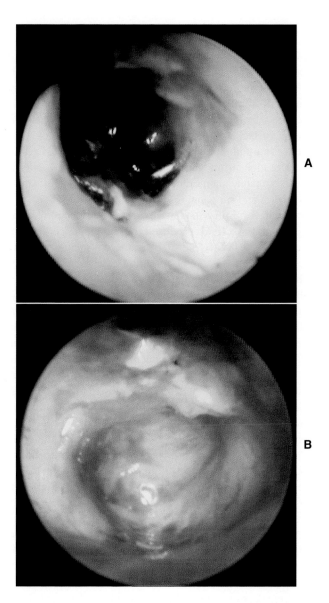

Figure 15-7

A, Chronic otitis media and ruptured eardrum in a 12-year-old Sheltie that was present for at least 6 months before treatment. **B,** Four months after treatment for the otitis media, the eardrum has healed.

Otitis Media Prevents Healing

Otitis media is a highly secretory condition. Copious mucus results from the increased number and activity of goblet cells lining the tympanic bulla. Purulent exudates result from inflammation within the middle ear. The fluid may be thin and serous or thick and mucopurulent. The accumulation of mucus and pus creates a high fluid pressure between the middle ear cavity and the horizontal canal of the external ear canal. When the eustachian tube is inflamed or the exudate is very viscous, the fluid escapes from the middle ear cavity along the path of least resistance, which is through any perforation in the eardrum, and moves into the external ear canal. For healing of the tympanic membrane to progress, the mucus and pus must be removed from the bulla and ear canal (Figure 15-8).

Effective treatment for otitis media diminishes production of mucopurulent fluid. Until the amount of fluid produced by the mucoperiosteum decreases, any attempt at eardrum healing is negated by the constant flow of fluid through the perforation. In addition, treatment for otitis externa reduces the quantity of exudates in the horizontal canal and alters the chemical composition of the exudates that move distally along the ear canal toward the eardrum. By properly treating the ear canal, the quantity of proteolytic enzymes decreases. The enzymes are not available to destroy the new epithelium that is attempting to heal the eardrum.

Depending on the severity of the otitis externa or otitis media, lysis of the malleus bone may be evident, and the germinal centers overlying this important structure destroyed. Extensive fibrosis may be present in the pars flaccida and around the annulus of the eardrum, occluding the vascular supply to the eardrum and leading to ischemia (Figure 15-9). In either case, the essential components for eardrum healing are removed and a chronic perforation remains.

Even if the otitis media is successfully treated and resolved, the eardrum may not heal completely closed. Often, a ring of hyperkeratotic epidermis surrounds the hole in the tympanic membrane; this condition represents a permanent perforation. Sometimes the eardrum will grow back only partially (Figure 15-10), and the middle ear is primed for inflammation. Any substance in the external ear canal, such as flush solution, exudates, loose hairs, epithelial cells, cerumen, or ototoxic otic drugs, can enter the middle ear and initiate an inflammatory response. Bacteria and yeasts gain access to the middle ear and provoke infection. Dogs with a permanent perforation of the tympanic membrane should not swim or get water in their ears. Veterinarians and groomers should be aware of this condition to ensure that no ototoxic ear cleaner or ototoxic topical medication enters the ears; otherwise, frequent flare-ups of otitis media result.

Chronic, persistent perforations of the tympanic membrane are common in dogs. In people with permanent holes in the tympanic membrane, the standard treatment is myringoplasty. This procedure is not performed in cats or dogs, however. An ongoing area of intense research is to identify substances that may be applied topically to the perforation to institute closure.

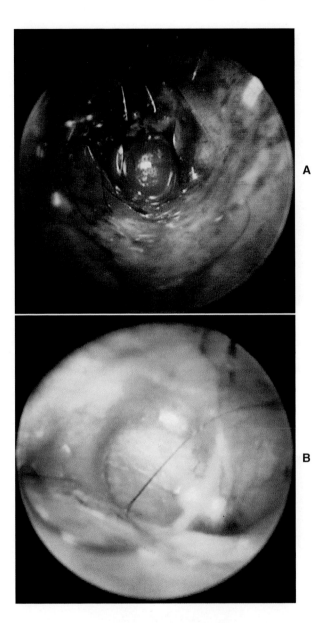

Figure 15-8

A, Severe mucopurulent discharge from the ear of an 8-year-old Shih-Tzu. The cytology revealed rods and neutrophils, and culture revealed *Pseudomonas.* The eardrum was not visible. **B,** After 6 months of treatment consisting of systemic and topical enrofloxacin, periodic middle ear flushes, tris-EDTA flushes by the owner at home, and topical and systemic corticosteroids, the eardrum healed.

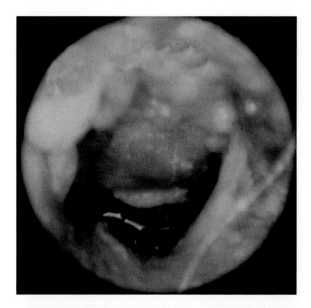

Figure 15-9

Chronic otitis media with extensive granulation tissue and fibrosis in the area of the pars flaccida, causing ischemia of the eardrum. The affected dog has permanent chronic otitis media, which requires total ear canal ablation and bulla osteotomy.

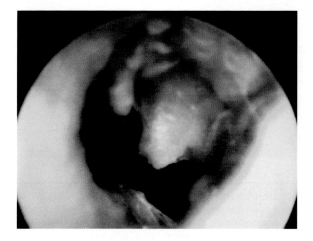

Figure 15-10

Chronic unstable otitis media. The eardrum has healed as much as it can. The middle ear mucosa is hyperemic, but no mucus or pus is seen. Any foreign substance that irritates the mucosa will result in otitis media.

Suggested Readings

Boedts D: Tympanic membrane perforations, *Acta Otorhinolaryngol Belg* 49:149-158, 1995.

Caye-Tomasen P: Changes in goblet cell density in rat middle ear mucosa in acute otititis media, *Am J Otol* 16:75-82, 1995.

Clymer MA: The effects of keratinocyte growth factor on healing of tympanic membrane perforations, *Laryngoscope* 106:280-285, 1996.

Gotthelf LN: Secondary otitis media: an often overlooked condition, *Canine Pract* 20:14-20, 1995.

Koba R: Epidermal migration and healing of the tympanic membrane: an immunohistochemical study of cell proliferation using bromodeoxyuridine labeling, *Ann Otol Rhinol Laryngol* 104:218-225, 1995.

Little CJL, Lane JG, Pearson GR: Inflammatory middle ear disease of the dog: the pathology of otitis media, *Vet Rec* 128:293-296, 1991.

Mattson C: Myringosclerosis caused by increased oxygen concentration in traumatized tympanic membranes: experimental study, *Ann Otol Rhinol Laryngol* 104:625-631, 1995.

Somers TH: Histology of the perforated tympanic membrane and its muco-epithelial junction, *Clin Otolaryngol* 22:162-166, 1997.

Steiss JE, Boosinger TR, Wright JC, et al: Healing of experimentally perforated tympanic membranes demonstrated by electrodiagnostic testing and histopathology, *J Am Anim Hosp Assoc* 28:307-310, 1992.

Truy E: Chronic tympanic membrane perforation: an animal model, *Am J Otol* 16:222-225, 1995.

16

Inflammatory
Polyps

Louis N. Gotthelf, DVM

Feline Polyps

The feline inflammatory polyp may be the most common non-neoplastic growth found in the ear canal. It is unclear whether polyps are truly congenital in origin or whether they are acquired as a result of otitis media secondary to upper respiratory infection. They are often found in young mature cats with an average age of 1.5 years, although they have been reported in cats of all ages. There seems to be no breed or sex predilection. There seems to be no relationship to feline leukemia virus (FeLV) or feline immunodeficiency virus (FIV) status.

Signalment and History

Nasopharyngeal or inflammatory polyps originate from the eustachian tube or from the middle ear mucosa. Most of these polyps have their origin in the middle ear; however, when they originate in the eustachian tube, growth is usually directed toward the throat. Nasopharyngeal polyps can be found exiting the eustachian tube on the lateral wall of the oropharynx, beneath the soft palate. Retraction of the soft palate with a spay hook reveals their presence. The cat with an oropharyngeal location of its polyp shows respiratory symptoms such as stertorous respiration, voice changes, wheezing, dyspnea, and dysphagia.[1]

The predominant clinical signs in a cat with an inflammatory polyp of the ear canal are discharge from the ear canal and head shaking and/or head tilt. Polyps are rarely bilateral. Nystagmus and vestibular disease may be present in severe cases of aural polyps, because pressure on the round and oval windows from the enlarging mass increases pressure in the endolymph within the semicircular canals.

Several presentations can be seen when a cat has a polyp in the ear canal. Some cats with an aural polyp are presented to the veterinarian with a waxy accumulation deep in the ear canal (Figure 16-1). This may look similar to a ceruminolith or wax plug. The polyp mass cannot be visualized because it is under the wax.

Some cats have dried, crusty material in the ear, similar to the discharge seen in *Otodectes* infections. The middle ear mucosa is a respiratory epithelium capable of producing copious amounts of mucus when it is inflamed. The mucus and pus that leak from the bulla into the external ear canal can dry out and become flaky, giving the impression that the cat has ear mites. More commonly, cats with polyps have a copious mucopurulent discharge in the affected ear due to liquid exudates filling the ear canal (Figure 16-2).

After cleaning the cat's ear, otoscopic examination reveals a pink to red, fleshy, mobile mass deep in the ear canal (Figures 16-3 and 16-4). When the mass is visible in the external ear canal, it has already protruded through the eardrum, having ruptured it as the polyp grew outward from the tympanic bulla. When this happens, a secondary otitis media can develop as bacteria gain access to the middle ear mucosa.

Manipulating the polyp mass often causes the release of material from the bulla into the external ear canal because the polyp acts as a seal for these middle

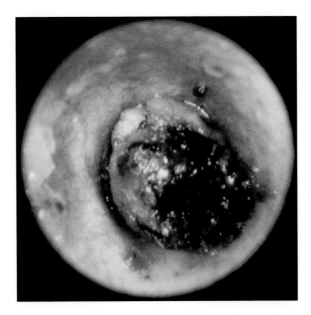

Figure 16-1

Cat with a waxy accumulation in the ear canal. This mass was located deep in the horizontal portion of the cat's ear canal. The cat was presented for a head tilt and ataxia.

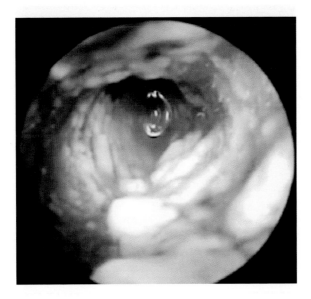

Figure 16-2

Liquid mucus and pus filling the ear canal of a kitten. After flushing the ear canal, the polyp was revealed (see Figure 16-4).

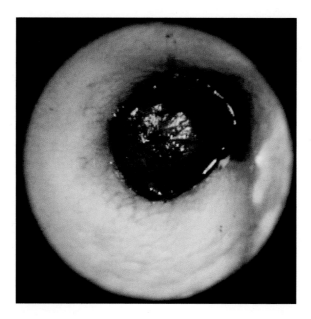

Figure 16-3

Nasopharyngeal polyp occluding the ear canal of a cat. The waxy accumulation in Figure 16-1 was removed to reveal this red, fleshy mass in the cat's ear canal.

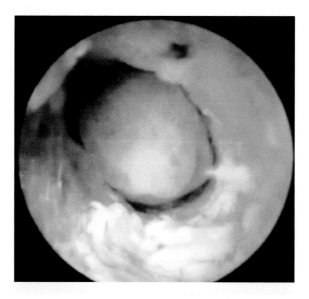

Figure 16-4

After the mucus and pus were removed from the ear canal from the cat in Figure 16-2, this fleshy mass was evident and could be pushed back into the middle ear. No eardrum is present in cats with polyps.

ear exudates. Polyps can become quite large and may reach the diameter of the ear canal, effectively forming a plug that seals in the secretions in the bulla under it.

Microbiology

Many kittens and grown cats have unrecognized middle ear disease often as a sequela to upper respiratory disease. Otitis media is a consistent feature when nasopharyngeal polyps are found in the ear canal. Many bacterial pathogens have been cultured from the middle ear after bulla osteotomy including *Pasteurella,* streptococci, staphylococci, and occasionally *Bacteroides* and *Pseudomonas.*[2] Some bacteria isolated from the middle ear in cats with polyps originate from the upper respiratory mucosa, and some pathogens originate from the external ear canal epithelium. Routine aerobic cultures for respiratory pathogens rarely include *Mycoplasma, Bordetella,* or *Chlamydia,* which may be involved in respiratory disease and middle ear disease of cats.[3] It was once thought that viruses played a role in development of polyps. In one study, tissues from inflammatory polyps were assayed for feline calicivirus and feline herpesvirus–1 by polymerase chain reaction (PCR). Failure to detect either of these viruses suggests that the persistence of these viruses is not associated with the development of inflammatory polyps.[4] In another study, polyps were induced in rats by placing type 3 pneumococci into one middle ear cavity of each rat. In 44% of the rats a polyp developed in the experimentally infected ear. None of the rats developed a polyp in the untreated ear.

The sequestered inflammation and infection lead to changes in the middle ear mucosa. It is theorized that the chronic irritation of the middle ear mucosa leads to the formation of polyps. Initially there is a rupture in the respiratory epithelium lining the tympanic bulla or the eustachian tube, followed by intraluminal protrusion of the lamina propria through the epithelial defect. Then the respiratory epithelium covers this protrusion. As the epithelium covering the polyp becomes damaged by infection or by the physical trauma of its own movement against the surrounding tissue, this process repeats a number of times, resulting in significant production of fibrous stroma and enlargement of the mass. Often the mass becomes lobulated (Figure 16-5).

Grossly, a nasopharyngeal polyp is pedunculated, having a narrow stalk at its origin and becoming a large fleshy mass as it grows. Histologically, a polyp is a hyperplastic inflammatory proliferation of the middle ear mucosa. A polyp is composed of well-vascularized fibrous tissue stroma covered with a respiratory epithelium, which is often ulcerated. The stroma is edematous, and the submucosa contains a mixed population of acute and chronic inflammatory cells, including neutrophils, macrophages, and plasma cells. Variable amounts of lymphocytes may also be present. It is difficult to determine the exact point of origin of a polyp histologically because the respiratory epithelium of the mucous membrane in the tympanic cavity, auditory tube, and nasopharynx is continuous.

Depending on their growth pattern, polyps can grow through the auditory tube toward the nasopharnx or they may grow through the tympanic membrane. When found in the external ear canal, the enlarging polyp mass has grown through the

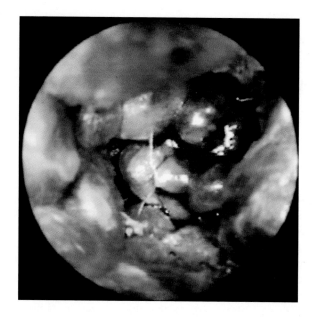

Figure 16-5

Multilobulated polyp in a cat. This type of polyp is usually more vascular than solitary-lobed polyps.

tympanic membrane, creating a permanent opening from the external ear canal to the middle ear. The middle ears of these cats have copious mucus and pus.

Treatment

Surgical Treatment

The most effective method for treating nasopharyngeal polyps is surgical because there is less chance of recurrence of the polyp. However, surgical treatment is associated with a high risk of postoperative complications. Veterinary surgeons recommend ventral bulla osteotomy to remove the origin of the polyp as well as to culture the inflamed mucosa and institute proper antibiotic therapy.[3,5] The cat has a double-chambered tympanic bulla. Exploration of the caudomedial portion, which is easily accessed through ventral bulla osteotomy, is relatively straightforward. However, exploration of the anterolateral portion requires breeching the septum that separates these two compartments. The sympathetic nerve fibers along the wall of the septum can be traumatized during this surgery. The interruption of these nerves results in Horner's syndrome, a common postoperative sequela to ventral bulla osteotomy in the cat. After ventral bulla osteotomy, most cases of Horner's syndrome resolve spontaneously. In addition, a branch of the facial nerve courses through the middle ear, and reversible facial neuropathy can occur as a result of trauma to this nerve. Vestibular signs such as head tilt, nystagmus, and ataxia can be associated with ventral bulla osteotomy; these signs may be irreversible.

Traction/Avulsion of Polyps

Polyps can be removed from a cat's ear canal with some type of grasping forceps through the otoscope cone. Special endoscopic tools or long alligator forceps can be used. The objective is to grasp the polyp mass and, using force, tear the attachment of the polyp away from the underlying mucosa. This is often accomplished by rotating the grasped mass 90 degrees and then applying traction. In this manner the entire polyp mass can often be removed from the mucosa lining the bulla. Increased exposure can be achieved by performing a lateral ear canal wall resection (Figure 16-6).[6] Traction works best in small, non-lobulated polyps. When removing some polyps using traction, only small pieces of the polyp can be removed. Visualization is difficult, and blood often oozes from the cut surface of the polyp mass. Repeated grasps and pulls are required to debulk the mass. This still leaves the polyp stalk in the middle ear, which may lead to regrowth of the polyp.

Endoscopic Removal of Polyps

Alternative methods for dealing with nasopharyngeal polyps in the ear canals of affected cats and kittens look promising. Removal of a polyp by traction may be easier when this procedure can be viewed endoscopically using the video otoscope and endoscopic instruments. A procedure called *perendoscopic trans-tympanic excision*

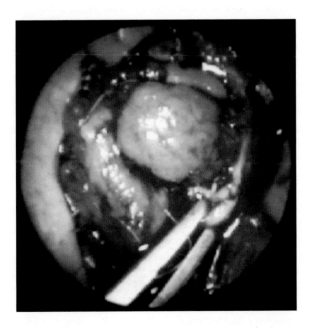

Figure 16-6

Lateral bulla osteotomy. When the polyp is inaccessible from the ear canal, an open procedure is required to excise the mass. In this cat, the polyp was not visible through the otoscope due to a stenotic condition in the vertical ear canal (a tumor) but was found during a total ear canal ablation.

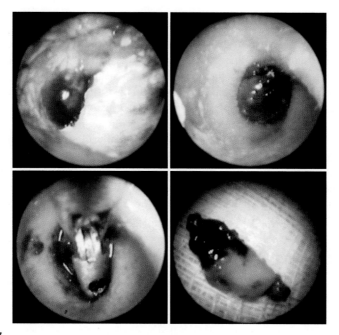

Figure 16-7

Removal of a polyp using perendoscopic trans-tympanic excision (PTTE). *Top left,* There is liquid in the ear canal of this cat. *Top right,* After cleaning, the fleshy polyp was revealed. Under direct video visualization, the polyp mass is grabbed with an endoscopic grasping forceps *(bottom left)* and rotated. A quick jerk on the forceps breaks the peduncle and the polyp is removed intact *(bottom right).*

(PTTE) has been described that uses a pinching technique with endoscopic forceps (Figure 16-7).[7] The major part of the polyp can be easily removed in this manner, and the lateral portion of the bulla can be explored to remove the remnants of the peduncle. In a study of PTTE, 10 cats with polyps were treated in this manner. With follow-up endoscopic evaluations from 3 to 24 months, eight of the cats had a complete remission; only two of the cats required a second PTTE. Two cats exhibited mild Horner's syndrome, which was temporary.

In another study of 22 cats with inflammatory polyps that were treated by traction alone, nine (41%) had recurrence. Because 59% of cats treated by traction alone had a successful outcome, these authors suggest that traction alone is a reasonable first treatment.[8] Eight of the cats in this study were treated with prednisolone (1 to 2 mg/kg per day for 2 weeks, followed by half the initial dose for 1 week, and then every other day for an additional 7 to 10 days) after traction removal of the polyp. None of the cats that received prednisolone had recurrence, whereas nine of 14 cats that did not receive prednisolone had recurrences. Because it is suspected that inflammation promotes the growth of polyps, it is reasonable to assume that controlling the mucosal inflammation after removal of the polyp would retard further growth. The author routinely treats cats that have had polyps removed by traction with a combination of

DMSO and a very potent corticosteroid, fluocinolone (Synotic, Fort Dodge), initially with bulla infusion through a 3½- or 5-Fr catheter placed into the bulla and then with eardrops administered by the owners twice daily for a minimum of 3 weeks. Recurrence of the polyp is rare in these cases. In addition, azithromycin (5 mg/lb orally every other day for two or three treatments) is prescribed to treat bacterial otitis media. Cats with only nasopharyngeal polyps were nearly four times more likely to be cured by traction alone than were cats with aural polyps.

Laser Ablation of Polyps

Another promising method for aural polyp removal is laser ablation under visualization with the video otoscope. The carbon dioxide laser has been used by the author and others in the treatment of nasopharyngeal polyps. There is a special rigid laser tip, 120 mm long, that can be placed through the 2-mm working channel of one video otoscope (MedRx, Inc., Largo, Florida), so that precise laser ablation can be performed while the entire procedure is viewed on a video monitor. Two techniques can be used in this manner.

For small polyps, the laser energy is applied to the polyp mass to vaporize cells and debulk the mass. The charred tissue is removed, and the ear is flushed. This procedure is repeated for several cycles to shrink the mass and seal off the blood vessels within the polyp. The laser procedure is continued until the stalk of the polyp can no longer be visualized.

If the polyp mass is large, the 120- × 0.8-mm tip can be extended through the 1.8-mm working channel of the endoscope into the tympanic bulla along the floor of the horizontal ear canal under the polyp mass. Laser energy is applied to vaporize portions of the polyp stalk, making traction removal easier. After the bulk of the polyp is removed from the bulla, the laser is placed into the bulla, and laser energy seals off the polyp stalk as previously described. Postoperative treatment includes the use of oral azithromycin for two or three treatments and fluocinolone/DMSO bulla infusion, followed by at-home ear drops for a minimum of 3 weeks.

Cats that have had their polyps removed rarely regrow their eardrums. Frequent reassessment of these cats is important to prevent secondary otitis media.

Canine Polyps

The dog only rarely develops a nasopharyngeal polyp originating from the mucosa of the tympanic bulla or from the eustachian tube. There have been reports of polyps occluding the airway as they grow through the eustachian tube into the nasopharynx. In one report, a canine nasopharyngeal polyp was so large that an incision into the soft palate was required to access it at the external opening of the auditory tube in order to grasp and remove it.[9] Other reports demonstrate that there are nasopharyngeal polyps that protrude through the eardrum into the ear canal in the same manner as the feline inflammatory polyp. Canine inflammatory polyps have been reported to occur bilaterally on occasion. One report indicated polyps only in older male dogs.

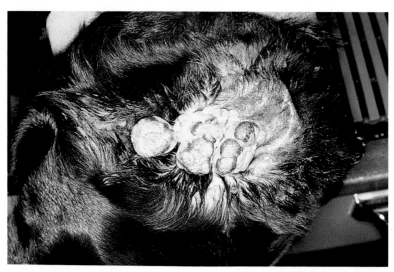

Figure 16-8

Canine inflammatory polyp. This Labrador Retriever was presented with both pinnae extending laterally from his head. Inflammatory polyps were present in both ears. The white polyp mass visible in this photo filled the external opening to the ear canal; as it grew, the polyp molded to the epithelial folds of the tragus of the pinna. The polyps were easily separated from the pinna. Each had a thick vascular stalk that extended through the entire ear canal to the middle ear. The polyps were easily removed by excision, and the stalks were removed using traction.

The significance of this is unclear.[10] The author has seen several canine aural polyps that grow very large, and they grow to the outside of the ear canal, often molding to the epithelial folds at the tragus (Figure 16-8).

Traction removal has been successful in canine polyps seen by the author, perhaps because they can be grasped with stronger forceps and can be visualized easier than feline polyps (Figures 16-9 and 16-10). Surgical treatment of canine polyps requires total ear canal ablation and lateral bulla osteotomy (TECA-LBO) rather than ventral bulla osteotomy, as in cats, because of the chronic nature of the external ear canal pathology that is found in most dogs with inflammatory polyps.

Most dog polyps are not true polyps but huge ceruminous gland adenomas. This type of tumor often has a broad base originating from the epithelial surface of the external ear canal. The eardrum is usually intact in these cases. The rapid growth and the position of this tumor mass in the ear canal make the diagnosis confusing. Pinch biopsies of these masses are sometimes reported as polyps, because there is an inflammatory stroma with inflammatory cells covered by epithelium. When the entire mass is submitted for histopathology, the dilated ceruminous glands become apparent.

This type of otic mass cannot be removed using traction because of its broad attachment. Lateral ear canal resection with excision from the ear canal at the base of the tumor is the preferred method of removing large ceruminous gland adenomas (Figure 16-11).

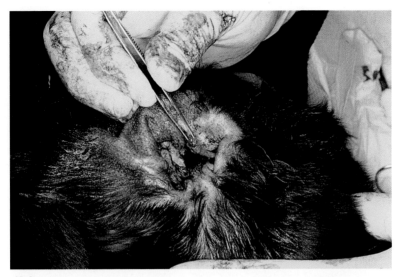

Figure 16-9

When the polyp is removed by excision, the peduncle remains (grasped in thumb forceps). Unless this vascular supply is removed at the time of surgery, the polyp is likely to grow back.

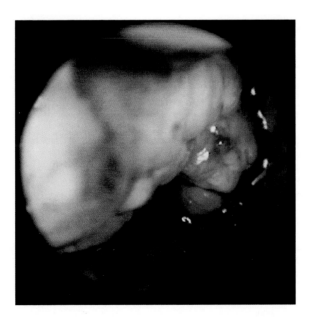

Figure 16-10

Endoscopic view of the stalk that remained in Figure 16-9. The long stalk, or peduncle, in this polyp extended from the middle ear mucosa through the external ear canal.

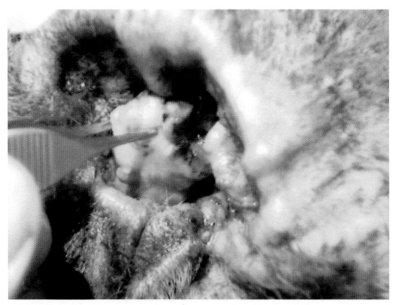

Figure 16-11

Cerumen gland adenoma in the vertical canal of a dog. This type of tumor is often confused with a true nasopharyngeal polyp. The difference is that these tumors are attached by a broad base to the ear canal epithelium. The eardrum in many of these dogs is normal, and there is no otitis media.

References

1. Allen HS, Broussard J, Noone K: Nasopharyngeal diseases in cats: a retrospective study of 53 cases (1991-1998), *J Am Anim Hosp Assoc* 35(6):457-461, 1999.
2. Faulkner JE, Budsberg SC: Results of ventral bulla osteotomy for treatment of ear polyps in cats, *J Am Anim Hosp Assoc* 26(5):496-499, 1990.
3. Trevor PB, Martin RA: Tympanic bulla osteotomy for the treatment of middle ear disease in cats: 19 cases (1984-1991), *J Am Vet Med Assoc* 202(1):123-128, 1993.
4. Veir JK, Lappin MR, Foley JE, et al: Feline inflammatory polyps: historical, clinical, and PCR findings for feline calicivirus and feline herpesvirus–1 in 28 cases, *J Feline Med Surg* 4(4):195-199, 2002.
5. Boothe HW: Surgery of the tympanic bulla (otitis media and nasopharyngeal polyps), *Prob Vet Med* 3(2):254-269, 1991.
6. Stanley BJ: *Management of nasopharyngeal polyps in cats,* Proceedings Waltham Feline Medicine Symposium, 1998.
7. Mortellaro CM, Alfieri C, DeFrancesco I, et al: *Perendoscopic trans-tympanic excision (PTTE) of ear canal polyps in cats: 10 case reports,* World Small Animal Veterinary Association Proceedings, 2001.
8. Anderson DM, White RAS, Robinson RK: Management of inflammatory polyps in 37 cats, *Vet Rec* 147(24):684-687, 2000.
9. Fingland RB, Gratzek A, Vorhies MW, et al: Nasopharyngeal polyp in a dog, *J Am Anim Hosp Assoc* 29:311-314, 1993.
10. Pratschke KM: Inflammatory polyps of the middle ear in 5 dogs, *Vet Surg* 32(3):292-296, 2003.

17

Ototoxicity

Louis N. Gotthelf, DVM

In human medicine, certain systemic drugs used to treat diseases can have profound negative effects on hearing and balance. Injectable antibiotics, mainly the aminoglycosides, and the cancer drug cisplatin seem to cause deafness in many children and adults. Some topical medications placed into the ear canals of children have caused hearing deficits and vestibular disease. In many of these cases there was eardrum damage, allowing these agents access to the nervous structures of the inner ear.

In human medicine, the symptoms of being dizzy or losing hearing can be detected very early in the course of treatment with ototoxic medications, so if an ototoxic reaction occurs, the drug can be stopped. In dogs and cats, these subtle signs cannot be easily detected, and ototoxicity is often only suspected when there is major neurologic damage to either the cochlea, manifesting in deafness, or the semicircular canals, resulting in vestibular signs.

The primary method of treatment of ear disease in dogs and cats is with topical products. It is well documented that more than 50% of dogs with chronic ear disease have absent or perforated eardrums, so an understanding of the potential for many of these drugs and/or chemicals to cause neurologic problems is necessary.[1,2]

Experimental Studies

Many reports have identified ototoxic substances in animals, including dogs and cats. Some of the ingredients found in topical preparations that are safely used on the skin in the external ear canal can cause damage to the respiratory tissues that line the middle ear cavity and to the nervous structures in the inner ear. Some drugs are ototoxic when used systemically but do not seem to have the same ototoxic potential when used topically. One example of this phenomenon is tobramycin. Numerous reports of ototoxicity have been published in regard to the injectable form; however, there are no published reports of ototoxicity from topical otic use of tobramycin.[3]

Many experimental trials demonstrating ototoxic potential are done in normal laboratory animals. They involve placing medication or ear cleaners directly into one of the tympanic bullae for several days. Usually saline is infused into the opposite bulla as a negative control. But for a positive contol, gentamicin infusion into the tympanic cavity of laboratory animals may be substituted. In ototoxicity studies, brain-auditory-evoked-response (BAER) testing is done to determine hearing loss prior to euthanizing the experimental animals. Cochlear damage occurs initially in the cells detecting high-frequency sounds, so these animals first lose the ability to detect high-pitched sounds. Neurologic examinations are used to assess the function of the vestibular system. Screening for ototoxicy using the BAER test during safety tests of any otic drug or chemical should be done before its release for use in animals.

Histopathologic analyses of the tympanic bulla and the inner ear from these experimental animals are used to verify evidence of damage to the epithelium of the bulla or to the neurologic structures in the inner ear.

Care is prudent in interpreting the studies done in laboratory animals and extrapolating the results to dogs and cats with diseased middle ears. Studies from normal experimental animals provide clues for potential ototoxicity concerns in dogs and cats; the results bear further investigation. For example, there have been many reported cases of acute deafness in dogs associated with the use of otic products containing gentamicin. One product containing gentamicin, clotrimazole, and betamethasone even warns on the drug label that the product "has been associated with deafness or partial hearing loss in a small number of sensitive dogs." However in a controlled experiment in 10 normal dogs, when low-dose aqueous gentamicin solution (3 mg/ml) was placed directly into one tympanic bulla twice daily for 21 days, neither cochlear nor vestibular function was affected.[4]

In another study that used juvenile guinea pigs to compare the ototoxicity of polymyxin and gentamicin directly instilled into the bullae, it was determined that the polymyxin group showed a 66% loss of cochlear hair cells compared with a 6.5% loss with gentamicin.[5] In human medicine, most people with gentamicin ototoxicity have vestibulotoxicity rather than deafness. It has been estimated that up to 1% of the human population has a genetic predisposition to gentamicin ototoxicity.[6]

Ticarcillin (Ticar, SmithKline, Beecham) and ticarcillin with clavulanate potassium (Timentin, SmithKline, Beecham) have been successfully used topically and parenterally for the treatment of refractory *Pseudomonas* otitis externa and media.[7] However, chinchilla studies using these compounds have demonstrated significant pathologic effects when they were injected as single applications into normal middle ears.[8]

Can a medication toxic to one species of animal also be ototoxic to another? Can a substance toxic to the cochlea in one species show toxicity to the vestibular apparatus in another species? It is possible that there are genetic differences among animals that confer susceptibility to certain drugs and chemicals, but most of these are undocumented.

Vehicles

Some of the studies done in animals reveal that other factors besides the active ingredient of the drug itself cause neurologic damage. For example, the alcohol bases of disinfectants, not the disinfectant itself, may cause the damage. Aqueous povidone iodine seems to be safe in the middle ear, but tincture of iodine contains alcohol, so it is not safe to use. Alcohol-containing products should be avoided if the status of the eardrum cannot be determined. Could it be that some of the carrier vehicles in ointment bases cause increased contact of the antibiotic with these sensitive epithelial and nervous tissues? Many topical otic products contain propylene glycol, which may cause some inflammation in the external ear canal. However, in the middle ear, it causes increased inflammation of the mucoperiosteum, leading to excessive granulation tissue and bony changes within the bulla.[9]

Dilutional Factors

Some topical products that are ototoxic if used as supplied may not be ototoxic at lower concentrations. Acetic acid at 5% seems to cause more problems than acetic acid at 2%. However, simply diluting a product may not render it safe.

In a series of studies done in cats, chlorhexidine gluconate was shown to cause degeneration of the hair cells in the labyrinthine vestibule of the vestibular apparatus. At a 2% concentration, chlorhexidine caused profound degeneration of these cells, but at a concentration of 0.05% there was less degeneration of these cells.[10] However, even in the dilute chlorhexidine group there were still clinical vestibular signs. Subsequent studies in cats showed loss of hair cells in the organ of Corti over a very wide range at both concentrations. This indicates a cause for hearing loss after the use of chlorhexidine gluconate.[11] Chlorhexidine gluconate also caused the loss of the mucociliary clearance function in the mucosa of the tympanic bulla as it produced subsequent cell destruction.[12]

The use of systemic drugs such as salicylates and furosemide causes increased concentrations of gentamicin in the endolymph in the cochlea within the inner ear, resulting in clinical ototoxicity.[13] Salicylates may actually increase the membrane conductance of the outer cochlear hair cells, increasing the amplification of sound. In human medicine, this results in tinnitus, a high-pitched ringing in the ears.[14] Other systemic drugs such as erythromycin, streptomycin, and cisplatin are also known ototoxins.

Mixing Drugs

Some nonototoxic medications can safely mix with dimethyl sulfoxide (DMSO) to enhance penetration of the drug into tissues. Enrofloxacin injectable (Baytril, Bayer) is frequently mixed with DMSO/fluocinolone (Synotic, Ft. Dodge) to treat otitis externa or media in the dog. However, mixing a known ototoxin with the non-ototoxic DMSO may potentiate the ototoxicity. Mixing the aminoglycoside drugs with DMSO may enhance their absorption into the inner ear and may increase the toxicity of the medication.[15]

Duration of Therapy

The duration of therapy with ototoxic medications can influence the amount of nervous tissue damage. Reversibility of clinical signs often depends on the duration of the treatment. In the case of neomycin applied to the middle ears of guinea pigs, the degree of cochlear damage and hearing loss worsens as the duration of its use increases.[16] Young animals seem to have a greater sensitivity to ototopical antibiotics. Neomycin, an aminoglycoside antibiotic, is contained in many commonly prescribed combination veterinary otic preparations. It is especially ototoxic in the ears of 2- or 3-week-old kittens.[17]

Delayed Ototoxicity

Delayed ototoxicity from topical gentamicin has been documented. It may persist within the inner ear of animals for more than 6 months. So gentamicin ototoxicity may continue for several months after the gentamicin therapy has stopped. Neomycin, streptomycin, and kanamycin are also known to be eliminated from the inner ear slowly.[18]

The duration of middle ear disease can affect the absorption of materials into the inner ear. The permeability of the round and oval windows increases early in the course of otitis media, allowing increased amounts of ototoxins to pass easily into the inner ear. With chronicity, granulation tissue and mucus accumulation within the middle ear may prevent the diffusion of the same medication into the inner ear. In a chinchilla study, when experimentally induced otitis media resolved there was less susceptibility to ototicity by polymyxin.[19] Some ototoxic medications and chemicals are also pro-inflammatory, causing thickening of the mucosa and the membranes of the round and oval windows, which limits absorption of these compounds into the inner ear.

With so many otic products available to veterinarians, it is prudent to look at the ingredients of an ear cleaner to see whether it may have ototoxicity potential. Many manufacturers are aware of the potential ototoxicity of the ingredients in their products and so they have been placing warnings on their labels stating "Caution: Do not use if the eardrum is ruptured."

Ear Cleaners

One study looked at four commonly used ear cleaners to determine what ototoxic effects could be determined. The ingredients tested included squalene, dioctyl sodium succinate, carbamide peroxide, and triethanolamine. These ear cleaners were instilled into the middle ears of both dogs and guinea pigs with a normal BAER. Each product was instilled into one bulla of each test animal, only one time, through a myringotomy incision. Neurologic function and BAER were assessed every week for 28 days. Then the animals were sacrificed, and the inner ears were examined histopathologically. The untreated ear (normal control) of the same animal was used for comparison. Only the ear cleaner containing squalene showed no morphologic or neurologic changes.[20] Another study comparing the vestibular and cochlear effects of the common topical antiseptics chlorhexidine, alcohol, and povidone iodine in sand rats showed that chlorhexidine and alcohol had a profound effect on both the vestibular and cochlear functions but that povidone iodine did not.[21]

Tables 17-1 through 17-3 list drugs that have known ototoxic potential as well as those agents generally recognized as safe. These lists should be used as guidelines based on sound scientific studies for making therapeutic decisions. Until we have answers to the questions regarding which compounds are known to cause ototoxicty in dogs and cats, we should attempt to preempt ototoxicity while treating otitis. We should base the use of these topical otic products on current evidence, including laboratory studies in animals other than dogs and cats. By learning which medications and ear cleaners may be potentially ototoxic if the eardrum cannot be seen or is ruptured, and avoiding their use, we will "do no harm."

TABLE 17-1   Potentially Ototoxic Systemic Agents

Aminoglycoside antibiotics	Amikacin
	Dactinomycin
	Dibekacin
	Dihydrostreptomycin
	Framycetin
	Gentamicin
	Kanamycin
	Netilmicin
	Ribostamycin
	Sisomicin
	Streptomycin
	Tobramycin
Nonaminoglycoside antibiotics	Erythromycin
	Ristocetin
Diuretics	Acetazolamide
	Bumetanide
	Ethacrynic acid
	Furosemide
	Mannitol
Antineoplastic agents	Actinomycin C and D
	Bleomycin
	Carboplatin
	Cisplatin
	Mechlorethamine
	Vinblastine
	Vincristine
Miscellaneous agents	Arsenic compounds
	Chloroquine
	Danazol
	Gold salts
	Pentobarbital
	Potassium bromide
	Quinidine
	Quinine
	Salicylates

TABLE 17-2 Potentially Ototoxic Topical Agents

Aminoglycoside antibiotics	All
Nonaminoglycoside antibiotics	Bacitracin*
	Chloramphenicol*
	Chlortetracycline*
	Colistin*
	Erythromycin
	Gramicidin*
	Hygromycin B
	Iodochlorhydroxyquinolone
	Minocycline
	Oxytetracycline*
	Pharmacetin
	Polymyxin B
	Tetracycline*
	Ticarcillin*
	Vancomycin
	Viomycin
Antiseptics	Acetic acid
	Benzalkonium chloride*
	Benzethonium chloride
	Cetrimide
	Chlorhexidine*
	m-Cresyl acetate
	Ethanol
	Iodine and iodophors
	Merthiolate
Antifungal agents	Amphotericin B*
	Griseofulvin*
Ceruminolytic agents and solvents	Carbamide peroxide*
	Dimethyl formamide
	Dioctyl sodium sulfosuccinate*
	Ethanol
	Propylene glycol*
	Polyethylene glycol 400
	Triethanolamine
	Toluene
Miscellaneous agents	Cyclophosphamide
	Dapsone
	Detergents
	Dimethyl sulfoxide
	Diphenylhydrazine
	Mercury
	Potassium bromide
	Triethyl tin bromide
	Trimethyl tin chloride

*Has an inflammatory effect on the middle ear.

TABLE 17-3   Safe Ototopical Agents*

Antibiotics	Carbenicillin
	Ceftazidime
	Cefmenoxime
	Ciprofloxacin
	Enrofloxacin
	Fosfomycin
	Ofloxacin
	Penicillin G
Antiinflammatory agents	Dexamethasone
	Triamcinolone
	Fluocinolone
Antifungal agents	Clotrimazole
	Nystatin
	Tolnaftate
Ceruminolytic agents and solvents	Isopropyl myristate
	Squalene

*Generally regarded as safe on the basis of published reports.

References

1. Little CLJ, Lane JG, Pearson GR: Inflammatory middle ear disease of the dog: the pathology of otitis media, *Vet Rec* 128:293-296, 1991.
2. Cole LK: Microbial flora and antimicrobial sensitivity patterns of the horizontal canal and middle ear in dogs with otitis media, *JAVMA* 212:1549-1553, 1997.
3. deHoog M, van Zanten GA, Hoeve LJ, et al: A pilot case control followup study on hearing in children treated with tobramycin in the newborn period, *Int J Pediatr Otorhinolaryngology* 65:225-232, 2002.
4. Strain GM, Merchant SR, Neer TM, et al: Ototoxicity assessment of a gentamicin sulfate otic preparation in dogs, *Am J Vet Res* 56(4):532-538, 1995.
5. Barlow DW, Duckert LG, Kreig CS, et al: Ototoxicity of topical otomicrobial agents, *Acta Otolaryngol* 115(2):231-235, 1995.
6. Hain TC: *Ototoxic medications,* Otoneurology Education Index: www.tchain/otoneurology/disorders/bilat/ototoxins.html.
7. Nuttall TJ: Use of ticarcillin in the management of canine otitis externa complicated by *Pseudomonas aeruginosa, J Sm Anim Pract* 39:1165-1168, 1998.
8. Jakob T, Wright CG, Robinson K, et al: Ototoxicity of topical ticarcillin and clavulanic acid in the chinchilla, *Arch Otolaryngol Head Neck Surg* 121(1):39-43, 1995.
9. Mansfield PD: Ototoxicity in dogs and cats, *Comp Cont Ed Pract Vet* 12(3):331-334, 336-337, 1990.
10. Igarashi Y, Suzuki, J: Cochlear ototoxicity of chlorhexidine gluconate in cats, *Arch Otorhinolaryngol* 242(2):167-176, 1985.
11. Igarashi Y, Oka Y: Vestibular ototoxicity following intratympanic applications of chlorhexidine gluconate in the cat, *Arch Otorhinolaryngol* 245(4):210-217, 1988.
12. Igarashi Y, Oka Y: Mucosal injuries following intratympanic applications of chlorhexidine gluconate in cats, *Arch Otorhinolaryngol* 245(5):273-278, 1988.
13. Pickerell JA, Oheme FW, Cash WC: Ototoxicity in dogs and cats, *Semin Vet Med Surg (Sm Anim)* 8(1):42-49, 1993.

14. Stypulkowski PH: Mechanisms of salicylate ototoxicity, *Hear Res* 46(1-2):113-145, 1990.
15. Brown RD, Daigneault EA: *Pharmacology of hearing,* New York, 1981, John Wiley and Sons.
16. Brummett RE, Harris RF, Lindgren JA: Detection of ototoxicity from drugs applied topically to the middle ear space, *Laryngoscope* 86(8):1177-1187, 1976.
17. Leake PA, Hradek GT: Cochlear pathology of long term neomycin induced deafness in cats, *Hear Res* 33(1):11-33, 1988.
18. Thomas J, Marion MS, Hinojosar: Neomycin ototoxicity, *Am J Otolaryngol* 13:54-55, 1992.
19. Ikeda K, Morizono T: Round window membrane permeability during experimental purulent otitis media: altered Cortisporin ototoxicity, *Ann Otol Rhinol Laryngol* suppl 148:46-48, 1990.
20. Mansfield PD, Steiss JE, Boosinger TR, et al: The effect of four commercial ceruminolytic agents on the middle ear, *J Am Anim Hosp Assn* 33:479-486, 1997.
21. Perez R, Freeman S, Sohmer H, et al: Vestibular and cochlear ototoxicity of topical antiseptics assessed evoked potentials, *Laryngoscope* 110(9):1522-1527, 2000.

18

Otitis Interna and Vestibular Disease

Todd W. Axlund, DVM, Dipl ACVIM

Otitis interna, or infection of the inner ear, is a relatively common disorder in the dog. It is usually a result of extension of middle ear infection (see Chapter 14) and results in a characteristic set of clinical signs. These signs reflect the dysfunction of the inner ear organs—namely, the cochlea and vestibular apparatus. Cochlear dysfunction manifests as decreased hearing acuity. This may be difficult to detect in the dog without electrodiagnostic testing, especially if it is unilateral. However, often the astute animal caregiver is able to detect the subtle signs of hearing loss in the animal's natural environment. This information can be elucidated by careful questioning of the caregiver. The vestibular system is responsible for the detection of acceleration and orientation in respect to the earth's gravitational field, and it is absolutely essential for an animal to be able to maintain normal balance and posture. It comprises components located in the bony labyrinth of the inner ear and nuclei located in the medulla oblongata.

Vestibular dysfunction results in a variety of readily visible clinical signs, including head tilt, small-radius circling, nystagmus, and strabismus. The primary concern of the examining veterinarian when presented with an animal with vestibular disease is to determine whether the problem lies within the bony labyrinth (peripheral vestibular disease [PVD]) or in the brainstem vestibular system (central vestibular disease [CVD]). This determination helps when forming a diagnostic differential list and also allows for some sense of prognostication. For the most part, CVD carries a grim prognosis, whereas PVD is often treatable and carries a much better prognosis.

Components of the Vestibulocochlear System

The peripheral vestibular apparatus lies within the bony labyrinth of the petrous temporal bone. Important structures of the labyrinth include the utriculus and saculus of the maculae, the semicircular canals, and the cochlea. The maculae detect the pull of gravity and linear acceleration, whereas the semicircular canals detect angular and rotational acceleration. The cochlea houses the cochlear membrane, which is the receptor organ for the sense of audition. Information from the vestibular and cochlear systems leaves the peripheral apparatus in the vestibulocochlear nerve (cranial nerve VIII), which terminates in the brainstem. Neurons emanating from the cochlear apparatus course into nuclei within the brainstem and eventually project to the cerebral cortex, where the auditory information is processed, resulting in the sense of audition. The majority of the neurons from the peripheral vestibular system synapse in one of the four divisions of the vestibular nuclei that are located on both sides of the medulla oblongata, adjacent to the fourth ventricle. The vestibular nerve also projects directly to the cerebellum, which in turn sends projections back to the vestibular nuclei. Numerous projections from the vestibular nuclei are sent to different areas within the central nervous system.

Projections from the vestibular nuclei to the motor nuclei of the oculomotor (CN III), trochlear (CN IV), and abducent (CN VI) nerves control reflex eye movement (Figure 18-1).

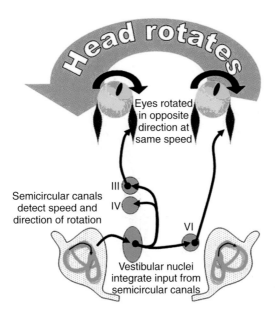

Figure 18-1

Vestibular control of eye movements. When the head rotates, the semicircular canals detect the direction and speed of the rotation. The vestibular nuclei integrate the information and direct the oculomotor (III), trochlear (IV), and abducens (VI) nuclei to move the eye in the opposite direction at the same speed. This maintains a fixed image on the retina even as the head moves. (From O'Brien DP: *Comparative neurology,* Columbia, MO, 2003, University of Missouri.)

Rotation of the head in one direction results in movement of the eyes in the opposite direction at the same speed. This reflex maintains a fixed image on the retina as the head moves. If the head is still moving when the eyes reach the furthest possible excursion in the opposite direction, the area of the pons that controls quick eye movements flicks the eyes quickly in the direction of the head movement, and the drift in the opposite direction begins again. Disease of the vestibular system creates the false perception of rotation, which produces a spontaneous drifting of the eyes in one direction with a quick reset in the opposite direction (spontaneous nystagmus). Projections to a separate area of the brainstem (the emetic center) are responsible for the nausea that may accompany vestibular disease.

Projections from the vestibular nuclei to the spinal cord maintain balance and support against gravity. They facilitate the ipsilateral large extensor muscle groups in all four limbs and the muscles of the neck that support the head (Figure 18-2).

Unilateral loss of this facilitation with vestibular disease produces the clinical signs of head tilt, leaning, and rolling toward the side of the lesion. The vestibular nuclei also send projections to the cerebral cortex, which mediates the conscious perception of movement and gravity.

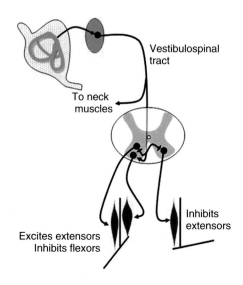

Figure 18-2

Vestibular control of posture. The vestibular nuclei give rise to the ipsilateral vestibulospinal tract. The medial vestibulospinal tract projects to the neck muscles supporting the head against gravity. The lateral vestibulospinal tract facilitates the extensor muscles of the ipsilateral limb. It also inhibits the ipsilateral flexor muscles and the contralateral extensor muscles. (From O'Brien DP: *Comparative neurology,* Columbia, MO, 2003, University of Missouri.)

Diagnosis: Otitis Interna (Otitis Media/Interna)

Otitis interna is a common cause of vestibular disease in dogs. It is almost always a result of infection of the middle ear (otitis media), but it must be noted that otitis media, in and of itself, does not cause vestibular disease. It is the extension of the infection into the petrosal bone, which houses the vestibular organs, that causes the signs associated with vestibular disease. Therefore, animals with signs consistent with PVD need to be thoroughly examined for evidence of middle ear disease. If present, it can usually be assumed that an otitis media/interna is causing the clinical signs, and treatment can begin.

Neurologic Examination

The first step in diagnosing animals with vestibular disease is the neurologic examination. Although patients with vestibular disease are often difficult to examine because of the severe clinical signs, the veterinarian can often get vital clues as to the location of the animal's problem by concentrating on certain aspects of the neurologic examination. Remember, the ultimate goal is to decide whether the animal is suffering from PVD or CVD. Animals with CVD have, by definition, brainstem dysfunction. Therefore, treating these animals for a presumptive diagnosis of otitis media/interna is ultimately unrewarding.

All animals with vestibular disease, regardless of whether they have PVD or CVD, have certain common clinical signs. They typically have a nystagmus, a strabismus that is more apparent when the animal is placed in dorsal recumbency (positional strabismus); a head tilt; a tendency to circle in one direction; and a generalized ataxia. Nystagmus, by convention, is named according to the direction of the fast phase of the ocular movement. For example, an animal with a nystagmus characterized by horizontal movement of the pupil with the fast phase to the right has a "right horizontal nystagmus." It is important to note that the fast phase is typically away from the side of the lesion; therefore the animal in the example above is likely to have a left-sided vestibular lesion. The head tilt, again by convention, is named according to the side of the head that is lower. In most cases the head tilt is directed toward the side of the lesion. The head tilt is often accompanied by a tendency to lean toward the side of the lesion. In severe cases the dog may roll toward the lesion. Circling, if present, should be described according to the direction of the circle (e.g., left circling) and by the radius of the circle (tight versus broad). Animals with vestibular dysfunction typically present with tight circles and circle toward the side of the lesion.

Peripheral Vestibular Disease

Animals with PVD may have either a horizontal or rotary nystagmus that does not change with the animal's head position. The nystagmus may not be constant, especially in more longstanding disease. In those cases, sudden head movements (e.g., quickly extending the head toward the ceiling) or rolling the animal onto its back may precipitate the nystagmus, but the direction of the nystagmus is constant. The head tilt is always directed toward the side of the lesion, whereas the fast phase of the nystagmus is away from the lesion. With severe, acute disease, the animal may not be able to stand, but if proprioception could be evaluated, it would be normal.

Animals with PVD as a result of otitis media or interna, in addition to the signs of vestibular dysfunction, may also have ipsilateral facial nerve paresis and Horner's syndrome. This is because the sympathetic fibers to the eye course through the middle ear, and the facial nerve (VII) courses through the petrosal bone in close proximity to the VIII nerve (Figure 18-3). Therefore an infection of the middle or inner ear often affects these two nerves as well as the vestibular system. Other cranial nerves should not be affected.

Central Vestibular Disease

Animals with CVD may have any type of nystagmus (horizontal, rotary, or vertical). However, if the animal has a vertical nystagmus, it must have CVD. Additionally, animals with CVD may have a nystagmus that changes in character or direction with a change in head position. Dysfunction of cranial nerves other than VII and VIII is suggestive of CVD, as is the presence of proprioceptive deficits. This is because any problem occurring in the brainstem that results in vestibular dysfunction may be large enough to affect the surrounding structures. These structures include the various nuclei of neighboring cranial nerves, the upper motor neuron fibers that course from

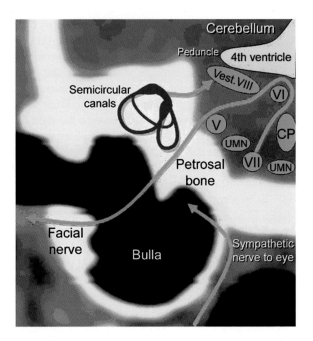

Figure 18-3

Structures of the middle and inner ear and brainstem superimposed on a computed tomography (CT) scan of the area. The facial nerve and sympathetic nerve to the eye run through the middle ear, where they can be damaged by otitis media. Structures in the brain that can be affected by CVD include the cerebellum, upper motor neuron *(UMN)* and conscious proprioception *(CP)* tracts, and other cranial nerves, including the facial *(VII)*, abducens *(VI)*, and trigeminal *(V)* nerves. (From O'Brien DP: *Comparative neurology,* Columbia, MO, 2003, University of Missouri.)

their origin in the cerebrum and brainstem to the spinal cord, and sensory fibers that carry proprioceptive information from the limbs to the cerebrum.

Lastly, animals with lesions affecting the cerebellar cortex, nuclei, or peduncles may show CVD. Such lesions may produce a paradoxical vestibular disease, in that the head tilt, ataxia, and strabismus are on the side opposite that of the lesion. In this instance the lesion can be localized by observing the side of the animal that shows proprioceptive deficits. For example, an animal with paradoxical vestibular disease may have a right head tilt and a left horizontal nystagmus, with prominent proprioceptive deficits on the left. The lesion would thus be localized to the left side of the brainstem. Other signs of cerebellar disease, such as dysmetria and intention tremors, would also be expected.

Diagnostic Tests

Animals with PVD should be thoroughly examined for evidence of otitis media or interna. Diagnostic procedures for this condition are discussed in depth elsewhere;

major points, however, are reviewed in this chapter. It is important to note that any animal with PVD should have a differential diagnosis list that includes otitis media and interna, inflammatory polyps (especially in cats), neoplasia, trauma (fracture of the petrosal bone), ototoxicity (drugs), congenital disease (rare), generalized polyneuropathy, hypothyroidism, and idiopathic disease. Diagnostic procedures, other than a thorough otic examination, may include advanced imaging procedures with computed tomography (CT) or magnetic resonance imaging (MRI), bulla radiographs, the Schirmer tear test (STT), and/or myringotomy.

Radiographs of the tympanic bulla (middle ear) may be used as a general screening test for middle ear disease. The presence of radiographically normal tympanic bulla, however, does not rule out the possibility of a middle ear infection because plain radiography is insensitive for detecting subtle soft tissue and bony abnormalities. Radiographs are most useful if oblique lateral, open-mouth, and ventrodorsal views are used and each side is examined for symmetry. Calcification of the external ear canals may be present in longstanding cases of otitis externa. Soft-tissue density within the bulla (such as exudates, granulation tissue, or neoplasia) is usually very difficult to visualize. However, in chronic cases of otitis media and interna, a thickening of the bulla or osteomyelitis of the petrous temporal bone or temporomandibular joint may be noted.

Advanced imaging should be performed in cases where otitis media or interna is suspected but not confirmed with the previous procedures and in all cases where CVD is suspected. Either CT or MRI can be used. An animal with exudate in the middle ear will have a soft-tissue opacity easily visualized using CT (Figure 18-4).

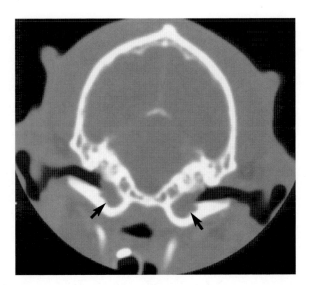

Figure 18-4

CT image of a dog with bilateral middle ear effusion *(arrows)*. (From O'Brien DP: *Comparative neurology,* Columbia, MO, 2003, University of Missouri.)

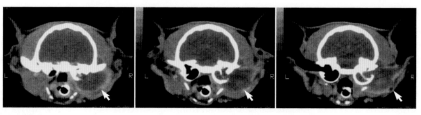

Figure 18-5

Serial CT images in a cat showing lysis of the right tympanic bulla and a large soft tissue mass associated with the right external ear canal *(arrows)*. (From O'Brien DP: *Comparative neurology*, Columbia, MO, 2003, University of Missouri.)

Erosive bone disease, such as in an animal with a bony neoplasia of the middle ear, appears as a mixed lytic and proliferative lesion (Figure 18-5).

CT is generally considered to be superior in the imaging of bone and MRI better at imaging soft tissue. This is even more marked when trying to image parts of the brain because a beam-hardening artifact (due to the thick and dense petrous temporal bone) prevents adequate visualization of the brainstem using CT. Therefore, when imaging the brainstem is important, as in cases of suspected CVD, an MRI would prove superior (Figure 18-6).

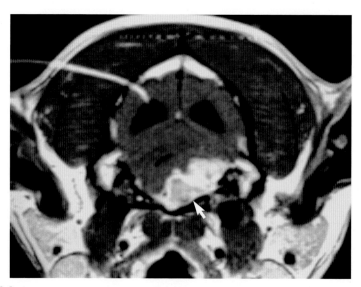

Figure 18-6

MRI of a dog with a tumor of the brainstem causing CVD *(arrow)*.

Myringotomy, or aspiration of middle ear contents, can be a useful diagnostic tool. This test is usually performed when the tympanic membrane is intact, but there is direct visual or imaging evidence of fluid accumulation. This procedure is performed on a heavily sedated or anesthetized animal. In short, the technique involves visualization of the tympanum with an otoscope, rupture of the tympanic membrane with a blunt probe caudal to the malleus, insertion of a 20-gauge spinal needle through the hole, and aspiration and culture/cytology of the middle ear contents, followed by gentle flushing of the tympanic bulla with warm sterile saline. Care is needed in this procedure to avoid damaging the auditory ossicles or nerves. This is best done by directing the flush caudally and ventrally.

A Schirmer tear test (STT) should also be performed in all animals with otitis media or interna. The major petrosal nerve, a branch of the facial nerve (VII), runs through the middle ear and often is damaged by the inflammatory process. The lacrimal gland is innervated by the major petrosal nerve, and denervation results in decreased secretion and the potential development of keratoconjunctivitis sicca (KCS). Also, certain antibiotics used to treat otitis interna and media can result in decreased tear production. Therefore, a baseline STT identifies dogs that may develop KCS; it can be used as a benchmark to determine whether the antibiotic is causing decreased tear production.

Evoked-response audiometry can yield valuable information in animals with suspected hearing loss. Brain-auditory-evoked-response (BAER) is a test that records the electrical activity of the auditory nerve and brainstem time-locked with an auditory stimulus that is delivered to the ear. In general, hearing loss can be attributed to either a conductive or sensorineural problem. Conductive hearing loss is dysfunction in the peripheral hearing mechanism as a result of external and/or middle ear disease. Exudate or waxy buildup in the external ear canal or middle ear, a ruptured tympanum, or auditory ossicle damage results in decreased transmission of airborne sound waves to the cochlear apparatus. This is reflected on the BAER by increased waveform latency (longer transmission time) and decreased amplitude for a given sound intensity.

Sensorineural hearing loss is caused by dysfunction of the cochlear apparatus, cochlear nerve, or portions of the auditory pathway in the central nervous system. BAER findings are variable, ranging from a complete absence of all waveforms (such as in the case of congenital deafness in white-coated breeds of dogs) to changes in amplitude and latency. It is important to note that the BAER tests auditory pathways, not the sense of audition. It is possible for an animal to have a normal BAER and be deaf.

Treatment

Treatment of otitis interna requires long-term oral antibiotics for most cases. A minority of cases also requires surgical drainage of the exudate in the middle ear. The choice of antibiotic is important because the clinician needs to consider both the organism causing the infection and the location of the infection. The organism can usually be identified by culturing the contents of the middle ear. The most common isolates include *Staphylococcus* spp., *Streptococcus* spp., and *Pseudomonas* spp. It is important to choose an antibiotic that has good penetration into areas with poor circulation because otitis interna involves infection of both soft tissue structures and bone. The drug of choice depends on the susceptibility pattern of the organism. If this is not available, a broad-spectrum antibiotic with good penetrability, such as a cephalosporin, chloramphenicol, or potentiated sulfonamide, should be used. Ototoxic drugs such as the aminoglycosides should be avoided. If trimethoprim/sulfa is used, monitoring of tear production is essential. Long-term antibiotic therapy of from 3 to 6 weeks is usually necessary to eradicate the infection. The animal should be examined periodically during the treatment period to evaluate recovery and monitor for the side effects of long-term antibiotic treatment.

Animals with severe signs of vestibular disease may benefit from the antihistamine meclizine. This drug helps to alleviate some of the signs of vestibular disease but does not affect the underlying pathology of the disease.

Prognosis

The prognosis for otitis media or interna is good if the disease is identified early and treated aggressively. The neurologic deficits—Horner's syndrome, facial paresis, head tilt, and hearing loss—may improve in time. However, it is not unusual for the animal to have permanent mild deficits.

Suggested Readings

deLahunta A: *Veterinary neuroanatomy and clinical neurology,* Philadelphia, 1983, Saunders.

O'Brien DP: Circling. In August JR, ed: *Consultations in feline internal medicine,* Philadelphia, 1994, Saunders.

O'Brien DP: *Comparative neurology,* Columbia, MO, 2003, University of Missouri, www.cvm.missouri.edu/academic/neurology/VM604/.

Oliver JE, Lorenz MD, Kornegay JN: *Handbook of veterinary neurology,* Philadelphia, 1997, Saunders.

19

Laser Ear Surgery

Jeffrey R. Moll, DVM

Peter H. Eeg, B.Sc, DVM

Noel Berger, DVM, MS

Common ear ailments of dogs and cats can be seen in up to 50% of patients in areas of humid climates during some or all of the patient's life. Dogs have a moderately higher incidence of ear disease than cats.

Treatment of the variety of inflammatory, infectious, neoplastic, and chronic connective tissue changes that can be observed in small animal patients is often very difficult, unrewarding, and frustrating. This is due to the restricted size of the external auditory meatus and tympanic bulla. The small size of these areas is often further restricted in the presence of disease due to excessive inflammation of the dermis and underlying tissues. Recurrences are common. This may be due to a failure to resolve the underlying pathology or incomplete treatment (resection) of the problem. Repeated treatments, assessments, and an extended duration of therapy are not uncommon. This often causes increased client concern and dissatisfaction.

Implementation of laser energy for the effective treatment of a variety of conditions can simplify both the therapeutic protocol and the recovery of the patient. Video otoscopy offers the opportunity to enhance the diagnostic ability of the veterinarian. Because tissues are visualized on a video monitor under magnification, the condition of the ear can be more accurately assessed. In combination with a surgical laser, many diseases of the ear canal and bulla can be treated in an aggressive, yet minimally invasive manner. The advent of advanced otoscopic equipment coupled with CO_2 and/or diode-wavelength laser energy can significantly improve the final therapeutic outcome for many diseases of the ear. This method of therapy can lead to shorter recovery times with less discomfort for the pet.

Video otoscopic equipment has greatly enhanced the veterinarian's ability to evaluate and treat diseases of the ear canal and middle ear (bulla). A variety of systems are available. These systems can be broadly categorized as diagnostic or therapeutic systems. The major difference is the presence of an operating channel in the therapeutic systems. For the purposes of this discussion, only therapeutic systems are considered.

Therapeutic endoscopic telescopes are usually either the 0 degree (directly forward) or 30 degree (oblique view). Video otoscopes are 0 degree. They are usually larger (around 4.75 mm [because of the presence of an operating channel]), have a larger field of view, and are more durable and less costly than other rigid endoscopes. The single working channel of the video otoscope allows access for suction, biopsy, irrigation, and laser devices. The 2-mm channel accepts instrumentation up to 5 Fr, or about 1.8 mm. The biopsy channel can provide for simultaneous irrigation, suction, and treatment with the use of a two- or three-port connector, as shown in Figure 19-1.

A 2.7- × 180-mm, 0-degree, or 30-degree rigid endoscopic telescope with a 14-Fr operating sheath can also be used in these procedures. The smaller overall diameter, longer length, and separate irrigation and operating channels make this endoscope an excellent choice for interventional otoscopy (Figure 19-2). The 30-degree endoscope is particularly useful in laser surgery and treating lesions of the middle ear. The 30-degree offset allows for visualization of the laser delivery system or surgical instrumentation as it exits the operating channel (Figure 19-3). This allows for more precise alignment of the instrument and decreases the possibility of iatrogenic damage.

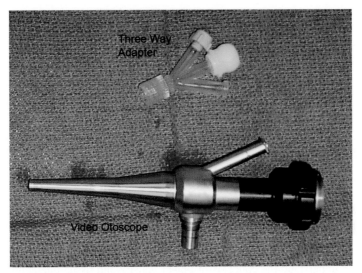

Figure 19-1

Video otoscope and three-way adapter.

Because of the higher cost and increased fragility of this equipment, it should not be used in conscious patients.

Lasers can both extend and enhance the therapeutic options for the treatment of aural disease. Two types of lasers are useful in the treatment of auricular pathology. They are the CO_2 laser (10,600-nm wavelength) and the diode laser (either 810- or 980-nm wavelength). It is beyond the scope of this chapter to discuss fully the physics involved with each of these wavelengths. The practitioner is strongly encouraged to

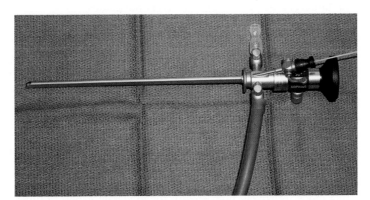

Figure 19-2

Rigid endoscope prepared for suction, irrigation, and laser surgery.

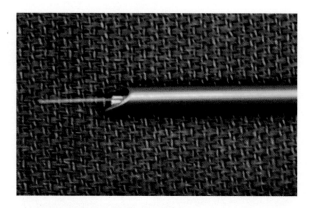

Figure 19-3

Treatment end of 30-degree rigid endoscope.

review and understand the concepts of power density and tissue interactions before using this technology. By combining lasers and video otoscopy, a wider range of problems can be corrected in a minimally invasive fashion. This often leads to a better outcome. Lasers can prove extremely useful in the following:

- Aural hematoma repair
- Removal of masses in the aural canal
- Controlling hemorrhage during video otoscopy
- Ear canal resection and ablation
- Removal of masses in and around the pinna
- Treatment of chronic otitis
- Myringotomies
- Cosmetic and therapeutic otoplasty (ear trims, correction of abnormal ear carriage, and treatment of neoplasia)

In general lasers can be used in three different modalities:

1. *Coagulation.* In this mode lasers are used to provide hemostasis. This is accomplished by providing laser energy at a lower power, usually with a longer exposure time. By using the laser in this manner, tissue contraction rather than vaporization is achieved. When the collagen in the end of a bleeding vessel is contracted, hemostasis is achieved.

2. *Incision.* By providing relatively high wattage with a small focal point, high power densities are achieved. This results in incision of the target tissue. This is particularly useful in situations where a mass is pedunculated and the base of the mass can be visualized. Depending on the power density, more or less hemostasis can be attained.

3. *Ablation.* Laser energy can also be applied to the surface of structures within the ear. In this mode, relatively high energy for moderate exposure times is introduced, and the surface of the targeted structure is vaporized. Through continuous appropriate application of energy, tumors can be removed from all parts of the aural canal and the middle ear.

A Comparison of CO_2 and Diode Laser Energy

CO_2 laser energy is primarily absorbed by water and must therefore be used in a relatively dry ear. When CO_2 laser energy interacts with tissue, the intracellular water is rapidly heated to boiling, and the cell ruptures. When this vaporization occurs, a smoke plume is generated that must be removed by an appropriate evacuation system.

The CO_2 laser energy is usually delivered through a semiflexible hollow tube (Figure 19-4) that guides the energy to the target through the operating channel of the endoscope. CO_2 laser energy is most useful in the ablation (vaporization) of abnormal tissue. It can also be effectively used to provide hemostasis. In cases where the base of the auricular mass is visible, the laser can be used in an incisional mode to remove these structures more quickly.

The limitations of CO_2 laser energy are primarily related to the wavelength itself. Because it is absorbed by water, it cannot be used in an ear that has been flooded with fluid (saline) to increase visualization.

Diode laser energy is absorbed by hemoglobin, oxyhemoglobin, and melanin. This selective absorption may aid in treatment if the abnormal area is more pigmented than the surrounding tissue. Lesions can be treated in a contact or noncontact mode. The noncontact mode is usually used only on pigmented lesions on the pinna. The noncontact mode has not been proven to be useful in a fluid environment. Diode laser energy is delivered by a shielded flexible quartz fiber (Figure 19-5). This system allows for the precise delivery of laser energy in a fluid environment in a contact mode. The fiber delivery system of the diode laser may become extremely hot when energized for a prolonged period. This depends on the fiber size, the energy setting (wattage), and the vascularity of the tissue (thermal diffusion). If the fiber becomes overheated, peripheral thermal damage results. It is vital to keep the fiber cool. This can be accomplished by limiting the exposure time (pulse duration) and by cooling the fiber with an irrigant such as saline. The ability to operate immersed in fluid makes the diode laser extremely useful in otoendoscopy. Continual irrigation during the procedure increases visualization and decreases unintentional iatrogenic damage. Irrigation also removes debris and helps control any heat from the laser or the endoscope.

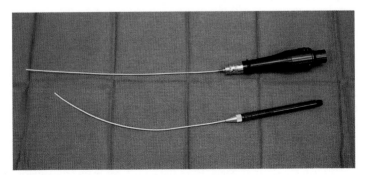

Figure 19-4

CO_2 delivery systems.

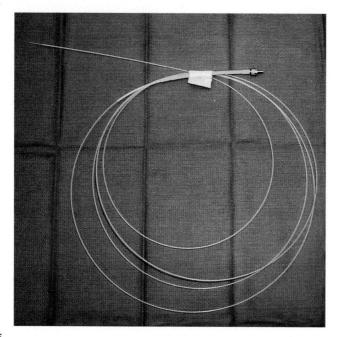

Figure 19-5

600-Micron diode laser fiber.

Specific Laser Therapy Goals

A treatment plan for the individual patient is based on the anatomic location and the suspected underlying etiology. These variables influence both the type and delivery method for the laser energy. In some cases multiple problems are present. These may require multiple wavelengths or delivery systems, which should be available in advance to facilitate the procedure.

CO_2 and diode laser energy allow for a more targeted removal or alteration of tissue. The ear canal is a confined space to work in and around, and the pinna has limited additional dermis with which to work. A laser can simplify a number of procedures, improve near-term recovery, and provide for more normal anatomy and return to function. This can be accomplished by incorporating laser-directed ablation (vaporization), incision, or excision of tissues. As discussed earlier, disease components in the ear that are predisposing to or perpetuating the disease can then be more efficiently removed with cleaning, medication, and evacuation.

The first step in the use of laser energy is to determine the way the energy is to be applied to the target tissue. Typically on the pinna, standard laser techniques can be used to accomplish the desired goals. Here the CO_2 laser is clearly superior because of its reduced peripheral thermal tissue interaction and noncontact application. Surgery of the pinna can be provided by laser energy, similar to techniques for other areas of the dermis. In the external ear canal the video otoscopic or fiberoptic tele-scope can be used to facilitate visualization and direction of the laser energy. This is usually accomplished by extending the direction of the laser energy through special tips that fit into and through working channels in the otoscopic equipment. Diode laser fibers are usually between 400 and 1000 microns and easily fit most working channels. This allows the clinician to visualize the area and provide treatment within the confined space of the external ear canal.

Treatment of Aural Hematomas

Aural hematomas occur when a vessel within the pinna ruptures and blood accumu-lates under the skin. Aural hematomas occur on the inner (concave) surface of the pinna and can occur in both dogs and cats (Figure 19-6). Because the skin is so firmly attached to the auricular cartilage on the concave surface, the hematoma actu-ally develops subparachondrally or intrachondrally, not subcutaneously.[1] Most aural hematomas are lined by cartilage; this suggests that damage to this cartilage may play a role in their occurrence.[2] The etiology of this condition is unknown. It may result from self-trauma or head shaking (secondary to otitis externa or media or to

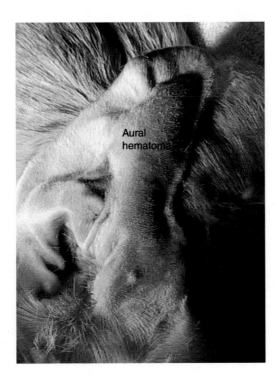

Figure 19-6

Canine aural hematoma.

external parasites), trauma, increased vascular fragility, hemorrhagic diathesis, or some form of immune-mediated disease.[3] Any underlying pathology should be addressed as part of the therapy. It may be wise to delay treatment in thrombocytopenic patients until any platelet abnormality has been corrected.

A variety of treatment methods have been published to repair aural hematomas. These treatments require various degrees of aftercare and some failures do occur. The CO_2 laser is extremely useful in the treatment of this condition. It reduces postoperative discomfort and the amount of aftercare required.

After the induction of anesthesia or heavy sedation, the affected ear is fully evaluated. Any evidence of otitis externa or media should be addressed at this time. If there has been a history of chronic otitis, ear swabs for cytology and culture and sensitivity should be obtained and a complete video otoscopic ear examination performed in both ears. Ear disease in one ear may result in an aural hematoma in the other ear from the constant head shaking. After the evaluation has been completed, the inner pinna of the affected ear is clipped and prepared for aseptic surgery. The patient is positioned in lateral recumbency with the affected side up.

Three or more round, partial-thickness circular skin incisions of approximately 0.3 to 0.7 centimeters are made in a triangular pattern (Figure 19-7). The size of the opening depends on the size of the patient. After this pattern has been made, one of the proximal incisions is continued to full thickness to penetrate the hematoma. At this time the fluid within the hematoma is removed. This fluid is usually hemorrhagic to serohemorrhagic, depending on the length of time the hematoma has been present. After the fluid has been removed, the remaining incisions are continued to full thickness. At this time any fibrin clots should be removed from the subcutaneous

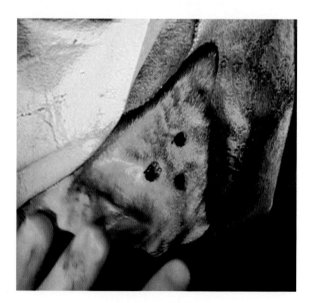

Figure 19-7

Ear pinna after creation of laser drain perforations.

space. It may be useful to lavage the space gently with normal saline or lactated Ringer's solution.

The skin is then sutured with stented 0 Prolene or nylon (3-0 Prolene for feline patients) to the underlying cartilage in a simple interrupted pattern. Only the inner pinna and the cartilage are sutured (Figure 19-8). The sutures should not penetrate the outer (dorsal) skin surface of the pinna. A taper needle is less likely to cause inadvertent bleeding and is preferred. The long axis of the individual sutures should be parallel to the long axis of the ear. This helps to preserve the normal blood supply to the pinna and avoid the three major branches of the auricular artery. After completion of the procedure, 0.006 mg/kg of buprenorphine (Buprenex) is given intravenously. Usually no additional pain control medication is required. An Elizabethan collar is placed to prevent self-trauma. Bandaging of the ear is not necessary or recommended. An alternative procedure that does not involve sutures has been published and may also be effective.[4]

Aftercare is performed at home by the client. This consists of twice-daily hot compresses applied to the ear for 5 to 10 minutes each. Any scab that forms should be removed, and the drain holes should be kept open for as long as possible. Any reaccumulation of fluid should be gently expressed during the process of compressing. Follow-up visits should be encouraged on a weekly basis. The drain holes

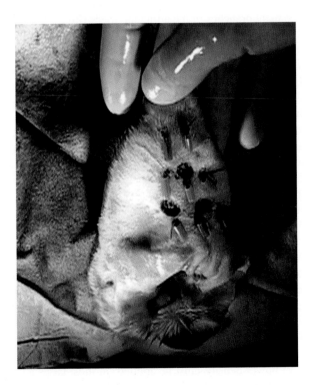

Figure 19-8

Postoperative appearance of the ear.

usually will close by the second postoperative week. Sutures should be left in place for approximately 7 days after they have closed. Any otitis that is discovered during the course of treatment must be fully and aggressively treated. It is recommended that the otitis be completely resolved for at least 5 days before suture removal.

This procedure is relatively easy to perform, has a low recurrence rate and a low degree of morbidity and mortality, and achieves excellent cosmetic results. Most patients have no noticeable deformity from the procedure and have excellent post-operative comfort.

Neoplasia of the Pinna

Tumors of the ear may originate from the skin, adnexa, or connective tissue. These tumors include papilloma, fibropapilloma, mast cell tumor, cutaneous hemangioma, cutaneous hemangiosarcoma, melanoma, histiocytoma, fibrosarcoma, apocrine gland cyst, rhabdomyoma, and plasma cell tumors.[2,5,6,7] Tumors can occur on either side of the pinna. Growths that occur on the outer (convex) surface of the ear are more likely to be centrally located and rarely penetrate the underlying cartilage. Excision of these masses is readily accomplished due to the loose attachment of the skin to the underlying cartilage. When removing these masses, it is important to identify the three main branches of the auricular artery (Figure 19-9). The CO_2 laser is useful in these cases. In cases where the mass is a small papilloma, the laser may be used to ablate the mass (Figure 19-10). In all other cases the laser should be used to excise the mass completely. The skin should be closed with 3-0 to 5-0 mono-filament nonabsorbable suture. Even in cases that require removal of auricular carti-lage, only the skin should be sutured. Deficits that cannot be closed without causing deformity to the ear should be allowed to heal by secondary intention or repaired by the use of a pedicle flap.[8] The excised tissue should undergo histopathologic evalu-ation. Malignant or incompletely excised neoplasia requires additional treatment, up to and including amputation of the pinna. Use of the CO_2 laser in these cases increases hemostasis and postoperative patient comfort, thus helping to prevent surgical complications.

Sharp excision with the CO_2 laser should be performed with a focal size of 0.4 mm or smaller and usually 7 to 9 watts of continuous-wave power. The power density should be great enough to incise the skin cleanly while controlling hemorrhage and causing minimal carbonization. Superpulse delivery of energy is ideal for excision but may have a decreased hemostatic effect. Any small bleeding vessels can usually be controlled by decreasing the power density. This may be accomplished by defo-cusing the laser or diminishing the power output. The hemostatic effect is usually better in a continuous-wave modality without superpulse.

Ablation of papillomas with the CO_2 laser may be accomplished with a larger focal size, usually 0.5 mm or larger (Figure 19-11). In order to ablate tissue effec-tively, a sufficient power density must be applied. In most cases a power setting of 8 to 15 watts is appropriate. If an insufficient power density is used, peripheral thermal damage may occur. Multiple passes are usually required to ablate the abnormal tissue.

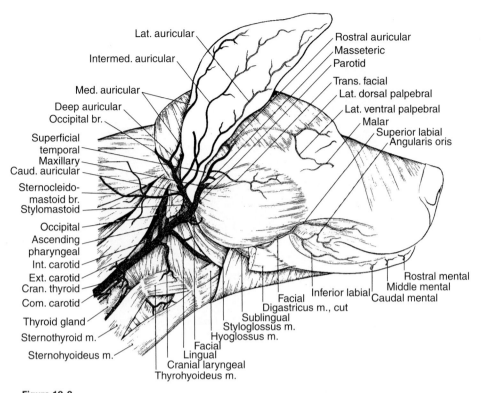

Figure 19-9

The vasculature of the canine ear. (From Evans: *Miller's Anatomy of the dog,* ed 3, Philadelphia, 1993, Saunders.)

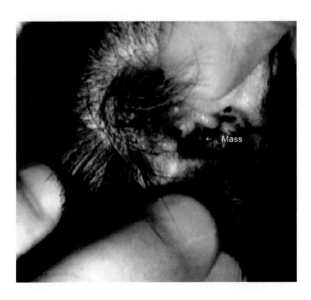

Figure 19-10

Mass on the pinna (feline).

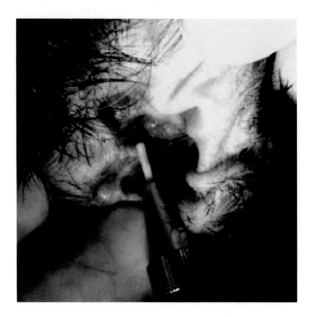

Figure 19-11

CO_2 treatment of a mass on the pinna (feline).

It is important to remove any carbonized tissue (char) that occurs between passes. Failure to remove char results in thermal injury to the surrounding tissue. If hemorrhage occurs during the ablation process, it can usually be controlled by decreasing the power density delivered to the tissue. This may be accomplished by decreasing the power setting (wattage) or defocusing the laser beam.

The diode laser may also be used. Diode laser energy is absorbed by hemoglobin, oxyhemoglobin, and melanin. This selective absorption results in excellent hemostasis and may help in the selective treatment of only the abnormal tissue. When the diode laser is used in an incisional mode, the tip of the fiber should be carbonized. Incision with the diode laser occurs through a thermal effect on the tissue. The carbonization of the tip ensures efficient thermal transfer. Caution must be used to prevent peripheral (unintended) thermal damage. The fiber delivery system of the diode laser becomes extremely hot when energized for a prolonged period. This depends on the fiber size, the energy setting (wattage), and the vascularity of the target tissue (thermal diffusion). If the fiber becomes overheated, peripheral thermal damage will result. It is vital to keep the fiber cool. This can be accomplished by limiting the exposure time (pulse duration) and by cooling the fiber with sterile saline. Pigmented lesions may be treated in a noncontact mode. Ablation of masses in this manner may be extremely effective because of the selective absorption of diode laser energy. It is imperative to rule out malignancy before treatment. Malignant masses should be treated by complete excision with an appropriate surgical margin. Peripheral thermal damage is still a concern in the noncontact mode, and cooling of the fiber is still important. Because the fiber is not in contact with the tissue, there is no thermal diffusion of the heat that is generated. If the fiber is not properly cooled, it will rapidly become white hot. This may damage tissue as well as the plastic sheath that surrounds the fiber.

Ceruminous Gland Hyperplasia

The lining of the external ear canal is stratified squamous epithelium with sebaceous and apocrine glands and hair follicles.[10] The apocrine glands in this area are also referred to as *ceruminous glands.* Springer Spaniels, Cocker Spaniels, and black Labrador Retrievers have an increased proportion of these ceruminous glands.[11] This may explain the higher incidence of otitis externa in these breeds. Patients with chronic otitis externa develop hyperplasia of the ceruminous and sebaceous glands (Figure 19-12).[12] Hyperplasia leads to decreased diameter of the ear canal as glandular tissue increases, and it also results in increased ceruminous secretions within the ear canal. Cocker Spaniels appear to develop primarily ceruminous gland hyperplasia with less fibrosis than other breeds.[13] In another study the quantity of sebaceous glands was found to be similar in dogs with and without otitis externa. In this study dogs with otitis externa were found to have a higher population of ceruminous glands.[14] It is important to remember that chronic otitis externa is usually not a primary disease. It is usually caused by some underlying allergy or unresolved chronic infection. As part of the therapy, it is important to address any underlying problem. Failure to resolve or at least control the underlying problem results in temporary palliation of the problem at best.

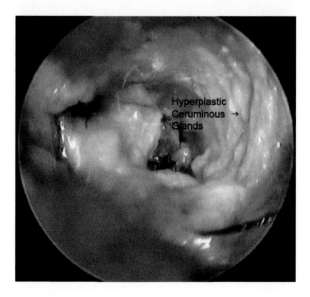

Figure 19-12

Hyperplasia of the ceruminous glands.

Before initiating treatment of the affected ear, swabs for cytology and bacterial culture should be obtained from just in front of the tympanic membrane (if present) or the middle ear if there is an obvious rupture of the membrane. Appropriate medications can then be prescribed and adjusted based on these results.

After the culture and cytology specimens have been obtained, the ear is thoroughly cleaned with a ceruminolytic agent and lavaged with copious amounts of saline. This should be done under direct visualization through the video otoscope. A complete evaluation of the ear canal may then be performed. Any hyperplastic areas within the ear canal should be easily visualized. Biopsies of the abnormal tissue should be taken for histopathology. The results of the histopathology may help to identify the underlying disease process. Hemostasis after the biopsy can be accomplished with the CO_2 or diode laser. The diode laser may be more clinically useful in this situation because it can be used in a fluid environment (Figure 19-13). A 600-micron fiber is used to deliver the diode laser energy. A setting of 3 to 4 watts in continuous wave mode usually rapidly accomplishes hemostasis.

The CO_2 laser may also provide hemostasis to the biopsy sites. The CO_2 laser's energy should be directed to the target site under direct visualization. This allows for accurate hemostasis and treatment with little iatrogenic damage to surrounding tissue. This is accomplished through a flexible, hollow waveguide. The CO_2 laser's energy must be directly applied to the hemorrhaging area. This means that adequate suction must be applied to the area for the laser energy to have the desired hemostatic effect. If sufficient suction cannot be obtained, the blood itself will be vaporized,

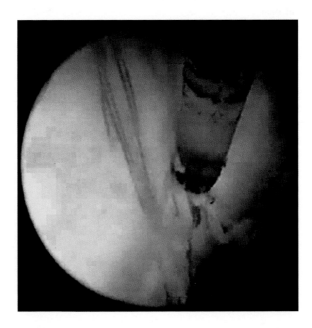

Figure 19-13

Diode laser coagulation.

producing significant char and possibly resulting in inadequate hemostasis and peripheral thermal damage. CO_2 laser hemostasis can usually be obtained with a power setting of 2 to 4 watts with a 0.8-mm focal size in a continuous-wave mode.

After hemostasis has been achieved, removal of the abnormal tissue can be accomplished; lasers are useful in this procedure. The laser is used to ablate the abnormal tissue. Removal of this tissue helps to increase the diameter of the ear canal and decrease the amount of secretions within the ear. Diode laser energy may be used for this procedure. The size of the fiber depends on the size of the operating channel in the video otoscope or therapeutic telescope or the size of the targeted area. Generally, fibers of 600 to 1000 microns are used. Because the laser is being used in a contact mode, the energy is precisely directed into the target tissue. Another advantage of the diode laser is its ability to operate in an aqueous environment. Continuous irrigation of the ear canal improves visualization by removing any blood or debris from the surgical field. It also diminishes or eliminates peripheral thermal damage. Power settings vary depending on the size of the fiber used and the size of the target. It is important to provide sufficient power to ablate the target tissue without causing peripheral damage. Diode laser energy penetrates more deeply than CO_2 laser energy, and care must be taken to avoid damaging the deeper structures. In general, a 600-micron fiber requires 6 to 12 watts of power to obtain the desired effect. A 1000-micron fiber requires 10 to 20 watts for a similar effect. The energy is delivered in continuous wave, and exposure times should generally be less than 3 seconds. The irrigant solution should not reach the boiling point. Bubbles will begin to form around the fiber if the solution is overheated. Prolonged exposure times increase the risk of peripheral thermal damage by overcoming the cooling effect of the irrigant and the thermal relaxation time of the tissue.

CO_2 laser energy can also be directed at the abnormal tissue as described previously (Figure 19-14). This energy vaporizes the abnormal tissue. CO_2 lasers cannot currently be used immersed in a fluid environment. Evacuation of the smoke (plume) produced during vaporization is vital. This allows for better visualization of the target tissue and is an important factor in the safety of operatory personnel. During the course of therapy a layer of char may form on the targeted tissue. It is essential to stop and remove this substance. If the carbonized layer is not removed, it absorbs the CO_2 laser energy and results in inadvertent peripheral thermal damage. The amount of carbonization and peripheral thermal damage is generally greater if an insufficient power density is used. A spot size of 0.8 mm with 8 to 14 watts of power in continuous-wave mode usually results in adequate vaporization with good hemostasis.

After the abnormal tissue has been removed, the ear canal should be lavaged with copious amounts of irrigant and any carbonized tissue gently removed. The ear is gently dried with suction and an appropriate topical antimicrobial with steroid instilled. It is important to evaluate fully the tympanic membrane because some medications may be ototoxic if the tympanic membrane is not intact. A myringotomy should be considered in cases of chronic otitis externa (see the section on Myringotomy later in this chapter). The short-term use of parenteral steroids may be indicated in some cases. Postoperatively most patients receive 0.006 mg/kg of buprenorphine (Buprenex) intravenously during the recovery period. Additional pain medication is usually

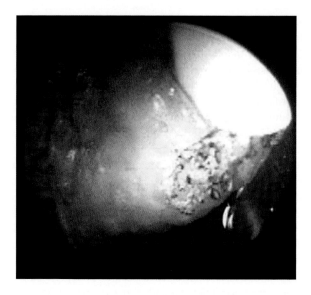

Figure 19-14

CO_2 ablation of hyperplastic ceruminous glands.

not required. Most patients seem markedly more comfortable postoperatively and are usually less resistant to the continued treatment of their ears.

Laser ablation often greatly improves the clinical outcome for cases of chronic otitis with ceruminous gland hyperplasia. Removal of the hyperplastic tissue increases the diameter of the ear canal, decreases the amount of discharge, helps remove some of the bacteria, and allows the owner to clean and maintain the ears more thoroughly. Postoperatively, most patients are very comfortable and readily allow the owner to treat the ears. Weekly follow-up visits that include otoscopic evaluation and ear swabs for cytology are imperative. Treatment should continue until the ears look normal and for 1 week after a negative swab is obtained. After healing, the ablated glandular areas are replaced with fibrous tissue covered by epithelium.

It is extremely important to use antibiotics based on culture and sensitivity in cases of bacterial infection. Many of these cases are a result of multidrug-resistant bacteria. Oral antibiotic or antifungal agents may be useful in the management of these cases. In addition, any underlying food allergy, inhaled allergy, contact dermatitis, or endocrinopathy should be properly evaluated and addressed.

Laser Polypectomy (Aural Tumor Removal)

Tumors can occur within the ear canals and middle ears of both dogs and cats. Tumors occur more frequently in dogs than in cats. The tumors that occur in dogs are usually less malignant than those that occur in cats.[15] Malignant tumors should be treated by total ear canal ablation and lateral bulla osteotomy. Both favorable and unfavorable long-term results from surgery alone have been reported.[16] The most common tumor found in the external ear canal of both dogs and cats arises from the ceruminous gland. Ceruminous gland adenomas are more common than ceruminous adenocarcinomas in the dog. In cats the tumors are more likely to be adenocarcinomas.[17] These masses can be an underlying cause or a result of chronic otitis.

In feline patients, inflammatory polyps can arise from the epithelium of the tympanic cavity or the eustachian tube.[18] Feline polyps can grow distally into the ear canal (Figure 19-15) or proximally into the retropharynx. It is therefore extremely important to evaluate the middle ear in cases of feline retropharyngeal polyps. Failure to remove this tissue from the middle ear may result in recurrence. Canine polyps can occur anywhere in the ear canal (Figure 19-16). These are usually cerumen gland adenomas and may occlude the entire ear canal. They may also grow into the middle ear. True retropharyngeal polyps in dogs are rare.

Before the advent of video otoscopy, complete excision of polyps within the ear canal often required a lateral ear canal resection to obtain the necessary access to the mass. This procedure, followed by laser excision of the mass(es) within the auditory canal, may still be necessary. The video otoscope allows improved identification and evaluation of these masses. Once identified and evaluated, they can usually be successfully removed by traction and/or laser vaporization.

Lasers offer significant improvements in the treatment of these lesions. The treatment of benign polyps in the ear canal is best accomplished as a two-step procedure. It is in the patient's best interest that the clinician obtain a biopsy and a definitive diagnosis before attempting to ablate any mass. As previously stated, malignancies

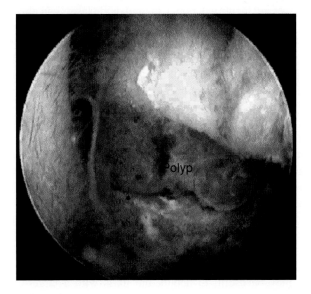

Figure 19-15

Feline polyp arising from the middle ear.

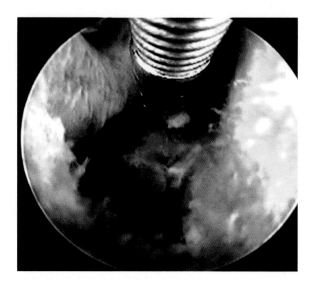

Figure 19-16

Canine polyp.

are best treated by resection of the entire ear canal. In addition, antibiotics can be started based on culture and sensitivity before mass removal.

In the first step cultures and biopsy specimens can be obtained through the operating channel of the video otoscope. Hemostasis is achieved with the CO_2 or diode laser, as explained in the previous section.

After the masses are identified, both CO_2 and diode lasers can ablate these masses within the ear canal. Diode laser energy may be superior in the removal of larger polyps. Diode lasers do not create carbonized tissue, and they operate in a fluid environment. This allows increased visualization of the target tissues and precise application of laser energy. In addition, simultaneous lavage prevents hemorrhage or plume from interfering with visualization. In most cases, any source of hemorrhage can be readily identified, and the diode laser can provide hemostasis.

When the diode laser is used, irrigation with saline is provided continuously. Irrigation is vital to visualization and essential to the prevention of peripheral thermal damage. Normal saline (0.9%) is currently the solution of choice. Depending on the size of the patient and the size of the mass, a 600- or 1000-micron fiber is used. The fiber is introduced into the center of the mass, and energy is provided until a majority of the abnormal-seeming tissue has a blanched appearance. This devitalized tissue is then removed with a biopsy forceps. It is often necessary to repeat this process in larger masses.

In some cases the tumor may be large enough to fill the entire auricular canal. It is possible to remove these masses with a laser and a video otoscope. To expedite the removal it may be useful to debulk the mass with a larger-diameter biopsy forceps placed alongside the endoscope. These forceps can then be positioned under direct visualization. Blakesley or Takahashi nasal forceps are well suited for this

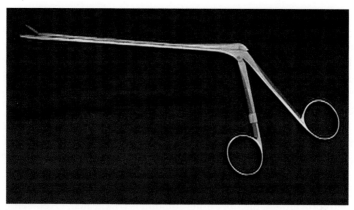

Figure 19-17

Nasal biopsy forceps.

procedure (Figure 19-17). In this manner, large masses can be rapidly reduced. Biopsy forceps of 3.5 to 5.0 Fr can also be introduced through the operating channel to debulk these masses (Figure 19-18). With this method, moderate hemorrhage is encountered. It is essential to provide adequate irrigation to allow visualization; irrigation is provided through the biopsy channel of the video otoscope. After debulking, hemostasis and removal of the remaining abnormal tissue is performed with the diode laser, as described previously. Rapid debulking can also be accomplished with an arthroscopic shaver. A hooded debrider blade provides rapid debulking while protecting the normal auricular canal. This system offers improved visualization because suction is provided by the shaver. Because irrigation is provided via the video otoscope, simultaneous irrigation and suction can occur.

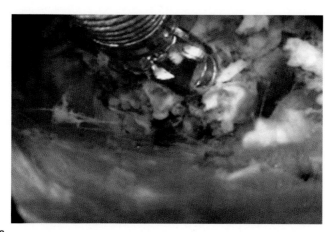

Figure 19-18

Debulking of a polyp with biopsy forceps.

By prepositioning the diode fiber in the operating channel of the video otoscope, hemostasis can be rapidly achieved, minimizing any blood loss. These debulking techniques can help to markedly reduce the surgical time required to remove larger masses. By using the laser to provide hemostasis and remove the final layer of abnormal tissue, the advantages of laser surgery can be preserved. Patients treated in this manner have minimal postoperative discomfort, edema, or hemorrhage. Power settings for the diode laser depend on the size of the fiber, the size of the mass, and whether ablation or hemostasis is desired. In general, a 600-micron fiber requires 6 to 12 watts of power for ablation (Figure 19-19) and 2 to 4 watts for hemostasis. A 1000-micron fiber requires 10 to 20 watts for ablation and 3 to 5 watts for hemostasis. As previously stated, the energy is delivered in a continuous wave, and exposure times should be limited to prevent the irrigant solution from reaching the boiling point. Bubbles will begin to form around the fiber if the solution is overheated. Overheating the irrigant increases the risk of peripheral thermal damage. Peripheral thermal damage markedly increases the patient's postoperative discomfort.

CO_2 lasers can also be used to remove large masses (Figure 19-20). In this procedure the mass is ablated in layers (Figure 19-21). Relatively high power is applied in a continuous-wave manner. Char must be removed between layers. Failure to remove this char will result in peripheral thermal damage. In some cases it may be possible to reduce the size of the mass by debulking. The hemorrhage that results from debulking can be difficult to control. In order to provide hemostasis, the CO_2 laser's energy usually must contact the end of the bleeding vessel. Due to the confined area of the auricular canal, blood can often fill the area, making it difficult to visualize the source of the hemorrhage. This limitation can sometimes be overcome by the use of a suction trap in the smoke evacuation line. The suction trap allows the smoke evacuator to function as a suction unit. The smoke evacuator should be directly connected to the otoendoscope; this may require a T or Y adapter so that both the laser and the suction unit can be active at the same time. In most CO_2 laser units, a

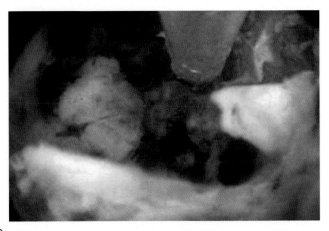

Figure 19-19

Treatment of a polyp with a diode laser.

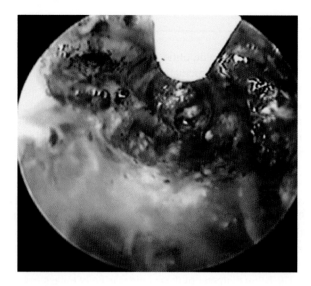

Figure 19-20

CO_2 laser ablation of a large mass.

column of air is produced and exits the laser aperture. This air is designed to keep the aperture free of debris, but it may also help in visualizing the source of the hemorrhage. In some cases the amount of hemorrhage is great enough to prevent laser coagulation. In these cases, hemostasis must be achieved in another manner before the procedure is continued; direct pressure or electrocautery is usually effective. Electrocautery should be used with caution. It may cause peripheral damage and can greatly reduce the potential benefits of laser surgery.

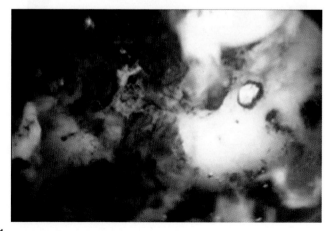

Figure 19-21

Middle ear after laser mass removal.

Myringotomy

In cases of otitis media or chronic otitis, the middle ear should be fully evaluated. Otitis media is an important perpetuating cause of recurrent otitis externa.[19] The evaluation should include radiography of the bulla, which may be accomplished with conventional radiology or with intraoral dental films. Intraoral films seem to provide better visualization. Magnetic resonance imaging (MRI) and computed tomography (CT) may also be useful in the evaluation of the middle ear.[20,21] In the future, ultrasound evaluation of the tympanic bulla may prove useful in the detection of fluid.[22]

After these imaging studies have been performed, the ear should be fully evaluated with the video otoscope. In order to evaluate the middle ear, a myringotomy must be performed. Both the diode laser and the CO_2 laser can be used for this procedure (Figure 19-22). The goal is to provide sufficient laser energy to ablate the tympanic membrane without damaging the underlying structures. This can be accomplished with the CO_2 laser by using a series of single pulses through a waveguide placed in the operating channel of the video otoscope aimed at the periphery of the pars tensa of the eardrum. The beam diameter of these guides usually ranges from 0.4 to 1.0 mm. In general a diameter of more than 0.5 mm and a power setting of 3 to 6 watts should be used. The higher power is usually necessary in cases with chronic disease. The diode laser is very useful in this procedure. A 600- to 1000-micron fiber is introduced into the video otoscope, and a myringotomy is performed in the contact mode. A setting of 4 to 7 watts is appropriate. This is performed while irrigating with sterile saline solution. This keeps the fiber cool, and peripheral damage is not an issue. In addition, any hemorrhage that occurs can be rapidly identified and controlled with

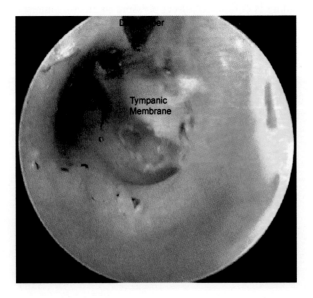

Tympanic Membrane

Figure 19-22

Diode laser myringotomy.

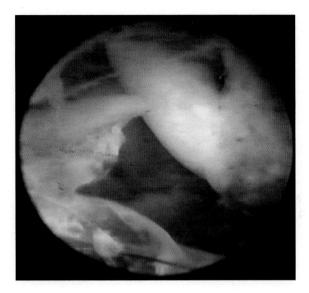

Figure 19-23

Normal middle ear after myringotomy.

this laser. Irrigation markedly increases visualization and allows for the removal of any matter within the bulla.

After the myringotomy has been performed, the middle ear should be carefully evaluated for any masses (Figure 19-23). These masses should be biopsied and then can be ablated with CO_2 or diode laser energy as described previously in this chapter.

Lateral Ear Canal Resection and Ear Canal Ablation

It is beyond the scope of this chapter to describe lateral ear canal resection and ear canal ablation fully; the reader is referred to a general surgery text. Lateral ear canal resection is indicated in cases where the management of chronic otitis externa has failed or the size and number of the masses within the auricular canal prevent their adequate removal with laser-assisted video otoscopy. In some cases it may be more time effective to perform a lateral ear canal resection and then use the laser to remove the masses under direct visualization.

Complete ear canal ablation and bulla osteotomy are indicated in cases where a malignant tumor has been diagnosed within the ear canal or tympanic cavity. It may also be performed as a salvage procedure in cases of refractory otitis externa (Figure 19-24).

The incisions and dissection required for these procedures are greatly enhanced by the use of the CO_2 laser. The hemostasis that can be achieved greatly increases the surgeon's visualization of vital structures, which in turn minimizes iatrogenic complications (Figure 19-25). In cases of chronic otitis externa, the ear canal is

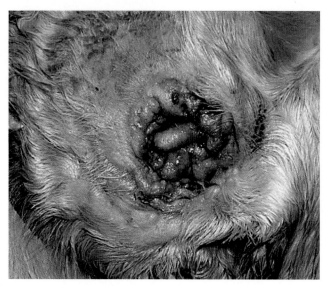

Figure 19-24

Preoperative total ear canal resection and bulla osteotomy.

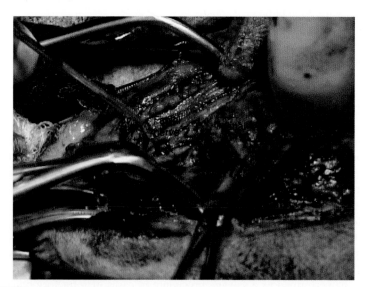

Figure 19-25

Intraoperative ear canal ablation.

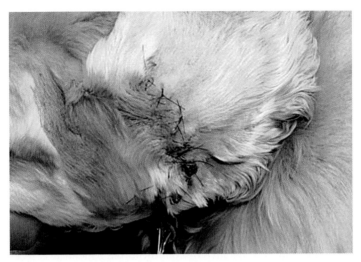

Figure 19-26

Postoperative total ear canal resection and bulla osteotomy.

markedly thickened and can be calcified and surrounded by a significant amount of fibrous tissue. The facial nerve can become entrapped in this tissue. Meticulous dissection is required to preserve this structure and its function. Facial nerve paralysis results if this nerve is damaged or severed. The use of the CO_2 laser for this procedure markedly increases postoperative comfort and seems to lead to a more rapid recovery (Figure 19-26).[23]

Cosmetic and Therapeutic Otoplasty

The dermis and auricular cartilage that make up the functional anatomic structure of the pinna are very responsive to CO_2 laser application. The great advantage of CO_2 laser energy in this region is the conservation of tissue.

Amputation of a specific area of the pinna using CO_2 laser energy can also be effectively accomplished. This technique should be used only when the mass or area of abnormal tissue cannot be effectively ablated. A tip of 0.4-mm spot size at a power setting of 10 watts efficiently incises both the dermis and the auricular cartilage. The tissue edges can then be sutured similarly to what occurs during ear-cropping techniques or by application of surgical-grade cyanoacrylic tissue adhesive.

Ear-cropping procedures have also been enhanced by the use of CO_2 laser energy. The pinna can be sculpted freehand or with a surgical guide. In either case the use of CO_2 laser energy significantly reduces the pain, swelling, and bleeding typically associated with standard scalpel technique. A spot diameter of 0.4 mm at a power setting of 10 to 15 watts produces excellent results. Small-diameter 3-0 or 4-0 nonabsorbable sutures on a small-cutting-edge needle are used to appose skin edges without involving the cut surface of the cartilage in the closure. Tissue adhesive cyano-acrylics also provide excellent closure and reduced maintenance.

Treatment of a pinna that does not stand correctly or that, due to technique, has an exaggerated curve after ear cropping is in some cases possible using CO_2 laser energy. The objective of this corrective surgery is to contract the overlying dermis so that the pinna either stands up more correctly or curves less severely. To accomplish this procedure, the hair should be shaved away completely over the area to be treated. A spot size of 0.8 mm or larger or a scanning attachment should be used to direct the laser energy. The power setting should be only high enough to produce collagen contraction of the dermis. Full-thickness incisions should be avoided. This technique may also require rigid taping of the pinna after the therapy to ensure that the underlying auricular cartilage learns the new position.

In cases where the pinna is badly damaged or neoplastic spread is too great, complete amputation of the pinna can be accomplished more effectively using CO_2 laser energy. In this area, laser energy allows for more efficient removal of the pinna with less bleeding and postoperative discomfort to the patient. It is recommended that after the pinna has been removed, the auricular cartilage edge be resected about 5 mm from the edge to allow for more complete cosmetic suturing of the incision.

Conclusion

The addition of laser energy for the treatment of abnormalities of the canine and feline ear can help to facilitate more rapid recovery, more effective subsequent treatment applications, and more cosmetically pleasing results for the patient and client. As with any use of laser energy, it is incumbent on the clinician to understand the laser tissue interaction and how it affects the outcome of cases related to the ear and ear canal.

References

1. Macy DW: *Textbook of veterinary internal medicine,* ed 3, 1989.
2. Henderson RA, Horne R: *Textbook of small animal surgery,* ed 3, Philadelphia, 2003, WB Saunders.
3. Macy DW: *Textbook of veterinary internal medicine,* ed 3, 1989, p 251.
4. Teresa LD, Teague HD, Ostwald DA, Jr, et al: Evaluation of a technique using the carbon dioxide laser for the treatment of aural hematomas, *J Am Anim Hosp Assoc* 38(4):385-390, 2002.
5. Miller MA, Ramos JA, Kreeger JM: Cutaneous vascular neoplasia in 15 cats: clinical, morphologic, and immunohistochemical studies, *Vet Pathol* 29(4):329-336, 1992.
6. Roth L: Rhabdomyoma of the ear pinna in four cats, *J Comp Pathol* 103(2):237-240, 1990.
7. Bensignor E: *A practical guide to feline dermatology,* 1999, pp 22-24.
8. Henderson RA, Horne R: *Textbook of small animal surgery,* ed 3, Philadelphia, 2003, WB Saunders, p 1742.
9. Cole LK: *Chronic otitis and otitis media,* Western Veterinary Conference 2002, Columbus, OH, 2002, Ohio State University, College of Veterinary Medicine.
10. Muller GH, Kirk RW, Scott DW: *Small animal dermatology,* ed 4, Philadelphia, 1989, WB Saunders, p 807.

11. Rosychuk RAW, Luttgen P: *Textbook of veterinary internal medicine,* ed 4, 1995, p 538.
12. McKeever PJ, Globus H: *Kirk's Current veterinary therapy XII small animal practice,* Philadelphia, 1995, WB Saunders, pp 647-655.
13. Angus JC, Lichtensteiger C, Campbell KL, et al: Breed variations in histopathologic features of chronic severe otitis externa in dogs: 80 cases (1995-2001), *J Am Vet Med Assoc* 221(7):1000-1006, 2002.
14. Stout-Graham M, Kainer RA, Whalen LR, et al: Morphologic measurements of the external horizontal ear canal of dogs, *Am J Vet Res* 51(7):990-994, 1990.
15. McKeever PJ, Globus H: In *Kirk's Current veterinary therapy XII small animal practice,* Philadelphia, 1995, WB Saunders, pp 647-655.
16. Henderson RA, Horne R: *Textbook of small animal surgery,* ed 3, Philadelphia, 2003, WB Saunders, p. 1755.
17. Rosychuk RAW, Luttgen P: *Textbook of veterinary internal medicine,* ed 4, Philadelphia, 1995, WB Saunders, p. 542.
18. White RAS: *Textbook of small animal surgery,* ed 3, p. 1760.
19. Cole LK: *Chronic otitis and otitis media,* Western Veterinary Conference 2002, Columbus, OH, 2002, Ohio State University, College of Veterinary Medicine.
20. Allgoewer I, Lucas S, Schmitz SA: Magnetic resonance imaging of the normal and diseased feline middle ear, *Vet Radiol Ultrasound* 41(5):413-418, 2000.
21. Dvir E, Kirberger RM, Terblanche AG: Magnetic resonance imaging of otitis media in a dog, *Vet Radiol Ultrasound* 41(1):46-49, 2000.
22. Griffiths LG, Sullivan M, O'Neill T, et al: Ultrasonography versus radiography for detection of fluid in the canine tympanic bulla, *Vet Radiol Ultrasound* 44(2):210-213, 2003.
23. Bartels KE: Lasers in medicine and surgery, *Vet Clin North Am Sm Anim Pract* 584-585, 2002.

20

Marketing Ear Service

Ronald E. Whitford, DVM

T he veterinary profession is undergoing major changes in the demographics of delivery of some services and products. Today's pet owner is more educated and pickier in decisions regarding pet care. Today's consumers are ever increasing their standards of "best value." Over the past several years, due to the introduction of new heartworm preventives and flea control products, many practices have seen the service/product mix of total revenues swing much more toward product sales as a major source of gross revenue. Recently I have evaluated practices with as much as 40% of total gross income coming from the sale of products. This in itself is not bad for as long as it lasts, but it does greatly increase the vulnerability of these practices to decreased income if and when these particular products become easily accessed over the counter (OTC). It is very disturbing to see that the vast majority of practices are showing more gross profit income coming from the sales of these products than true bottom-line profit in the practice, as defined by taking the true net income reported and deducting a fair investment return for land, building, and equipment, as well as 25% of gross income product by owners, as which is the fair compensation paid to another veterinarian for performing services for the practice. After these statistics are reviewed, sadly, many practice owners would be better off working as associates in another practice, eliminating the risk they are taking for the very poor returns they currently receive.

It is crucial for long-term survival that practices immediately change to a major emphasis on providing professional services rather than merely being vendors selling products. Fortunately, there is significant pathology in the majority of patients we see every day. The problem in most practices today that minimizes the detection and treatment of pathology is complacency—being satisfied with less than maximizing the potential of every patient seen.

From a profit perspective, it is better to select potential profit center services that offer minimal competition from sources other than licensed veterinarians. Placing major emphasis on marketing services rather than products greatly reduces our risk of competition, limiting it to veterinarians committed to at least the same level of quality veterinary medicine as ourselves.

Marketing of professional services also has definite financial bearings as well. Typically products are priced simply by doubling the cost to determine retail price. Therefore approximately 50% of the selling price is "hard costs." That 50% is all that is left to help pay the daily clinic overhead. However, when professional services are charged, the percentage of gross margin profits over "hard costs" of materials needed to provide those services is much greater, typically being at least 80% of the fee charged. A rule of thumb in pricing professional services is that the fee should be at least five times the costs of materials needed. The result of this strategy is that 80% of the fee charged now becomes available to help pay daily clinic overhead, as well as leave some bottom-line profit as well.

More Bad News

Latest surveys show that pet populations have stabilized. Fewer people are adopting pets. A primary reason for this is thought to be the "inconvenience" associated with taking care of pets with today's hectic lifestyles. Due to the fact that the number of veterinarians continues to increase as a result of new graduates entering practice and current practitioners choosing to remain in the profession longer, one can assume that the number of pets available to be seen by a veterinarian is decreasing. It also is a known statistic that many pet owners are choosing not to replace deceased pets. All these factors underscore the importance of retaining as many clients as possible in the practice as well as maximizing the number of services provided for each pet presented. It is estimated that the typical practice in a relatively stable community with minimal transient populations loses 30% of its clients annually through normal attrition—owners moving, pets dying, etc. Survival of this profession depends on finding as many problems as possible and making appropriate recommendations for pets to live the longest quality life possible for every pet presented to the practice.

There Is Some Good News

Pets are predisposed to many conditions because of specific breed predilection or environmental conditions. This is especially true for ear conditions and disease. Fortunately, there is more pathology out there than would be needed to keep every veterinarian busy 24 hours per day, 52 weeks per year. The biggest problem, however, in capitalizing on this fact is complacency—many veterinarians seem to be disenchanted with the current financial situation and feel hopeless about reversing current trends.

The human-pet bond continues to grow tighter and stronger. Many pets are no longer considered "disposable." Pet owners who value their pets as four-legged family members want the same high quality of veterinary care as they expect for their own human health care. There are now more than 6,000,000 dogs and 6,000,000 cats in the United States older than 6 years. As pets age, in most cases they become even more cemented in the human family. Fortunately, as these pets grow into the "senior years," the aging process initiates many medical conditions, including ear problems. Therefore ear care programs can be developed to help catch problems earlier, allowing the practitioner to either prevent, minimize, or slow the progression of the particular problem.

Even though the United States economy has been weakened over the past few years, pet owners who consider their pets to be true "family members" have proven with their pocketbooks that they still expect and are willing to pay for quality pet health care.

Of all the marketing strategies and options currently open to the practitioner today, none is more professional, more restricted to services provided only by licensed veterinarians, or has more potential to grow both gross and net income than the professional marketing of services related to ear care. These services are not easily duplicated by sources outside our profession because of the expertise required to diagnose and prescribe the appropriate treatment to resolve abnormal conditions. Clients often relate ear infections to the very painful conditions seen in human ear problems. A veterinarian's best clients—those who want and can afford high-quality pet health care—readily accept ear care services. Pet owners in need of these services cannot readily price-shop for comparison, leading to the potential for higher gross margin profits, resulting in higher bottom-line nets. Unfortunately, a survey of practitioners today would show that only a very small percentage of practices are currently placing a significant emphasis on ear care as a major profit center.

Other reasons the practitioner should seriously consider placing more emphasis on ear hygiene, diagnostics, and treatment include the following:

- Pets have two ears, thereby doubling the potential for problems over singular internal organs.
- The ear canals of dogs and cats are anatomically formed in such a way as to increase the potential for medical problems.
- People do not put a price on pain control. Ear infections are perceived to, and often do, hurt—and the pain is perceived by the owner who observes a bad odor coming from the ears as well as the pet scratching, shaking its head, or whining when the ears are touched.
- Ear infections are often lifelong problems. Unfortunately, however, a major reason for chronic otitis is a failure to treat long enough as well as to determine the underlying problem creating the environment conducive to otitis (e.g., allergies). It is not all the fault of the practitioner; many owners fail to return on time for rechecks or to treat according to the recommended treatment schedule or for sufficient periods of time to gain total resolution. It is human nature (coupled with today's busy lifestyles) to avoid placing ear treatment at a high-enough priority to effect a long-term cure.
- People often feel guilty when their pet has a recurrence after they understand that it has occurred because of a failure to continue treatment long enough. The feeling of guilt may make the client more willing to seek more extensive treatment at a later time.
- Clients often leave one veterinary practice for another because the first veterinarian failed to diagnose, explain, or treat the pet's ear disease adequately. A failure to do the job correctly the first time often causes a practitioner to lose all other potential services for the duration of the pet's life. Therefore there is a bright future for practices willing to give ear care the respect it is due and to work diligently to resolve problems and help pets lead healthier, longer lives.

What Is Marketing, Anyway?

Marketing is nothing more than communication. It is simply providing facts and benefits about the services recommended so clients can make educated decisions. Therefore marketing, as strictly defined, is not enough. We must market assertively. This means being the "pet's spokesperson/advocate." We wish only for the pet to have the opportunity to receive the best that veterinary medicine has to offer. Marketing assertively is not only providing facts and benefits about the recommendations but doing it in such a way that the client wants to accept those recommendations.

We must first know what pets need and what we can provide. We must then consistently find the problems with thorough medical history-taking and comprehensive physical "nose-to-tail" examinations. We must take time to develop trusting relationships with our clients so they perceive that we are making recommendations that are truly in the pet's best interest. We must also take the time to understand our clients and what is most important to them, learning how to stimulate each individual client to the positive response we desire. The marketing strategy of the 1990s was to listen to the client and then give them what they wanted. However, it has changed today to "listen to the client and then *lead* them to what the pet needs." This is accomplished by learning the "hot buttons" for each individual client. Each client is an individual with unique perspectives and desires.

Some marketing fundamentals to remember:

- Be prepared. You must know the "whys" and "whats" as well as the "hows" for the services and products you recommend.
- Avoid creating the impression of high-pressure selling. Clients love to buy but hate to "be sold." Few people buy from pushy sales personnel, at least not more than once.
- Marketing is not manipulative or unethical; it is simply providing facts and benefits so the consumer makes an educated buying decision.
- Clients must first trust us and have confidence in us as medical professionals rather than merely vendors selling "stuff."
- We must discover the needs of each client in order to make the appropriate recommendations in the form of solutions. The key is assisting the client in finding the right solution for the specific problem.
- Clients must believe we care. We must develop friendships before clients will trust us and allow us to gain client compliance with our recommendations. People don't care how much we know until they know how much we care. We show we care by being sincerely interested, listening, asking good questions, and knowing what to recommend by correctly interpreting what the client wants along with what the pet needs.

Much research has been conducted on the "buying process." People buy to feel better or to solve a problem. We want solutions that lead to "peace of mind." Owners request veterinary services to make the pet feel better, which in turn makes them feel better, or to solve a problem with the pet, which again makes them feel better. Eighty percent of all purchases are based on emotional issues rather than logic. Therefore it is important to first determine the emotional needs of the client. Emotional buying requires emotional selling. Marketing is nothing more than a battle of perceptions. We must position ourselves as caring, concerned pet health care professionals interested in providing the best that veterinary medicine has to offer.

Clients must first trust us before they will accept our recommendations. Some principals to understand include the following:

- People are interested in themselves and want to be noticed.
- People crave to feel important and be appreciated.
- People want to deal with other people whom they can trust.
- People tend to judge other people and organizations on the basis of first impressions.

We must never forget that every time clients have any interaction with the clinic, they are reassessing the perceptions they have of the value received. The sum total of these assessments forms the basis of the "new" overall impression of a practice. Perception is reality. For clients to accept our recommendations readily, they must believe we are professionally competent. Because almost no clients are capable of judging true competence, this perception is grounded in areas in which they can make comparisons. Such things as friendliness, cleanliness, professionalism, state-of-the-art equipment, and time efficiency are common factors that enter into the final overall impression perceived by the client of the veterinary practice.

We therefore gain clients' trust by making them feel important and confident they have made the right decisions for their pets. Treating the client as an individual, giving frequent compliments, respecting the client's opinion, using the client's name and pet's name often, being a good listener, respecting the client's time, and expressing appreciation are all ways to make the client feel important.

Successful marketing depends on communicating with the client. Communication is incomplete without comprehension. We must talk in language that the client understands. One of the biggest obstacles we must overcome is thinking the client understands what we are talking about. Most clients will never tell a veterinarian when they don't understand something due to embarrassment. We must never assume a client knows what services the pet needs or what we can provide.

Children are great teachers of successful marketing tactics. All we really need to know about marketing successfully can be learned by watching toddlers who want something:

- They are persistent. They know it takes six to eight interactions just to get someone to think about something. They know it may take 16 to 18 interactions to get to the "yes."
- "No" always means "maybe." "No" means they did not provide enough facts and benefits about what they want for daddy to give it to them!
- They are never embarrassed to ask over and over again. They know the average sale in America only occurs after the consumer has said "no" four times. They know that only one in four salespersons persists through the four "nos" to get to the "yes."
- They know that most sales are based on emotions rather than logic—and that emotional selling requires emotional buying. Crying works!

Clients have three types of needs that the veterinarian must solve to gain compliance. These needs include the following:

- Professional needs: Making the pet well or keeping it well.
- Emotional needs: Making the client feel good about owning a pet, seeking veterinary attention, and choosing a particular clinic to provide those services. Meeting these emotional needs is the number-one reason that clients return to the clinic.
- Consumer needs: These needs are most often the reason a client visits for the first time. They include convenience, costs, and so on.

Successful marketing is an accumulation of many different strategies. First and foremost is the creation of a perceived high medical competence. Trust results when the client believes the veterinarian and staff really know what they are talking about and are committed to high-quality care. After this barrier has been broken, our marketing efforts become much easier and must be directed toward "emotional" selling.

Our success depends on using the following basic strategies to persuade clients of their need for the services we are recommending:

- Show how the pet benefits.
- Show how the client benefits.
- Detail the consequences of failing to accept the recommendation now.
- Communicate the consequences of failing to accept the recommendation at all.
- Show how others (pets or people) might benefit from acceptance of the recommendation.

Enthusiasm is crucial for marketing professional services successfully. Enthusiasm can be generated only when there is a genuine belief in the value of the recommended services. The last four letters in the word *enthusiasm* can be defined as standing for "I Am Sold Myself!" The best salesman is the one sold on the product. This creates a more enthusiastic selling approach. One should remember that the only thing more contagious than enthusiasm is apathy.

An enthusiastic response to your recommendations by the client comes from *involvement.* We must do everything possible to involve the client in making the diagnosis as well as instituting treatment. Some ways to involve the client include the following:

- Show the problem on the pet.
- Explain the importance of preventing and treating potential problems.
- Show the client how to administer medications properly.
- Observe and praise the client's efforts to use the medications.
- Schedule telephone progress reports and frequent rechecks to help the client perceive the progress being made.

Smiling is one of the best ways to show enthusiasm. Smiling breaks down barriers, drops defenses, increases credibility, shows we care, and defuses anger. The most important thing we can wear is a smile. We cannot afford to "have a bad day." Clients don't really care what kind of day we are having—only how we affect their day!

Rejection is a normal part of successful marketing. The Coca-Cola Company sold only 400 bottles the first year. Marketing research has determined that (as mentioned previously) it takes six to eight interactions just to enter the subconscious mind of a consumer. Additionally, it may take 16 to 18 interactions to get them to agree to the recommendation. The average consumer says "no" four times before finally agreeing. Sadly, as we've noted, only one in four salespersons is persistent enough to make it through the four "nos." Everyone hates rejection, and the tendency is just to drop the subject to avoid confrontation. However, a mission statement of being the pet's advocate does not allow us simply to forget about offering what the pet really needs for the best life possible.

Specific Strategies for Successfully Marketing Preventive and Therapeutic Ear Care

Believe In Its Importance. Understand that preventing and resolving ear problems is very important to the pain-free life of the pet.

Educate Yourself. As in all other facets of our veterinary education, we must first understand both normal and abnormal conditions, including disease processes of the ear. The veterinarian must become proficient with physical examination techniques and appropriate laboratory evaluation of ear specimen cytology and cultures. Surprisingly, the investment of a very small amount of additional study time can greatly enhance one's professional abilities in the diagnostics and therapeutics of ear care. Many professional reference textbooks and journals now include in-depth information on ear care. This book, for example, can greatly enhance our visual perception of abnormalities that occur within the ear. Almost all regional and national continuing education programs now have full-day programs devoted to ear pathology.

It is also important for the veterinarian to keep abreast of the numerous products now available for both preventive care and therapeutics for the ear. The formulary contained in the appendix of this book lists many drugs, along with specific ingredients. The chapter on ototoxicity has a helpful guide to ingredients contained in products that may potentially cause additional problems if used in pets compromised with a ruptured tympanum. It is crucial to understand not only what products are available but also their uses and contraindications. Many of today's pet owners are better educated than ever before—and sadly, with the help of the Internet, may be better versed in particular products than the veterinarian who has not taken the time to study each product introduced to this profession.

Educate the Staff. Clients relate better and therefore talk more openly with your staff members than to the veterinarians in the practice. Therefore the veterinary staff may be in the best position to "plant the seeds" of potential ear problems that should be brought to the attention of the veterinarian during the examination. Since this is the case, it is crucial that all staff members be educated in the importance of ear care as well as looking in the ears of every pet at every opportunity. Staff should be taught the consequences of failing to catch ear disease early and of being persistent to resolve ear problems before treatment is discontinued completely.

Staff must understand the importance of *not* making a telephone diagnosis or examination table–side diagnosis until appropriate confirmation diagnostics are performed, so that all recommendations are made based on confirmed and documented diagnoses. It is very difficult for any veterinarian or other staff member to overcome wrong information that has been provided by an uneducated staff member without destroying some credibility of the practice as a whole. Every staff member must fully appreciate the power of each interaction with the client and the potential consequences of giving out wrong information. Every staff member interaction with the client has a positive or negative effect on every client decision.

Seeing is believing and one of the best staff education tools. Teaching staff members what a normal horizontal and vertical canal looks like allows them to know what is abnormal. The use of videoscopes such as the MedRX Video Vetscope (MedRx, Inc., Largo, Florida) allows the veterinarian to teach many staff members at the same time, by generating a visual image on a video monitor that all can watch. The educated staff is far more capable of selling clients on the need for thorough ear examinations when clients call with questions about a problem, as well as when medical history indicates the possibility of aural pathology.

It is impossible for anyone to market successfully anything he or she does not understand. All educational tools available should be used to teach both staff and clients about ear care. This might include wall pictures and charts (excellent ones are available from several suppliers of ear products, as well as MedRx, Inc.), pamphlets, handouts, and ear models. Most people learn much more easily and retain more information when visual aids are used.

Equip Yourself. Much of the instrumentation needed for ear disease diagnostics and therapeutics is already present in the typical veterinary clinic. Client perception of overall medical competence is influenced by the equipment seen and used in the examination room. Otoscopes must be in *every* examination room, ready for use, if one expects to gain 100% compliance in thorough examination of each and every ear, each and every time. Battery-operated otoscopes provide portability but also are prone to become inoperable due to low battery charge. Wall-mounted transformers (Welch-Allyn) eliminate the embarrassment of dead batteries—and the resulting perception of incompetence. These units typically also have a much brighter light, allowing better visualization.

Particular attention should be paid to sanitation and cleanliness of the otoscope specula so they are always ready for use when a new patient enters the room. A new, innovative specula-cleaning device is available, consisting of a brush within a stainless cylinder, which can be filled with disinfectant. Having the cleaner instrument on the counter in every room maximizes time efficiency and guarantees specula are kept clean. A cheap alternative would be to place a small bristle brush used for cleaning test tubes in each examination room—or having two sets of specula in each room so the soiled one can be removed from the room during the cleaning process before the next client is called in. Staff should also be educated on the possibility of spreading infectious organisms from one pet to another when using an uncleaned specula, even though it may not appear dirty.

The expense of new equipment is relatively unimportant relative to the immediate cash flow that can be generated from the use of such medical instrumentation. Gross revenue enhancement is much more effective in increasing profits than trying to minimize expenses by purchasing only minimal equipment—and the best way to decrease the cost of equipment per use is to use it more often. Never underestimate the potential that exists in every ear canal you have the opportunity to examine thoroughly. Most practices quickly find that after new equipment is purchased, the caseload of use for that equipment increases substantially, if only for the reason that now it is there, it needs to be paid for! The end results are better client service, more pets with otitis treated earlier, and the satisfaction that comes from providing quality medicine.

New video otoscopes now available not only allow the practitioner to do a better job with diagnostics but also educate the client at the same time and treat more thoroughly and effectively. Adequate visualization, a clear view of the inner lining of canine and feline ear canals and tympani, can be very difficult owing to the limits of standard diagnostic otoscopy instruments. Showing clients, staff, students, and other practitioners ear canal abnormalities through a standard otoscope can be awkward, even using the "teaching otoscope" heads that are available.

The video otoscope employs new technology to expose the hidden world of ear pathology. Because the instrument is attached to a miniature video camera and video display, otic examinations can be visualized in real time on a video monitor. A color video printer allows "before and after" pictures of ear canal conditions that can be shown to the client later. The photographs generated can provide pathologic information in a way that is perceived much more seriously by the client; the client is more willing to request needed procedures because it has now become a much more informed (educated) decision.

Failure to look is much more often the problem in clinic income than is a lack of knowledge. It should become standard protocol that every ear of every anesthetized pet in the clinic for any procedure, related to ear disease or not, be examined using the videoscope; doing so often results in the discovery of many additional medical problems in the ear that would otherwise go unnoticed until they became much more severe. These problems can be photographed to be shown to the client later as "proof" of the problem, which often must be discussed with the client on the phone after discovery when the client is not present to witness it. This photograph then becomes factual evidence and documentation of the findings; they can even be converted into digital images in the pet's medical record. If the client refuses the initial treatment recommendation when communicated via the phone call, these pictures increase the chance that the client will allow later treatment after the pet is presented for dismissal and the case discussed with the client.

"Before and after" pictures can also be kept on file to use in educating other clients about ear disease and the reason for appropriate preventive ear hygiene. These pictures can also be added to the reminders sent out to the client for various procedure updates.

Adapters allow other hospital instruments to generate video images for both the practitioner and client. Such instruments as microscopes, rigid endoscopes, and flexible endoscopes can be enhanced via the videoscope.

Although many practices have purchased videoscopes, most greatly underuse them. Why? They are not convenient to use. For that reason, I have installed a new videoscope system called Vet Dock (MedRx, Inc., Largo, Florida) that is economical enough to be placed in all examination rooms. This has allowed videoscope visualization of all ears during every examination to become habitual. The client is able to visualize the ear examination at the same time as the veterinarian does. Involvement breeds interest, and interest generates additional requests for appropriate services.

Look for Problems. The foundation of a successful wellness program includes both a thorough medical history and comprehensive physical examination of the patient, with the goal of catching signs of potential disease before it becomes clinically evident. Time is required for thoroughness. Staff delegation is an important tool in optimizing the time available for the veterinarian to concentrate and perform these nose-to-tail examinations. A thorough medical history form can be used to ensure that nothing is overlooked when obtaining the medical history. Many times the client does not know the subtle signs of pain. Asking the right questions can provide insight into observations by the client assumed to be "normal." A pet examination report card noting both the normal and abnormal findings becomes tangible proof to the client of the thoroughness of the examination. Abnormalities noted on the report card may serve as a reminder to the client later at home of the problems discovered and recommendations refused. Most clients do not like to make hasty decisions and may request appropriate services after they have had time to think about it. Standardized protocols for handling ear diagnostics are very useful in maintaining consistency. Standardization of procedures allows the staff to have all needed supplies ready when the pet is presented for a specific problem. Standard protocol for all examinations should include evaluation of the eardrum and middle ear.

Educate the Client. People do not buy what they do not understand. A lack of client education reduces the choices by the client to a matter of price. Because a large amount of ear disease lies deep in the ear, the pet owner may not even perceive a problem. The old adage "show and tell to sell" is still true. As mentioned, every client is a unique individual having different "hot buttons" and different desires. The particular "hot button" (stimulus triggering the client to take action) may be visual, auditory, tactile, or olfactory. Clients learn in different ways. It is crucial that the practitioner take the time not only to be thorough in the examination but also to discover the "hot button" of each client to determine what is the most important to them. Clients want to know: What is wrong? Can we solve it? Will it hurt? How long will it take? How much will it cost?

Never assume the client is aware of all the services/products the pet needs or you can provide! Increasing the client's perception of all abnormalities may be accomplished by the following:

- Show the problem to the client via the standard otoscope, teaching otoscope, or video otoscope. Reddened, inflamed ears are quite easy to understand when they are observed.
- Have the client smell the odor.
- Have the client feel the swollen or bony ear canals.
- Explain to the client that the resistance by the pet to having the ears examined or whining during manipulation or insertion of the otoscope specula indicates that the ear is painful. Use the analogy of how painful human ear infections may be.

Other visual aids that are available and should be used include the following:

- Diagrams of the ear's anatomy. These should be framed to enhance the professional image and placed on the wall of each examination room close to the examination table so they can be referred to when discussing ear disease.
- Wall posters of photographs of dog and cat ear disease conditions
- Loose-leaf notebooks in each examination room showing pictures of ear disease and therapeutic/surgical procedures
- Brochures from product suppliers
- Ear models
- Personalized handouts on clinic letterhead, including a diagram of the ear, so that the area of the problem can be identified. It should be standard policy that no client ever leaves the examination room without a handout detailing the specific conditions diagnosed. Handouts become miniature billboards marketing both the practice as a whole and the specific problem being explained.

Visual aids are good, but the most important educational tool is staff and veterinarian interaction with the client! Staff training in ear disease conditions, therapy, and prevention is essential. After appropriate staff members are properly trained, much of the client education time can be delegated to them. Everyone must understand the "hows" and "whys" of ear disease. Staff must comprehend that the number-one reason for chronic otitis is lack of client compliance, which is most commonly a result of a lack of perceived importance to the long-term quality of life of the pet. To market ear recommendations most effectively, relate otitis to the following:

- *Otitis hurts!* It can be very painful, as is often evident from the swelling and redness. Many pets with painful ear infections may show behavioral changes such as aggression from the pain. Compare it with human ear infections.
- *Otitis stinks!* A stinky pet may well not remain inside the house for long. Pets relegated to the backyard most often no longer get the best care.
- *Otitis includes infection!* Any infection can be a "seed" for infection elsewhere in the body. Infection can rupture the eardrum and even move on to the nervous system. The inner ear is a direct route to the brain!
- *Otitis can cause loss of hearing!*

Successful client education requires an environment conducive to learning. Client anxiety limits concentration. Do you think it is fun to put a pet in the car and come to the veterinary hospital? Do we make it easy for them to do business with us? Think of all the barriers we throw up to the client, making it inconvenient for them. Waiting time is the number-one de-marketing problem in almost all practices. Today's client does not have time to wait. Today, instant service takes too long! When we feel hassled, we are not in the best state for listening attentively. Minimizing client anxiety allows the client to concentrate more on what you are saying and showing. Such things as striving to see appointments on time and minimizing confusion in the reception area can improve client relations. Offering to assist the client with the pet both on arrival and when paying says a lot about the value the practice places on its clientele.

Methods for entertaining children, such as a TV showing pet movies and quiet toys, can be quite useful in distracting them so they do not distract the parents.

Anxiety can also occur from a perception that the pet is being hurt during the examination or treatment. The best way to show you care is to be gentle. Sedatives are greatly underused in veterinary medicine and result in poor examinations and missed diagnoses. Any resistance to a thorough examination should result in sedation of the pet.

Clients must also be educated about the many products available that have the potential for enhancing the ear's resistance to infection. These products should be evaluated by the veterinarian, who should make appropriate recommendations to the client, including the facts and benefits of the particular product. Recommendations should be provided in the form of "the pet *needs*—" rather than merely "I recommend—."

Most treatment failures are a result of poor client compliance with prescribed home-care therapy. Successful outcomes require that the client understand both the importance of following the treatment protocol and how to do it. Written home-care instructions should always be provided after discussion in the examination room. Using treatment regimens that clients can actually do and that fit their lifestyles are the cornerstones of successful treatment. Proper administration should always be demonstrated and then observed as the client attempts to mimic your demonstration. If the client cannot perform it satisfactorily, it would be appropriate either to hospitalize the pet or have it brought to the clinic daily for treatment. Remember that you will be judged by your results. If the problem does not resolve, even though it may be due to the client's lack of appropriate treatment, you will be blamed. That's not fair—but that is reality! After a few days of appropriate treatment, ideally, the pet will feel more comfortable and the pain reduced so the owner can take over treatment. It is crucial that the practitioner understand the importance of resolving the pain as quickly as possible so the pet will accept treatment readily. Everyone should praise the client's efforts. Everyone loves compliments and being made to feel important. Compliance with home-care recommendations should always be assessed during telephone progress checks.

Make Your Services Convenient! Convenience rules the world today. The astute practitioner offers such services as pet drop-off and late pickup. Treatment procedures such as topical medication application should be initiated during the initial visit to better ensure client compliance. All needed services should be scheduled for a time most convenient for the client—which in most cases is the initial time of presentation for the problem or routine examination. The veterinary practice demonstrates respect for the client's time when appointments are behind schedule by offering an opportunity to leave the pet at the clinic for a few hours while complete diagnostic evaluation and therapeutic procedures are performed. The client will appreciate the explanation that it would be more convenient for them to have all work performed now that the pet is already there. Staff should be trained to schedule a specific dismissal appointment time to minimize client waiting, frustration, and anxiety.

Price for Your Market! There are two types of fools: those who charge too much and those who do not charge enough! Fee schedules vary tremendously due to practice philosophy, locale, and financial status of the typical client in the practice. Different clinics attract different types of clients. The key to success is being sure that the level of service exceeds the fees charged.

Pricing is no longer based on what it costs to provide a service but rather what the client perceives the service is worth. My rule of thumb is that the fee for any service should be a minimum of five times the hard costs of materials. In other words, drugs and materials needed to provide the service should be no more than 20% of the total fee.

The major cause of relapsing otitis is failure to recheck and treat long enough. A line item on a client's bill entitled "otitis recheck package" may be established to include the medical progress examination, sedation, ear swab and staining, and flushing. This is preferable to listing all services at a standard fee and then providing a discount. Discounting merely hints to the client that the veterinary practice's services are overpriced. Bundling these services into one line-item fee enables the practice to set an appropriate fee for the group of services, which may allow a lower total fee than if the fees are individually itemized and are perceived as too much by the client. It is always better to adjust fees to an acceptable level and still provide "best care" whenever possible. When procedures start to be deleted because of client resistance to the total fee, quality medicine begins to suffer quickly. This group of bundled services may then be lumped into one total fee and the package given a separate treatment computer number. The total fee is the same as it would have been with some discount given at the bottom of the invoice, but this strategy avoids the flavor of being merely another retail outlet. It is important to look at long-term practice revenues rather than short-term gratification. The key is to keep pets healthy and coming back for years to come.

The fee charged for individual components of ear problems must be based on client perception of the importance and difficulty of each service. Some of the line items include examination, cytology, cultures, cleaning, flushing, biopsy, sedation, corticosteroid injections, antibiotic injections, and medications dispensed, including pain management. The practice manager must look at the total as well as the individual line-item fees and make a determination as to what is acceptable to the client to maintain a high level of compliance with recommendations.

Fees must always be related to value. Clients should always leave with tangible evidence of the intangible services provided. Examples would be client handouts, pet examination report cards, pictures of the individual pet's problem, and brochures. If clients are to return, they must perceive the services as worth the fees charged. Unfortunately, clients constantly reevaluate everything they encounter while visiting the clinic, and the sum total of these evaluations determines the overall practice's image of competence and compassion—and it continues to improve or decline on every new encounter.

Remind Clients! Clients hate making hasty decisions. Spending money causes the same stages as the death of a family member: anger, denial, grief, acceptance. Even a pet's chronic renal failure may be an acute diagnosis to the client—which requires time for mental adjustment. Some tips for better compliance include the following:

- Go slowly. Give the client time to weigh the potential disadvantages of *not* accepting the recommendations.
- Give the client a reason to act promptly, such as better chance of complete resolution.
- Show the client how the pet will benefit, such as pain resolution.
- Show the client how he or she will personally benefit (healthier pet, lower future costs).
- Detail the consequences of noncompliance with the recommendations.

Today's client has an absolute right to be demanding. It is important that all staff members understand that every client must always be given the opportunity to provide the best care available for their beloved family member. Sometimes financial constraints do not allow all pets to receive this highest level of care. We must, however, always be thankful that every client and pet encounter gives us an opportunity to recommend the best course of treatment. Clients unable to accept this "best care" level should not be made to feel bad but rather given options for treatment. In my own practice, the first option is to finance the difference in "best care" and "OK" care. If the client can pay at least a significant portion of the total fee, it may be wise to consider financial arrangements. Financing will always be more profitable than discounting. The sad fact is that we all discount every day by not charging what our human-care counterparts do for anything we do! Veterinarians should make medical decisions, not financial decisions. Clients do not pay us to be financial counselors. Whenever we do not offer the best, we are prejudging the value of the particular pet to the client—and we do not have the right to do that.

Computer searches of the practice's client base can produce lists of patients with past otitis problems that can be targeted for marketing efforts. Even offering complimentary rechecks of this client base can result in significant findings of additional pathology, allowing the recommendation of additional services and products. The real key is simply finding a way to get these pets presented for examination—which is then followed by thorough medical history-taking and comprehensive physical examinations, with the goal being to discover every potential medical problem with every pet every time it is presented. After the problems are found, a commitment to assertive marketing is essential to help pets live the longest, highest-quality life possible.

Follow Up! It is surprising how many veterinarians are willing to allow a client to spend large sums of money on ear diagnostics and therapy but then rely on the client's impression of the response to treatment. A phone call to the client to check on the pet's progress in 24 to 48 hours impresses the client by reflecting a caring attitude and stressing the importance the doctor places on complete resolution of the problem.

Clients respond better when they are treated nicely from the start and are made to feel that they are an important part of their pet's future well-being. Scheduling and charging for follow-up examinations and diagnostic testing greatly enhance the client bonding rate to the practice, build client trust, and ensure administration of appropriate therapy. Staff should *always* schedule the recheck appointment and ensure that needed reminders are entered into the computer before the client leaves the clinic. The veterinarian should also consider sending reminder notes to clients for procedures recommended that were not accepted at the time of the initial diagnosis and recommendation. Patients with severe wax accumulation in the ear canals should receive a reminder for rechecking and ear flushing at an appropriate interval. All pets receiving long-term medications should receive periodic rechecks.

Become Creative! The practice wishing to improve or grow the practice should consider the following strategies:

- Plan a staff meeting to discuss ear care and ask staff for ways to improve compliance.
- Write an article for a local newspaper on proper ear care.
- Position the clinic as an ear care clinic.
- Place messages on the outside marquee reader board to generate questions about ear care.
- Develop relationships with local groomers and other pet care professionals to increase the number of referrals for ear disease.

Why is client compliance with ear care recommendations so low?

- They do not perceive the significance of catching problems early and treating them to get complete resolution.

- They do not realize that the normal ear anatomy predisposes pets to external ear disease.
- Clients often do not recognize the early, subtle signs of pain from ear disease.
- Clients have financial issues. Sufficient money is most likely not the problem but rather the client's priorities in spending discretionary funds. Your goal is to raise that priority through client education.
- Fear of anesthesia. Clients do not understand the advances in anesthesia safety of the past few years. Everyone must be careful not to create unnecessary anxiety by overemphasizing the "risks" of anesthesia required for appropriate treatment. Clients must definitely be informed of the inherent risks of all anesthetic events and appropriate consent documentation completed, but they should also perceive that the risk of anesthesia is much less than the damage an untreated ear infection can cause. Consider using the term *sedation* rather than *anesthesia,* when deep surgical planes of anesthesia are not needed. Emphasize all the precautions, such as vital-sign monitoring, that are performed to make the procedure as safe as humanly possible.
- Owner forgetfulness of the recommendation. It pays to develop a system of consistent reminders for needed procedures.

Marketing ear care is one of the most professional services a veterinary practice can offer. Clients perceive the veterinarian as the pet health care professional. We must not disappoint them. More ear disease is missed because we don't look than because we don't know. We must look for it consistently and thoroughly in every pet presented for examination. Current estimates are that 15% to 20% of all canine patients and 4% to 6% of all feline patients presented have some type of ear abnormality. A little quick arithmetic reveals that the income potential for marketing ear care is not insignificant:

Typical client base: 2500 canine patients + 1000 feline patients = 3500 patients
10% to 20% of canine patients with ear disease = 250 to 500 patients
4% to 6% of feline patients with ear disease = 40 to 60 patients
Total possible patients = 290 to 560
   Minimum services needed and suggested fees to perform thorough ear examinations:

Office visit and physical examination	$35
Ear swab and cytologic evaluation	$22
Sedation and reversal	$35
Ear flushing and suction	$28
Total	$120

NOTE: The potential income from examination and minimal treatment only is $37,700 (290 patients) to $72,800 (560 patients).
   Add fees for any other treatments, drugs, additional testing, surgical procedures, follow-up visits, and so on, and the income stream continues to increase substantially.

There is probably sufficient ear pathology in our current patient base to keep a veterinarian busy full time. The real question is whether practitioners are willing to dedicate themselves to examinations thorough enough to find all the problems present and then have the time needed to educate the client so that every recommendation is borne out by an educated decision by the client. Assertive marketing is nothing more than providing all the facts and benefits of the recommendations in such a way that the clients *desire* to accept those recommendations. Assertive marketing requires persistence, consistency, passion, and credibility. Veterinarians who maintain the trust of their clients see a high level of compliance in the acceptance of recommendations. That is all there is to successfully marketing high-quality ear care in the veterinary practice.

It is the veterinarian's professional, ethical, and moral duty to recommend everything the pet needs. Never assume that the client is aware of all the services the pet needs or you can provide. Good medicine is great business!

Appendix
Ear Product Formulary

This formulary is presented as a guide to products available for treating ear disease. The products listed are for *topical use* in the ear canal unless indicated otherwise. Many topical formulations are compounded mixtures containing ingredients that may be potentially ototoxic when there is no eardrum. Consult the manufacturer for the recommendation for use when the eardrum is perforated.

The organization of the formulary is by function or mode of action. Ingredients are categorized as antiinflammatory, antibacterial, antifungal, miticidal, ear cleaners, and drying agents. Some formulations have more than one function and may be listed again in the appropriate sections. Under each category, the generic ingredient, the trade name, and the manufacturers are listed. The proprietary names and active ingredients of products are listed after the ingredients.

Active Ingredients of Ear Products, Listed by Function

POTENT ANTIINFLAMMATORY AGENTS

Betamethasone 0.1%	Genta-Otic	Vetus
	Gentaved Otic	Vedco
	Gentocin Otic	Schering-Plough
	Otomax	Schering-Plough
	Tri-Otic	Med-Pharmex
Betamethasone 0.64 mg	Lotrisone	Schering-Plough
Dexamethasone 0.1%	Decadron Phosphate	Merck
	Tobradex	Alcon
	Tresaderm	Merial
Fluocinolone 0.01%	Synotic Otic	Ft. Dodge

MODERATE ANTIINFLAMMATORY AGENTS

Isoflupredone acetate 0.1%	Neo-Predef	Upjohn and Pharmacia
	Tritop	Upjohn and Pharmacia
Triamcinolone acetonide 0.1%	Animax	Pharmaderm
	Coly-Mycin S Otic	Parke-Davis
	Cortisporin Otic	Glaxo Wellcome
	Derma 4 Ointment	Pfizer
	Dermalone	Vedco
	Derma-Vet	Med-Pharmex
	Forte Topical	Upjohn and Pharmacia
	Neo-Predef	Upjohn and Pharmacia
	Panolog	Solvay

MILD ANTIINFLAMMATORY AGENTS

Hydrocortisone acetate 0.2%	Forte Topical	Upjohn and Pharmacia
Hydrocortisone 1%	Bur-O-Cort	Q.A. Labs
	Burotic HC	Allerderm
	Cipro HC Otic	Bayer Pharmaceutical
	Clear X Ear Drying Solution	DVM

Active Ingredients of Ear Products, Listed by Function—cont'd

	Coly-Mycin S Otic	Parke-Davis
	CORT/ASTRIN	Vedco
	Cortisporin Otic	Glaxo Wellcome
	Epiotic HC	Allerderm
	VoSol HC Otic	Wallace
Prednisolone 0.17%	Chlora-Otic	Vetus
	Liquichlor	Evsco

ANTIBACTERIALS

Acetic acid–boric acid	DermaPet Ear/Skin Cleanser	DermaPet, Inc.
Chloramphenicol	Chlora-Otic	Vetus
	Chloromycetin Otic	Parke-Davis
	Liquichlor	Evsco
Ciprofloxacin	Cipro HC Otic	Bayer Pharmaceuticals
Colistin	Coly-Mycin S Otic	Parke-Davis
Enrofloxacin	Baytril Injection	Bayer Pharmaceuticals

(Mix 2 ml in 13 ml of artificial tears or saline)

Gentamicin	Genta-Otic	Vetus
	Gentaved Otic	Vedco
	Gentocin Otic	Schering-Plough
	Otomax	Schering-Plough
	Topagen Ointment	Schering-Plough
	Tri-Otic	Med-Pharmex
Neomycin	Animax	Pharmaderm
	Coly-Mycin S Otic	Parke-Davis
	Cortisporin Otic	Glaxo Wellcome
	Derma 4 Ointment	Pfizer
	Dermalone	Vedco
	Derma-Vet	Med-Pharmex
	Forte Topical	Upjohn and Pharmacia
	Neo-Predef	Upjohn and Pharmacia
	Panolog	Solvay
	Quadritop	Vetus
	Tresaderm	Merial
	Tritop	Upjohn and Pharmacia
Ofloxacin	Floxin Otic	Daiichi
Polymyxin B sulfate	Cortisporin	Glaxo Wellcome
	Forte Topical	Upjohn and Pharmacia
Silver sulfadiazine 0.1%	Silvadene Crème	Marion

(Mix 1.5 ml of cream in 13.5 ml of distilled water)

Ticarcillin	Ticar 1 g vial	SmithKline Beecham

Active Ingredients of Ear Products, Listed by Function—cont'd

(Mix with 2 ml of sterile water. Add 0.5 ml of this solution to 15 ml of artificial tears or saline. Keep refrigerated. Use as ear drops for 1 week, then discard remaining solution.) Freeze the remainder in 0.5-ml increments for future use; good for 90 days frozen.

Tobramycin	Tobradex Ophthalmic	Alcon
Tris-EDTA	TrizEDTA	DermaPet, Inc.
	T8 Solution Ear Rinse	DVM

ANTIFUNGALS

Acetic acid–boric acid	DermaPet Ear/Skin Cleanser	DermaPet, Inc.
Clotrimazole 1%	Lotrimin AF	Schering-Plough
	Lortisone	Schering-Plough
	Otomax	Schering-Plough
	Tri-Otic	Med-Pharmex
Miconazole 1%	Conofite	Mallinckrodt
	Micazole	Vetus
	Miconosol	Med-Pharmex
Nystatin 100,000 U/ml	Animax	Pharmaderm
	Derma-4	Pfizer
	Dermalone	Vedco
	Derma-Vet	Med-Pharmex
	Panolog	Solvay
	Quadritop	Vetus
Zinc undecylenate	Fungi-dry-ear	Q.A. Labs

MITICIDALS

Fipronil	Frontline Top Spot	Merial
Ivermectin 1% injectable	Ivomec 1%	Merial

(0.1 ml/10 lb subcutaneously every 2 weeks for three injections)

Pyrethrins	Aurimite	Schering-Plough
	Cerumite	Evsco
	Eradimite	Solvay
	Mita-Clear	Pfizer
	Nolvamite with Nolvasan	Ft. Dodge
	Oticare-M Ear Mite Treatment	ARC
	Otomite Plus	Allerderm
Rotenone 0.12%	Mitaplex-R	Tomlyn
Rotenone 0.12% and cube resins 0.16%	Ear Mite Lotion	DurVet
	Ear Miticide	Vedco
	Ear Miticide	Phoenix
Thiabendazole	Tresaderm	Merial

Ear Products Listed by Trade Names

Animax Ointment (Pharmaderm)

Active ingredients: Nystatin, neomycin sulfate, thiostrepton, and triamcinolone acetonide in a nonirritating polyethylene and mineral oil base.

Aurimite (Schering-Plough)

Active ingredients: Dioctyl sodium sulfosuccinate 1.952%, benzocaine 1.952%, technical piperonyl butoxide 0.49%, pyrethrins 0.04%. Inert ingredients 95.566%.

Baytril Injection Solution (Bayer)

Active ingredients: Each milliliter of injection solution contains enrofloxacin 22.7 mg, n-butyl alcohol 30 mg, potassium hydroxide for pH adjustment, and water for injection, q.s. (quantum sufficiat).

Bur-O-Cort 2:1 (Q. A. Labs)

Active ingredients: Each milliliter contains Burow's solution (astringent) 20 mg, hydrocortisone (antiinflammatory, antipruritic) 10 mg.

Burotic HC (Q. A. Labs)

Active ingredients: Hydrocortisone 1%. Other ingredients: Propylene glycol, water, Burow's solution, acetic acid, benzalkonium chloride.

CERUMITE (Evsco)

Active ingredients: Squalane (hexamethyltetracosane) 25.00%, pyrethrins 0.05%, technical piperonyl butoxide 0.50%. Inert ingredients 74.45%.

Chlora-Otic

Active ingredients: Each milliliter contains chloramphenicol 4.2 mg, prednisolone 1.7 mg, tetracaine 4.2 mg, squalane 0.21 ml.

Chloromycetin Otic

Active ingredients: Each milliliter contains 5 mg (0.5%) chloramphenicol in propylene glycol.

Cipro HC Otic (Bayer)

Active ingredients: Each milliliter contains ciprofloxacin HCl (equivalent to 2 mg ciprofloxacin), 10 mg hydrocortisone, and 9 mg benzyl alcohol as a preservative.

Clear X Ear Drying Solution (DVM)

Active ingredients: Acetic acid 2.5%, colloidal sulfur 2%, hydrocortisone 1%.

Coly-Mycin S Otic

Active ingredients: Each milliliter contains colistin base activity 3 mg (as the sulfate), neomycin base activity 3.3 mg (as the sulfate), hydrocortisone acetate 10 mg (1%), thonzonium bromide 0.5 mg (0.5%), with polysorbate 80, acetic acid, sodium acetate buffered at a pH of 5.

Conofite Lotion (Mallinckrodt)

Active ingredients: 1.15% miconazole nitrate (equivalent to 1% miconazole base by weight), polyethylene glycol 400, and ethyl alcohol 55%.

CORT-ASTRIN Solution (Vedco)

Active ingredients: Each milliliter contains Burow's solution 20 mg, hydrocortisone 10 mg in a water-miscible propylene glycol base.

Cortisporin Otic Solution

Active ingredients: Each milliliter contains polymyxin B sulfate 10,000 units, neomycin sulfate 3.5 mg neomycin base, and hydrocortisone 10 mg (0.1%). The vehicle contains potassium metabisulfate 0.1% and the inactive ingredients cupric sulfate, glycerin, hydrochloric acid, propylene glycol, and water for injection.

Decadron Phosphate 0.1% (Merck)

Active ingredients: Each milliliter contains 1 mg dexamethasone phosphate. Inactive ingredients: Creatinine, sodium citrate, sodium borate, polysorbate 80, disodium edentate, hydrochloric acid to adjust pH, and water for injection.

Derma 4 Ointment (Pfizer)

Composition: Each milliliter contains 100,000 units of nystatin, neomycin sulfate (equivalent to 2.5 mg of neomycin base), 2500 units of thiostrepton, and 1.0 mg of triamcinolone acetonide. Inert ingredients: Plastibase* 50-weight, 20%; mineral oil USP, 80%.

*Plastibase trademark of E.R. Squibb & Sons, Princeton, N.J.

Dermalone Ointment (Vedco)

Active ingredients: Each milliliter contains nystatin 100,000 units, neomycin sulfate (equivalent to neomycin base) 2.5 mg, thiostrepton 2500 units, triamcinolone acetonide 1.0 mg, polyethylene and mineral oil gel base.

Derma-Vet Ointment

Active ingredients: Each milliliter contains nystatin 100,000 units, neomycin sulfate (equivalent to neomycin base) 2.5 mg, thiostrepton 2500 units, triamcinolone acetonide 1.0 mg.

Epi-Otic HC (Virbac)

Active ingredients: Hydrocortisone 1%, lactic acid, and PCMX in a surface-acting vehicle.

Ear Mite Lotion (Durvet)

Active ingredients: Rotenone 0.12%, cube resins 0.16%. Inert ingredients 99.72%.

Ear Miticide (Vedco)

Active ingredients: Rotenone 0.12%, cube resins 0.16%. Inert ingredients 99.72%.

Ear Miticide (Phoenix)

Active ingredients: Rotenone 0.12%, cube resins 0.16%. Inert ingredients 99.72%.

Eradimite (Solvay)

Active ingredients: Pyrethrins 0.15%, piperonyl butoxide technical 1.50%. Inert ingredients 98.35%.

Floxin Otic (Daiichi)

Active ingredients: 0.3% (3 mg/ml) ofloxacin with benzalkonium chloride 0.0025%, sodium chloride 0.9%, and water for injection. Hydrochloric acid and sodium hydroxide are added to adjust the pH to 6.5.

Frontline Top Spot (Merial)

Active ingredients: Fipronil: 5-amino-1-(2,6-dichloro-4-[trifluoromethyl]phenyl)-4-([1<R,S]-[trifluoromethyl]sulfinyl)-1-H-pyrazole-3-carbonitrle 9.7%. Inert ingredients 90.3%.

Fungi-Dry-Ear (Q. A. Labs)

Active ingredients: Isopropyl alcohol, deionized water, silicon dioxide, zinc unde-cylenate (undecylenic acid), methyl salicylate, PEG 75 lanolin oil, sucrose octyl acetate, polysorbate 60, propylene glycol, acetic acid, FD & C blue #1.

Genta-Otic Solution (Vetus)

Active ingredients: Each milliliter contains gentamicin sulfate equivalent to 3 mg gentamicin base, betamethasone valerate equivalent to 1 mg betamethasone, 1.0 mg hydroxyethylcellulose, 2.5 mg glacial acetic acid, 200 mg purified water, 19% ethanol, 9.4 mg benzyl alcohol as preservative, 300 mg glycerine and propylene glycol q.s.

Gentaved Otic Solution (Vedco)

Active ingredients: Each milliliter contains gentamicin sulfate equivalent to 3 mg gentamicin base, betamethasone valerate equivalent to 1 mg betamethasone, 1.0 mg hydroxyethylcellulose, 2.5 mg glacial acetic acid, 200 mg purified water, 19% ethanol, 9.4 mg benzyl alcohol as preservative, 300 mg glycerine and propylene glycol q.s.

Gentocin Otic Solution (Schering-Plough)

Active ingredients: Each milliliter contains gentamicin sulfate equivalent to 3 mg gentamicin base, betamethasone valerate equivalent to 1 mg betamethasone, 1.0 mg hydroxyethylcellulose, 2.5 mg glacial acetic acid, 200 mg purified water, 19% ethanol, 9.4 mg benzyl alcohol as preservative, 300 mg glycerine and propylene glycol q.s.

Ivomec 1% Injection for Cattle and Swine (Merck)

Active ingredients: 1% ivermectin, 40% glycerol formal, and propylene glycol, q.s. at 100%.

Liquichlor (Evsco)

Active ingredients: Each milliliter contains chloramphenicol 4.2 mg, prednisolone 1.7 mg, tetracaine 4.2 mg, squalane 0.21 ml.

Lotrisone (Schering-Plough)

Active ingredients: Each gram contains 10.0 mg clotrimazole, 0.64 mg betametha-sone diproprionate (equivalent to 0.5 mg betamethasone) in a hydrophilic emollient cream consisting of purified water, mineral oil, white petrolatum, cetostearyl, alcohol, cetareth-30, propylene glycol, sodium phosphate, monobasic, and phosphoric acid.

Micazole Lotion 1% (Vetus)

Active ingredients: 1.15% miconazole nitrate (equivalent to 1% miconazole base by weight), polyethylene glycol 400, and ethyl alcohol 55%.

Miconosol Lotion 1%

Active ingredients: 1.15% miconazole nitrate (equivalent to 1% miconazole base by weight), polyethylene glycol 400, and ethyl alcohol 55%.

Mita-Clear

Active ingredients: Pyrethrin 0.15%, piperonyl butoxide technical 1.50%, N-octyl bicycloheptene dicarboximide 0.50%, di-n-propyl isocinchomeronate 1.00%. Inert ingredients 96.85%.

Neo-Predef (Upjohn and Pharmacia)

Active ingredients: Each gram contains isoflupredone acetate 1 mg (0.1%), neomycin sulphate 5 mg (0.5%) (equivalent to 3.5 mg neomycin), anhydrous lanolin, white petrolatum, mineral oil. Chlorobutanol (chloral derivative) 0.65% added as a preservative.

Nolvamite (Ft. Dodge)

Active ingredients: Pyrethrin 0.10%, piperonyl butoxide technical 1.05%. Inert ingredients 99.85%. Contains Nolvasan as a preservative.

Oticare-M Ear Mite Treatment (ARC)

Active ingredients: Pyrethrin 0.15%, piperonyl butoxide technical 1.50%. Inert ingredients 98.35%.

Otomax (Schering-Plough)

Active ingredients: Each gram contains gentamicin sulfate veterinary equivalent to 3 mg gentamicin base; betamethasone valerate USP equivalent to 1 mg betamethasone; and 10 mg clotrimazole USP in a mineral oil–based system containing a plasticized hydrocarbon gel.

Otomite Plus (Virbac)

Active ingredients: Pyrethrin 0.15%, piperonyl butoxide technical 1.50%, N-octyl bicycloheptene dicarboximide 0.5%, di-n-propyl isocinchomeronate 1.0%. Inert ingredients 96.85%.

Panalog Ointment (Solvay)

Active ingredients: Nystatin, neomycin sulfate, thiostrepton, and triamcinolone acetonide in a nonirritating protective vehicle, Plastibase (plasticized hydrocarbon gel), a polyethylene and mineral oil gel base.

Quadritop Ointment (Vetus)

Ingredients: Each milliliter contains nystatin 100,000 units neomycin sulfate (equivalent to neomycin base 2.5 mg), thiostrepton 2500 units, triamcinolone acetonide 1.0 mg.

Silvadene Creme 1%

Active ingredients: Each gram contains 10 mg micronized silver sulfadiazine. The cream vehicle consists of white petrolatum, stearyl alcohol, isopropyl myristate, sorbitan monooleate, polyoxyl 40 stearate, propylene glycol, and water.

Synotic Otic Solution (Ft. Dodge)

Active ingredients: Each milliliter contains 0.01% fluocinolone acetonide (6a, 9a-difluoro-11b, 16a, 17, 21-tetrahydroxypregna-1, 4-diene-3, 20-dione, cyclic 16, 17-acetal with acetone) and 60% dimethyl sulfoxide in propylene glycol and citric acid.

Ticar Sterile Powder for Intramuscular or Intravenous Injection (Smithkline Beecham)

Active ingredients: Ticarcillin is a semisynthetic injectable penicillin derivative supplied as a white to pale yellow powder for reconstitution.

Tobradex Suspension (Alcon)

Active ingredients: Each milliliter contains tobramycin 0.3% (3 mg) and dexa methasone 0.1% (1 mg). Preservative: Benzalkonium chloride 0.01%. Inactive ingredients: Tyloxapol, edentate disodium, sodium chloride, hydroxyethyl cellulose, sodium sulfate, sulfuric acid and/or sodium hydroxide (to adjust pH), and purified water.

Topagen Ointment (Schering-Plough)

Active ingredients: Each gram contains gentamicin sulfate veterinary equivalent to 3 mg gentamicin base, betamethasone valerate equivalent to 1 mg betamethasone, and sesame oil in a special gel base composed of polyethylene and mineral oil. Benzyl alcohol is the preservative.

Tresaderm (Merial)

Active ingredients: Each milliliter contains thiabendazole 40 mg, dexamethasone 1 mg, neomycin (from neomycin sulfate) 3.2 mg. Inactive ingredients: Glycerin propylene glycol, purified water, hypophosphorous acid, calcium hypophosphite, about 8.5% ethyl alcohol, and about 0.5% benzyl alcohol.

Tri-Otic

Active ingredients: Each gram of gentamicin-betamethasone-clotrimazole ointment contains gentamicin sulfate USP equivalent to 3 mg gentamicin base, betamethasone valerate USP equivalent to 1 mg betamethasone, 10 mg clotrimazole USP in a mineral oil–based system containing a plasticized hydrocarbon gel.

Tritop (Upjohn and Pharmacia)

Active ingredients: Each gram contains the potent antiinflammatory agent isoflupredone acetate 1 mg (0.1%), the antibiotic neomycin sulfate 5 mg (0.5%) (equivalent to 3.5 mg neomycin), and the topical anesthetic tetracaine hydrochloride 5 mg (0.5%).

VoSol HC Otic

Active ingredients: Solution of acetic acid 2% in a propylene glycol vehicle containing propylene glycol acetate (3%) and hydrocortisone (1%).

Ear Cleaners, Listed by Trade Name

Ace-Otic (Vetus)

Active ingredients: Acetic acid 2.0%, lactic acid 2.7%, salicylic acid 0.1%. In a pH-buffered at 2.3 surface-active vehicle containing docusate sodium (DSS) and propylene glycol.

Adams Pan-Otic (Pfizer)

Active ingredients: Purified water USP, isopropyl alcohol, aloe vera, diazolidinyl urea, methylparaben, propylparaben, dioctyl sodium sulfosuccinate, octoxynol, sodium lauryl sulfate, parachlorometaxylenol, propylene glycol USP, fragrance, tetrasodium EDTA, FD&C blue #1.

Aloacetic Ear Rinse (DVM)

Ingredients: Water, acetic acid, nonoxynol-12, fragrance, methylparaben, DMDM hydantoin, aloe vera gel, FD&C yellow #5, FD&C blue #1.

Burotic (Allerderm)

Active ingredients: Propylene glycol, water, Burow's solution, acetic acid, benzalkonium chloride.

Cerulytic (Allerderm)

Active ingredients: Benzyl alcohol and butylated hydroxytoluene in a propylene glycoldicaprylate base with fragrance.

Cerumene (Evsco)

Active ingredients: Cerumene (squalane) 25% in an isopropyl myristate liquid petrolatum base.

Clear X Ear Cleansing Solution (DVM)

Active ingredients: Dioctyl sodium sulfosuccinate 6.5%, urea peroxide 6%.

Corium 20 (VRx)

Active ingredients: Purified water USP, SDA-40B 23%, glycerol tri-esterified with fatty acids, glycerine USP, fragrance, and B.H.A.

Corium TX (VRx)

Active ingredients: Pramoxine HCI (1%). Also contains purified water USP, SDA-40B 23%, glycerol tri-esterified with fatty acids, glycerine USP, Tween 80, fragrance, B.H.A.

DermaPet Ear/Skin Cleanser (DermaPet, Inc.)

Active ingredients: A multicleanse, acetic and boric acid solution with surfactants.

EarMed Cleansing Solution & Wash (Davis)

Active ingredients: 50A 40B alcohol, propylene glycol, cocamidopropyl phosphatidyl and PE dimonium chloride.

EarOxide Ear Cleaner (Tomlyn)

Active ingredients: Carbamide peroxide 6.5% in a stabilized glycerin base.

Epiotic Ear Cleanser (Allerderm)

Ingredients: Lactic acid and salicylic acid are present in encapsulated (spherulites) and free forms. Chitosanide is present in encapsulated form. PCMX propylene glycol and sodium docusate are present in free form. Also contains water, fragrance, and FD&C blue #1.

Fresh-Ear (Q.A. Labs)

Active ingredients: Deionized water, isopropyl alcohol, propylene glycol, glycerine, fragrance, salicylic acid, PEG 75 lanolin oil, lidocaine hydrochloride, boric acid, acetic acid, FD&C blue #1.

Gent-L-Clens (Shering)

Active ingredients: Lactic acid and salicylic acid in a propylene glycol surface-acting vehicle preserved with PCMX.

Nolvasan Otic (Ft. Dodge)

Active ingredients: Special solvent and surfactant.

Oticalm Cleansing Solution (DVM)

Active ingredients: Benzoic acid, malic acid, salicylic acid, and oil of eucalyptus in a soothing solubilizing vehicle.

Otic Clear (Butler)

Active ingredients: Deionized water, isopropyl alcohol, propylene glycol, glycerine, fragrance, salicylic acid, PEG 75 lanolin oil, lidocaine hydrochloride, boric acid, acetic acid, FD&C blue #1.

Oticlean A Ear Cleaning Solution (ARC)

Active ingredients: 35% isopropyl alcohol, boric acid, salicylic acid, fragrance, PEG 75, lanolin oil, acetic acid, propylene glycol, glycerine, and FD&C blue #1.

Oticlens (Pfizer)

Active ingredients: A clear, colorless liquid with an approximate pH of 2.3 prepared from the following active ingredients: propylene glycol, malic acid, benzoic acid, and salicylic acid.

Otipan Cleansing Solution (Harlmen)

Active ingredients: Propylene glycol, hydroxypropyl cellulose, octoxynol, and a phosphate buffer system (phosphoric acid and potassium hydroxide). The pH is adjusted to 2.5 or less.

Otisol (Wysong)

Active ingredients: Copper chelate of chlorophyll, essential oils of eucalyptus, peppermint, cajeput, juniper, wintergreen, clove, jojoba oil, aloe vera extract, benzocaine, carbolic acid, and natural oleoresins, menthol in a coconut soap, sodium metasilicate, isopropanol base. Stabilized with rosemary extract and vitamin E.

Otisol O (Wysong)

Active ingredients: Copper chelate of chlorophyll, jojoba oil, aloe vera, arnica, and essential oils of eucalyptus, peppermint, cajeput, juniper, wintergreen, clove, and menthol in a base of extra virgin olive oil stabilized with Wysong oxherphol (tocopherol epimers of vitamin E, botanical oleoresins, ascorbate oxidase, and glutathione peroxidase).

Otocetic Solution (Vedco)

Active ingredients: 2% acetic acid with surfactants.

T8 Solution Ear Rinse (DVM)

Ingredients: Purified water, USP, benzyl alcohol, nonoxynol-12, PPG-12/PEG-50, lanolin, tromethamine base, tromethamine HCl, and tetrasodium edetate.

TrizEDTA Aqueous Flush or Crystals (DermaPet)

Ingredients: Each 4-ounce bottle contains 112 ml distilled water, 533 mg tromethamine (tris) USP, 141 mg edetate disodium dihydrate (EDTA) USP, buffered to pH 8 with tromethamine HCl.

Wax-O-Sol (Life Science)

Active ingredients: 25% hexamethyltetracosane in mineral oil.

Zymox (Pet King Brands)

Ingredients: Lactoperoxidase, lysozyme, lactoferrin, hydrocortisone 1%.

Ear-Drying Products

CLEARX Ear Drying Solution (DVM)

Active ingredients: Acetic acid 2.5%, colloidal sulfur 2%, hydrocortisone 1%.

Oticare B Drying Creme (ARC)

Active ingredients: 70% isopropyl alcohol, silicon dioxide, salicylic acid, boric acid, fragrance, polysorbate 60, zinc oxide, talc, PEG 75 lanolin oil, sucrose octyl acetate, acetic acid, propylene glycol, FD&C blue #1.

Index*

*Page numbers followed by *f* indicate figures; *t*, tables; *b*, boxes.